THIRD EDITION

CASE FILES®
Surgery

Eugene C. Toy, MD
The John S. Dunn, Senior Academic Chair and Program Director
The Methodist Hospital Ob/Gyn Residency Program
Houston, Texas

Vice Chair of Academic Affairs
Department of Obstetrics and Gynecology
The Methodist Hospital
Houston, Texas

Associate Clinical Professor and Clerkship Director
Department of Obstetrics and Gynecology
University of Texas Medical School at Houston
Houston, Texas

Associate Clinical Professor
Weill Cornell College of Medicine

Terrence H. Liu, MD
Clinical Professor of Surgery
University of California San Francisco School of Medicine
San Francisco, California

Program Director
University of California San Francisco East Bay Surgery Residency
San Francisco, California

Attending Surgeon, Alameda County Medical Center
Oakland, California

Andre R. Campbell, MD, FACS
Professor of Clinical Surgery
Endowed Chair of Surgical Education

Department of Surgery
University of California San Francisco School of Medicine
San Francisco General Hospital
San Francisco, California

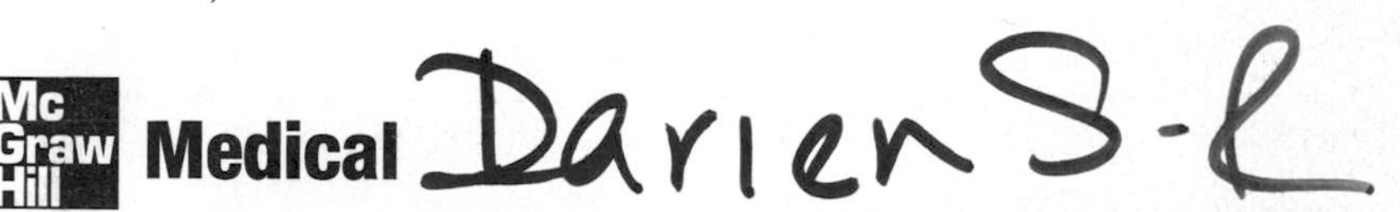

New York Chicago San Francisco Lisbon London Madrid Mexico City
Milan New Delhi San Juan Seoul Singapore Sydney Toronto

The McGraw-Hill Companies

Case Files®: Surgery, Third Edition

2 3 4 5 6 7 8 9 0 DOC/DOC 12 11 10

ISBN 978-0-07-159897-2
MHID 0-07-159897-9

Notice

Medicine is an ever-changing science. As new research and clinical experience broaden our knowledge, changes in treatment and drug therapy are required. The authors and the publisher of this work have checked with sources believed to be reliable in their efforts to provide information that is complete and generally in accord with the standard accepted at the time of publication. However, in view of the possibility of human error or changes in medical sciences, neither the editors nor the publisher nor any other party who has been involved in the preparation or publication of this work warrants that the information contained herein is in every respect accurate or complete, and they disclaim all responsibility for any errors or omissions or for the results obtained from use of the information contained in this work. Readers are encouraged to confirm the information contained herein with other sources. For example and in particular, readers are advised to check the product information sheet included in the package of each drug they plan to administer to be certain that the information contained in this work is accurate and that changes have not been made in the recommended dose or in the contraindications for administration. This recommendation is of particular importance in connection with new or infrequently used drugs.

This book was set in Goudy by International Typesetting and Composition.
The editors were Catherine A. Johnson and Cindy Yoo.
The production supervisor was Catherine H. Saggese.
Project management was provided by Gita Raman, International Typesetting and Composition.
The designer was Janice Bielawa; the cover designer was Aimee Nordin.
RR Donnelley was printer and binder.

This book is printed on acid-free paper.

Library of Congress Cataloging-in-Publication Data

Toy, Eugene C.
Case files. Surgery / Eugene C. Toy, Terrence H. Liu, Andre R. Campbell.—3rd ed.
p. ; cm.
Includes bibliographical references and index.
ISBN-13: 978-0-07-159897-2 (pbk. : alk. paper)
ISBN-10: 0-07-159897-9 (pbk. : alk. paper) 1. Surgery—Case studies.
I. Liu, Terrence H. II. Campbell, Andre R. III. Title. IV. Title: Surgery.
[DNLM: 1. Surgical Procedures, Operative—methods—Case Reports. 2. Surgical Procedures, Operative—methods—Examination Questions. WO 500 T756c 2009]
RD34.T69 2009
617—dc22 2008052506

McGraw-Hill books are available at special quantity discounts to use as premiums and sales promotions, or for use in corporate training programs. To contact a representative please e-mail us at bulksales@mcgraw-hill.com.

International Edition ISBN 978-0-07-163904-0; MHID 0-07-163904-7

DEDICATION

To my dear parents Chuck and Grace who taught me the importance of pursuing excellence and instilled in me a love for books, to my sister Nancy for her compassion and unselfishness, her husband Jason and their beautiful daughters Madison and Peyton, and to my brother Glen for his friendship and our fond memories growing up and his wife Linda who are expecting their first child.

—ECT

To my wife Eileen for her love, friendship, support, and encouragement. To my parents George and Jackie for their constant loving support, and to my sons Andrew and Gabriel who show to me the importance of family values, everyday. To all my teachers and mentors, who took the time and effort to teach and serve as role models.

—THL

To the wonderful medical students of the University of Texas Medical School at Houston for whom this curriculum was developed.

—THE AUTHORS

CONTENTS

CONTRIBUTORS

Gildy V. Babiera, MD
Associate Professor
Department of Surgical Oncology
University of Texas—MD Anderson Cancer Center
Houston, Texas
Breast Cancer
Breast Cancer Risk and Surveillance

Gregory J. Beilman, MD
Professor of Surgery and Anesthesia
Chief of Surgical Critical Care
University of Minnesota
Minneapolis, Minnesota
The Hypotensive Patient

Karen J. Brasel, MD, MPH
Professor of Surgery
Division of Trauma and Critical Care
Department of Surgery
The Medical College of Wisconsin
Milwaukee, Wisconsin
Closed Head Injury
Hernia

M. Kelley Bullard, MD
Assistant Professor
Department of Surgery
University of California, San Francisco
San Francisco, California
Attending Surgeon
Division of Trauma and Critical Care
University of California, San Francisco—East Bay Surgery Program
Oakland, California
The Hypotensive Patient

Eileen T. Consorti, MD, MS
Chief of General Surgery
Alta Bates Medical Center
Berkeley, California
Chief of Surgery
Alameda Community Hospital
Alameda, California
Breast Cancer
Breast Cancer Risk and Surveillance
Esophageal Carcinoma
Gallstone Disease
Nipple Discharge (Serosanguineous)

Charles S. Cox Jr., MD
Professor
Division of Pediatric Surgery
University of Texas Medical School at Houston
Surgeon
Division of Pediatric Surgery
Memorial Hermann Children's Hospital
Houston, Texas
Neonatal Jaundice (Persistent)

Anthony L. Estrera, MD
Associate Professor
Department of Cardiothoracic and Vascular Surgery
University of Texas Medical School at Houston
Houston, Texas
Esophageal Perforation
Chest Trauma (Blunt)
Pneumothorax (Spontaneous)
Thymoma and Myasthenia Gravis

Lillian S. Kao, MD, MS
Associate Professor
Department of Surgery
University of Texas Medical School at Houston
Houston, Texas
Gastroesophageal Reflux Disease
Diverticulitis

Karen L. Kwong, MD
Medical Student Surgery Clerkship Director
Oregon Health Sciences University
Portland, Oregon
Thermal Injury
Nipple Discharge (Serosanguineous)

Christopher R. McHenry, MD
Professor of Surgery
Case Western Reserve University School of Medicine
Vice Chairman
Department of Surgery
Director
Division of General Surgery
MetroHealth Medical Center
Cleveland, Ohio
Adrenal Incidentoloma and Pheochromocytoma
Thyroid Mass
Hyperparathyroidism

David W. Mercer, MD
Professor and Vice Chairman
Division of General Surgery
University of Texas Medical School at Houston
Houston, Texas
Upper Gatrointestinal Tract Hemorrhage
Peptic Ulcer Disease

Kenric M. Murayama, MD
Professor of Surgery
University of Pennsylvania School of Medicine
Chief
Department of Surgery
Penn Presbyterian Medical Center
Philadelphia, Pennsylvania
Pancreatitis (Acute)
Immune Thrombocytopenia Purpura (Splenic Disease)

Ming Pan, MD, PhD
Associate Professor
Division of General Surgery
Penn State University College of Medicine
Milton S. Hershey Medical Center
Hershey, Pennsylvania
Staff Surgeon
Department of Surgery
Veteran's Affairs Medical Center
Lebanon, Pennsylvania
Short Bowel Syndrome

Martin A. Schreiber, MD, FACS
Professor of Surgery
Chief of Trauma Critical Care
Oregon Health Sciences University
Portland, Oregon
Penetrating Abdominal Trauma

Ara A. Vaporcyan, MD
Associate Professor
Department of Thoracic and Cardiovascular Surgery
University of Texas–MD Anderson Cancer Center
Houston, Texas
Pulmonary Nodule

Gregory P. Victorino, MD
Associate Professor of Clinical Surgery
Department of Surgery
University of California, San Francisco—East Bay
Chief
Division of Trauma
Alameda County Medical Center
Oakland, California
Postoperative Acute Respiratory Insufficiency

PREFACE

We appreciate all the kind remarks and suggestions from the many medical students over the past three years. Your positive reception has been an incredible encouragement, especially in light of the short life of the *Case Files* series. It was rewarding to work together with Andre Campbell, the endowed chair of surgical education at the University of California, San Francisco. In this third edition of *Case Files: Surgery*, the basic format of the book has been retained. Improvements were made by updating many of the chapters, with three completely new cases: Esophageal Cancer, Renal Failure and Transplant, and Diabetic Foot Disease. We reviewed the clinical scenarios with the intent on improving them; however, their real-life presentations patterned after actual clinical experience were accurate and instructive. The multiple-choice questions have been carefully reviewed and rewritten to ensure that they comply with the National Board and USMLE formats. By reading the third edition, we hope that you will continue to enjoy learning surgical management through the simulated clinical cases. It is certainly a privilege to be a teacher for so many students, and it is with humility that we present this edition.

The Authors

ACKNOWLEDGMENTS

The curriculum that evolved into the ideas for this series was inspired by two talented and forthright students, Philbert Yao and Chuck Rosipal, who have since graduated from medical school. It has been a tremendous joy to work with my friend since medical school: Terry Liu, a brilliant surgeon, and the many excellent contributors. I am greatly indebted to my editor, Catherine Johnson, whose exuberance, experience, and vision helped to shape this series. I appreciate McGraw-Hill's believing in the concept of teaching through clinical cases. I am also grateful to Catherine Saggese for her excellent production expertise and Cindy Yoo for her wonderful editing. I cherish the ever-organized and precise Gita Raman, senior project manager, whose friendship and talent I greatly value; she keeps me focused, and nurtures each of my books from manuscript to print. At Methodist Hospital, I appreciate the great support from Drs Marc Boom, Dirk Sostman, Alan Kaplan, and Karin Larsen-Pollock. Likewise, without Ayse McCracken, Reggie Abraham, and Marla Buffington for their advice and support, this book may never have been completed. Without my dear colleagues, Drs Konrad Harms, Jeané Holmes, Priti Schachel, and Christopher Hobday, this book could not have been written. Most of all, I appreciate my loving wife, Terri, and my four wonderful children, Andy, Michael, Allison, and Christina, for their patience and understanding.

Eugene C. Toy

INTRODUCTION

Mastering the cognitive knowledge within a field such as general surgery is a formidable task. It is even more difficult to draw on that knowledge, procure and filter through the clinical and laboratory data, develop a differential diagnosis, and finally form a rational treatment plan. To gain these skills, the student often learns best at the bedside, guided and instructed by experienced teachers and inspired toward self-directed, diligent reading. Clearly, there is no replacement for education at the bedside. Unfortunately, clinical situations usually do not encompass the breadth of the specialty. Perhaps the best alternative is a carefully crafted patient case designed to stimulate the clinical approach and decision making. In an attempt to achieve this goal, we have constructed a collection of clinical vignettes to teach diagnostic or therapeutic approaches relevant to general surgery. Most importantly, the explanations for the cases emphasize the mechanisms and underlying principles rather than merely rote questions and answers.

This book is organized for versatility to allow the student "in a rush" to go quickly through the scenarios and check the corresponding answers, and to provide more detailed information for the student who wants thought-provoking explanations. The answers are arranged from simple to complex: a summary of the pertinent points, the bare answers, an analysis of the case, an approach to the topic, a comprehension test at the end for reinforcement and emphasis, and a list of resources for further reading. The clinical vignettes are purposely arranged randomly in order to simulate the way that real patients present to the practitioner. A listing of cases is included in Section III to aid the student who desires to test his or her knowledge of a certain area or to review a topic, including basic definitions. Finally, we intentionally did not primarily use a multiple-choice question format because clues (or distractions) are not available in the real world. Nevertheless, several multiple-choice questions are included at the end of each scenario to reinforce concepts or introduce related topics.

HOW TO GET THE MOST OUT OF THIS BOOK

Each case is designed to simulate a patient encounter and includes open-ended questions. At times, the patient's complaint differs from the issue of most concern, and sometimes extraneous information is given. The answers are organized into four different parts:

PART I

1. **Summary:** The salient aspects of the case are identified, filtering out the extraneous information. The student should formulate his or her summary from the case before looking at the answers. A comparison with the summation in the answer helps to improve one's ability to focus on the important data while appropriately discarding irrelevant information, a fundamental skill required in clinical problem solving.
2. A **straightforward answer** is given to each open-ended question.
3. An **analysis of the case,** which consists of two parts:
   a. **Objectives:** A listing of the two or three main principles, which are crucial for a practitioner in treating a patient. Again, the student is challenged to make educated "guesses" about the objectives of the case after an initial review of the case scenario, which helps to sharpen his or her clinical and analytical skills.
   b. **Considerations:** A discussion of the relevant points and a brief approach to a **specific** patient.

PART II

An **approach to the disease process,** consisting of two distinct parts:

a. **Definitions:** Terminology pertinent to the disease process
b. **Clinical approach:** A discussion of the approach to the clinical problem in general, including tables, figures, and algorithms.

PART III

Comprehension questions: Each case includes several multiple-choice questions, which reinforce the material or introduce new and related concepts. Questions about material not found in the text are explained in the answers.

PART IV

Clinical Pearls: A listing of several clinically important points, which are reiterated as a summation of the text and to allow for easy review, such as before an examination.

SECTION I

How to Approach Clinical Problems

- Part 1. Approach to the Patient
- Part 2. Approach to Clinical Problem Solving
- Part 3. Approach to Reading

Part 1. Approach to the Patient

The transition from textbook or journal article learning to an application of the information in a specific clinical situation is one of the most challenging tasks in medicine. It requires retention of information, organization of the facts, and recall of a myriad of data with precise application to the patient. The purpose of this text is to facilitate this process. The first step is gathering information, also known as establishing the database. This includes recording the patient's history; performing the physical examination; and obtaining selective laboratory examinations, special evaluations such as breast ductograms, and/or imaging tests. Of these, the historical examination is the most important and most useful. Sensitivity and respect should always be exercised during the interview of patients.

Clinical Pearl

> The history is usually the single most important tool in reaching a diagnosis. The art of obtaining this information in a nonjudgmental, sensitive, and thorough manner cannot be overemphasized.

HISTORY

1. Basic information:
   a. Age: must be recorded because some conditions are more common at certain ages; for instance, age is one of the most important risk factors for the development of breast cancer.
   b. Gender: some disorders are more common in or found exclusively in men such as prostatic hypertrophy and cancer. In contrast, women more commonly have autoimmune problems such as immune thrombocytopenia purpura and thyroid nodules. Also, the possibility of pregnancy must be considered in any woman of childbearing age.
   c. Ethnicity: some disease processes are more common in certain ethnic groups (such as diabetes mellitus in the Hispanic population).

Clinical Pearl

> The possibility of pregnancy must be entertained in any woman of childbearing age.

2. Chief complaint: What is it that brought the patient into the hospital or office? Is it a scheduled appointment or an unexpected symptom such as

abdominal pain or hematemesis? The duration and character of the complaint, associated symptoms, and exacerbating and/or relieving factors should be recorded. The chief complaint engenders a differential diagnosis, and the possible etiologies should be explored by further inquiry.

Clinical Pearl

> The first line of any surgical presentation should include **age, ethnicity, gender,** and **chief complaint.** Example: A 32-year-old Caucasian male complains of lower abdominal pain over an 8-hour duration.

3. Past medical history:
   a. Major illnesses such as hypertension, diabetes, reactive airway disease, congestive heart failure, and angina should be detailed.
      i. Age of onset, severity, end-organ involvement.
      ii. Medications taken for a particular illness, including any recent change in medications and the reason for the change.
      iii. Last evaluation of the condition. (eg, When was the last echocardiogram performed in a patient with congestive heart failure?)
      iv. Which physician or clinic is following the patient for the disorder?
   b. Minor illnesses such as a recent upper respiratory tract infection may impact on the scheduling of elective surgery.
   c. Hospitalizations no matter how trivial should be detailed.
4. Past surgical history: Date and type of procedure performed, indication, and outcome. Laparoscopy versus laparotomy should be distinguished. Surgeon, hospital name, and location should be listed. This information should be correlated with the surgical scars on the patient's body. Any complications should be delineated, including anesthetic complications, difficult intubations, and so on.
5. Allergies: Reactions to medications should be recorded, including severity and temporal relationship to administration of medication. Immediate hypersensitivity should be distinguished from an adverse reaction.
6. Medications: A list of medications, including dosage, route of administration and frequency, and duration of use should be developed. Prescription, over-the-counter, and herbal remedies are all relevant.
7. Social history: Marital status, family support, alcohol use, use or abuse of illicit drugs, and tobacco use, and tendencies toward depression or anxiety are important.
8. Family history: Major medical problems, genetically transmitted disorders such as breast cancer, and important reactions to anesthetic medications, such as malignant hyperthermia (an autosomal dominant transmitted disorder) should be explored.

9. Review of systems: A system review should be performed focusing on the more common diseases. For example, in a young man with a testicular mass, trauma to the area, weight loss, neck masses, and lymphadenopathy are important. In an elderly woman, symptoms suggestive of cardiac disease should be elicited, such as chest pain, shortness of breath, fatigue, weaknesses, and palpitations.

Clinical Pearl

> Malignant hyperthermia is a rare condition inherited in an autosomal dominant fashion. It is associated with a rapid rise in temperature up to 40.6°C (105°F), usually on induction by general anesthetic agents such as succinylcholine and halogenated inhalant gases. Prevention is the best treatment.

PHYSICAL EXAMINATION

1. General appearance: Note whether the patient is cachetic versus well nourished, anxious versus calm, alert versus obtunded.
2. Vital signs: Record the temperature, blood pressure, heart rate, and respiratory rate. Height and weight are often included here. For trauma patients, the Glasgow Coma Scale (GCS) is important.
3. Head and neck examination: Evidence of trauma, tumors, facial edema, goiter and thyroid nodules, and carotid bruits should be sought. With a closed head injury, pupillary reflexes and unequal pupil sizes are important. Cervical and supraclavicular nodes should be palpated.
4. Breast examination: Perform an inspection for symmetry and for skin or nipple retraction with the patient's hands on her hips (to accentuate the pectoral muscles) and with her arms raised. With the patient supine, the breasts should be palpated systematically to assess for masses. The nipples should be assessed for discharge, and the axillary and supraclavicular regions should be examined for adenopathy.
5. Cardiac examination: The point of maximal impulse should be ascertained, and the heart auscultated at the apex as well as at the base. Heart sounds, murmurs, and clicks should be characterized. Systolic flow murmurs are fairly common in pregnant women because of the increased cardiac output, but significant diastolic murmurs are unusual.
6. Pulmonary examination: The lung fields should be examined systematically and thoroughly. Wheezes, rales, rhonchi, and bronchial breath sounds should be recorded.
7. Abdominal examination: The abdomen should be inspected for scars, distension, masses or organomegaly (ie, spleen or liver), and discoloration. For instance, the Grey Turner sign of discoloration on the flank areas may

indicate an intra-abdominal or retroperitoneal hemorrhage. Auscultation should be performed to identify normal versus high pitched, and hyperactive versus hypoactive bowel sounds. The abdomen should be percussed for the presence of shifting dullness (indicating ascites). Careful palpation should begin initially away from the area of pain, involving one hand on top of the other, to assess for masses, tenderness, and peritoneal signs. Tenderness should be recorded on a scale (eg, 1 to 4, where 4 is the most severe pain). Guarding and whether it is voluntary or involuntary should be noted.

8. Back and spine examination: The back should be assessed for symmetry, tenderness, or masses. The flank regions are particularly important in assessing for pain on percussion that may indicate renal disease.
9. Genital examination:
   a. **Female:** The external genitalia should be inspected, and the speculum then used to visualize the cervix and vagina. A bimanual examination should attempt to elicit cervical motion tenderness, uterine size, and ovarian masses or tenderness.
   b. **Male:** The penis should be examined for hypospadias, lesions, and infection. The scrotum should be palpated for masses and, if present, transillumination should be used to distinguish between solid and cystic masses. The groin region should be carefully palpated for bulging (hernias) on rest and on provocation (coughing). This procedure should optimally be repeated with the patient in different positions.
   c. **Rectal examination:** A rectal examination can reveal masses in the posterior pelvis and may identify occult blood in the stool. In females, nodularity and tenderness in the uterosacral ligament may be signs of endometriosis. The posterior uterus and palpable masses in the cul-de-sac may be identified by rectal examination. In the male, the prostate gland should be palpated for tenderness, nodularity, and enlargement.
10. Extremities and skin: The presence of joint effusions, tenderness, skin edema, and cyanosis should be recorded.
11. Neurologic examination: Patients who present with neurologic complaints usually require thorough assessments including evaluation of the cranial nerves, strength, sensation, and reflexes.

Clinical Pearl

➤ A thorough understanding of anatomy is important to optimally interpret the physical examination findings.

12. Laboratory assessment depends on the circumstances:
    a. A complete blood count: to assess for anemia, leukocytosis (infection), and thrombocytopenia.

b. Urine culture or urinalysis: to assess for hematuria when ureteral stones, renal carcinoma, or trauma is suspected.
c. Tumor markers: for example, in testicular cancer, β-human chorionic gonadotropin, α-fetoprotein, and lactate dehydrogenase values are often assessed.
d. Serum creatinine and serum urea nitrogen levels: to assess renal function, and aspartate aminotransferase (AST) and alanine aminotransferase (ALT) values to assess liver function.

13. Imaging procedures:
    a. An ultrasound examination is the most commonly used imaging procedure to distinguish a pelvic process in female patients, such as pelvic inflammatory disease. It is also very useful in diagnosing gallstones and measuring the caliber of the common bile duct. It can also help to discern solid versus cystic masses.
    b. Computed tomography (CT) is extremely useful in assessing fluid and abscess collections in the abdomen and pelvis. It can also help determine the size of lymph nodes in the retroperitoneal space.
    c. Magnetic resonance imaging identifies soft tissue planes and may assist in assessing prolapsed lumbar nucleus pulposus and various orthopedic injuries.
    d. Intravenous pyelography uses dye to assess the concentrating ability of the kidneys, the patency of the ureters, and the integrity of the bladder. It is also useful in detecting hydronephrosis, ureteral stones, and ureteral obstructions.

Part 2. Approach to Clinical Problem Solving

There are typically four distinct steps that a clinician takes to systematically solve most clinical problems:

1. Making the diagnosis
2. Assessing the severity or stage of the disease
3. Proposing a treatment based on the stage of the disease
4. Following the patient's response to the treatment

MAKING THE DIAGNOSIS

A diagnosis is made by a careful evaluation of the database, analyzing the information, assessing the risk factors, and developing the list of possibilities (the differential diagnosis). Experience and knowledge help the physician to "key in" on the most important possibilities. A good clinician also knows how to ask the same question in several different ways and use different terminology. For example, a patient may deny having been treated for "cholelithiasis" but answer affirmatively when asked if he has been hospitalized for "gallstones." Reaching a diagnosis may be achieved by systematically reading about each possible cause and disease.

Usually a long list of possible diagnoses can be pared down to two or three that are the most likely, based on selective laboratory or imaging tests. For example, a patient who complains of upper abdominal pain *and* has a history of nonsteroidal anti-inflammatory drugs use may have peptic ulcer disease; another patient who has abdominal pain, fatty food intolerance, and abdominal bloating may have cholelithiasis. Yet another individual with a one-day history of periumbilical pain localizing to the right lower quadrant may have acute appendicitis.

Clinical Pearl

➤ The first step in clinical problem solving is **making the diagnosis.**

ASSESSING THE SEVERITY OF THE DISEASE

After establishing the diagnosis, the next step is to characterize the severity of the disease process, in other words, describing "how bad" a disease is. With malignancy, this is done formally by staging the cancer. Most cancers are categorized from stage I (least severe) to stage IV (most severe). With some diseases, such as with head trauma, there is a formal scale (the GCS) based on the patient's eye-opening response, verbal response, and motor response.

Clinical Pearl

➤ The second step in clinical problem-solving is to **establish the severity or stage of the disease.** There is usually prognostic or treatment significance based on the stage.

TREATING BASED ON THE STAGE

Many illnesses are stratified according to severity because the prognosis and treatment often vary based on the severity. If neither the prognosis nor the treatment were affected by the stage of the disease process, there would be no reason to subcategorize the illness as mild or severe. For example, obesity is subcategorized as moderate (body mass index [BMI] 35 to 40 kg/m^2) or severe (BMI greater than 40 kg/m^2), with different prognoses and recommended interventions. Surgical procedures for obesity such as gastric bypass are only generally considered when a patient has severe obesity and/or significant complications such as sleep apnea.

Clinical Pearl

➤ The third step in clinical problem-solving is, in most cases, tailoring the treatment to the extent or stage of the disease.

FOLLOWING THE RESPONSE TO TREATMENT

The final step in the approach to disease is to follow the patient's response to the therapy. The "measure" of response should be recorded and monitored. Some responses are clinical, such as improvement (or lack of improvement) in a patient's abdominal pain, temperature, or pulmonary examination. Other responses can be followed by imaging tests such as a CT scan to determine the size of a retroperitoneal mass in a patient receiving chemotherapy, or with a tumor marker such as the level of prostate-specific antigen in a male receiving chemotherapy for prostatic cancer. For a closed head injury, the GCS is used. The student must be prepared to know what to do if the measured marker does not respond according to what is expected. Is the next step to treat again, to reassess the diagnosis, to pursue a metastatic workup, or to follow up with another more specific test?

Clinical Pearl

➤ **The fourth step in clinical problem-solving is to monitor treatment response or efficacy,** which can be measured in different ways. It may be symptomatic (the patient feels better) or based on a physical examination (fever), a laboratory test (prostate-specific antigen level), or an imaging test (size of a retroperitoneal lymph node on a CT scan).

Part 3. Approach to Reading

The clinical problem-oriented approach to reading is different from the classic "systematic" research of a disease. A patient's presentation rarely provides a clear diagnosis; hence, the student must become skilled in applying textbook information to the clinical setting. Furthermore, one retains more information when one reads with a purpose. In other words, the student should read with the goal of answering specific questions. There are several fundamental questions that facilitate **clinical thinking:**

1. What is the most likely diagnosis?
2. How can you confirm the diagnosis?

3. What should be your next step?
4. What is the most likely mechanism for this disease process?
5. What are the risk factors for this disease process?
6. What are the complications associated with this disease process?
7. What is the best therapy?

Clinical Pearl

> ➤ Reading with the purpose of answering the seven fundamental clinical questions improves retention of information and facilitates the application of book knowledge to clinical knowledge.

WHAT IS THE MOST LIKELY DIAGNOSIS?

The method of establishing the diagnosis has been covered in the previous section. One way of attacking this problem is to develop standard approaches to common clinical problems. It is helpful to understand the most common causes of various presentations, such as "The most common cause of serosanguineous nipple discharge is an intraductal papilloma."

The clinical scenario might be "A 38-year-old woman is noted to have a 2-month history of spontaneous blood-tinged right nipple discharge. What is the most likely diagnosis?"

With no other information to go on, the student notes that this woman has a unilateral blood-tinged nipple discharge. Using the "most common cause" information, the student makes an educated guess that the patient has an **intraductal papilloma.** If instead the patient is found to have a discharge from more than one duct and a right-sided breast mass is palpated, it is noted: "The bloody discharge is expressed from multiple ducts. A 1.5-cm mass is palpated in the lower outer quadrant of the right breast."

Then student uses the clinical pearl: "The most common cause of serosanguinous breast discharge in the presence of a breast mass is breast cancer."

Clinical Pearl

> ➤ The most common cause of serosanguinous unilateral breast discharge is intraductal papilloma, but **the main concern is breast cancer.** Thus, the first step in evaluating the patient's condition is careful palpation to determine the number of ducts involved, an examination to detect breast masses, and mammography. If more than one duct is involved or a breast mass is palpated, the most likely cause is breast cancer.

HOW CAN YOU CONFIRM THE DIAGNOSIS?

In the preceding scenario, it is suspected that the woman with the bloody nipple discharge has an intraductal papilloma, or possibly cancer. Ductal surgical exploration with biopsy would be a confirmatory procedure. Similarly, an individual may present with acute dyspnea following a radical prostatectomy for prostate cancer. The suspected process is pulmonary embolism, and a confirmatory test would be a ventilation/perfusion scan or possibly a spiral CT examination. The student should strive to know the limitations of various diagnostic tests, especially when they are used early in a diagnostic process.

WHAT SHOULD BE YOUR NEXT STEP?

This question is difficult because the next step has many possibilities; the answer may be to obtain more diagnostic information, stage the illness, or introduce therapy. It is often a more challenging question than, "What is the most likely diagnosis?" because there may be insufficient information to make a diagnosis and the next step may be to obtain more data. Another possibility is that there is enough information for a probable diagnosis and that the next step is staging the disease. Finally, the most appropriate answer may be to begin treatment. Hence, based on the clinical data, a judgment needs to be rendered regarding how far along one is in the following sequence.

(1) Make a diagnosis → (2) Stage the disease →
(3) Treat based on stage → (4) Follow the response

Frequently, students are taught to "regurgitate" information that they have read about a particular disease but are not skilled at identifying the next step. This talent is learned optimally at the bedside in a supportive environment with the freedom to take educated guesses and receive constructive feedback. A sample scenario might describe a student's thought process as follows:

1. **Make a diagnosis:** "Based on the information I have, I believe that Mr Smith has a small bowel obstruction from adhesive disease *because* he presents with nausea, vomiting, and abdominal distension and has dilated loops of bowel on radiography."
2. **Stage the disease:** "I do not believe that this is severe disease because he does not have fever, evidence of sepsis, intractable pain, leukocytosis, or peritoneal signs."
3. **Treat based on stage:** "Therefore, my next step is to treat with nothing per mouth, nasogastric tube drainage, and observation."
4. **Follow the response:** "I want to follow the treatment by assessing his pain (asking him to rate the pain on a scale of 1 to 10 every day), recording his temperature, performing an abdominal examination, obtaining a serum bicarbonate level (to detect metabolic acidemia) and a leukocyte count, and reassessing his condition in 24 hours."

In a similar patient, when the clinical presentation is unclear, perhaps the best next step is a diagnostic one such as performing an oral contrast radiologic study to assess for bowel obstruction.

Clinical Pearl

> ➤ The vague question, "What is your next step?" is often the most difficult one because the answer may be diagnostic, staging, or therapeutic.

WHAT IS THE LIKELY MECHANISM FOR THIS DISEASE PROCESS?

This question goes further than making the diagnosis and requires the student to understand the underlying mechanism of the process. For example, a clinical scenario may describe a 68-year-old male who notes urinary hesitancy and retention and has a large, hard, nontender mass in his left supraclavicular region. This patient has bladder neck obstruction due to benign prostatic hypertrophy or prostatic cancer. However, the indurated mass in the left neck area is suggestive of cancer. The mechanism is metastasis in the area of the thoracic duct, which drains lymph fluid into the left subclavian vein. The student is advised to learn the mechanisms of each disease process and not merely to memorize a constellation of symptoms. Furthermore, in general surgery it is crucial for students to understand the anatomy, function, and how a surgical procedure will correct the problem.

WHAT ARE THE RISK FACTORS FOR THIS DISEASE PROCESS?

Understanding the risk factors helps the practitioner to establish a diagnosis and to determine how to interpret test results. For example, understanding the risk factor analysis may help in the treatment of a 55-year-old woman with anemia. If the patient has risk factors for endometrial cancer (such as diabetes, hypertension, anovulation) and complains of postmenopausal bleeding, she likely has endometrial carcinoma and should undergo endometrial biopsy. Otherwise, occult colonic bleeding is a common etiology. If she takes nonsteroidal anti-inflammatory drugs or aspirin, peptic ulcer disease is the most likely cause.

Clinical Pearl

> ➤ A knowledge of the risk factors can be a useful guide in testing and in developing the differential diagnosis.

WHAT ARE THE COMPLICATIONS OF THIS DISEASE PROCESS?

Clinicians must be cognizant of the complications of a disease so that they can understand how to follow and monitor the patient. Sometimes, the student has to make a diagnosis from clinical clues and then apply his or her knowledge of the consequences of the pathologic process. For example, a 26-year-old male complains of a 7-year history of intermittent diarrhea, lower abdominal pain, bloody stools, and tenesmus and is first diagnosed with probable ulcerative colitis. The long-term complications of this process include colon cancer. Understanding the types of consequences also helps the clinician to become aware of the dangers to the patient. Surveillance with colonoscopy is important in attempting to identify a colon malignancy.

WHAT IS THE BEST THERAPY?

To answer this question, the clinician not only needs to reach the correct diagnosis and assess the severity of the condition but also must weigh the situation to determine the appropriate intervention. For the student, knowing exact dosages is not as important as understanding the best medication, route of delivery, mechanism of action, and possible complications. It is important for the student to be able to verbalize the diagnosis and the rationale for the therapy.

Clinical Pearl

- Therapy should be logical based on the severity of the disease and the specific diagnosis. An exception to this rule is in an emergent situation such as shock, when the blood pressure must be treated even as the etiology is being investigated.

Summary

1. There is no replacement for a meticulous history and physical examination.
2. There are four steps in the clinical approach to the patient: Making the diagnosis, assessing the severity of the disease, treating based on severity, and following the patient's response.
3. There are seven questions that help to bridge the gap between the textbook and the clinical arena.

REFERENCES

Doherty GM. Preoperative care. In: Doherty GM, Way LE, eds. *Current Surgical Diagnosis and treatment*. 12th ed. New York, NY: McGraw-Hill Publishers; 2005:6-13.

Englebert JE, Way LW. Approach to the surgical patient. In: Doherty GM, Way LE, eds. *Current Surgical Diagnosis and treatment*. 12th ed. New York, NY: McGraw-Hill Publishers; 2005:1-5.

SECTION II

Clinical Cases

Case 1

A 33-year-old woman presents to the outpatient clinic for the evaluation of a painless breast mass that has been slowly enlarging over the past 3 months. Her past medical history is unremarkable. She has no prior history of breast complaints or trauma. The findings from the physical examination are unremarkable except for the breast examination. A hard, nontender 3-cm mass is noted in the upper outer quadrant of her left breast. The left axilla is without abnormalities. Examination of the right breast reveals no dominant mass or axillary adenopathy.

- What is your next step?
- What is the likely therapy for this patient if she is concerned about breast cosmetic appearance and preservation?

ANSWERS TO CASE 1:
Breast Cancer

Summary: A 33-year-old woman has a 3-cm palpable left breast mass. The findings from an examination of the left axilla and of her right breast are normal. Her presentation is highly suspicious for left breast carcinoma.

- **Next step:** Obtain tissue for diagnosis, and if a malignancy is confirmed, proceed with cancer staging, which should include bilateral mammography.
- **Likely therapy:** If the biopsy confirms breast carcinoma, the disease is likely to be clinical stage IIa (Table 1–1), which is generally best managed by (1) first surgery and then adjuvant therapy or (2) initially systemic therapy (chemotherapy) to shrink the tumor, followed by locoregional surgical therapy (neoadjuvant). Neoadjuvant therapy is probably the best choice in this case because the patient has concerns regarding the cosmetic appearance and desires breast conservation.

ANALYSIS

Objectives

1. Learn the initial workup and staging process for a patient with newly diagnosed breast cancer.
2. Learn the options for locoregional and systemic therapy of breast cancer and the basis for selecting neoadjuvant therapy for certain patients.

Considerations

The initial workup for this patient requires confirmation of breast cancer, including core needle biopsy and bilateral mammography. If carcinoma is confirmed, her metastatic workup should include a complete blood count (CBC), liver function tests, and chest radiography (CXR). If a biopsy confirms breast carcinoma, it is likely to be stage IIa because the lesion is between 2-5 cm in size (Table 1–1), which is best managed by surgery and adjuvant therapy or by systemic therapy (neoadjuvant) prior to locoregional therapy. Mastectomy and breast conservation therapy (BCT) are both viable options because the extent of local surgery generally does not impact overall survival. Because this patient desires breast conservation therapy, neoadjuvant therapy is probably the best choice because clinical trials have showed increased success with BCT following neoadjuvant therapy. Breast MRI should be obtained to help delineate the local extent of cancer prior to considering breast conservation therapy.

Table 1–1 BREAST CANCER STAGING

Stage 0	Tis	N0	M0
Stage I	T1	N0	M0
Stage IIA	T0-T1	N1	M0
	T2	N0	M0
Stage IIB	T2	N1	M0
	T3	N0	M0
Stage IIIA	T0-T2	N2	M0
	T3	N1-N2	M0
Stage IIIB	T4	N0-N2	M0
	T_{any}	N3	M0
Stage IV	T_{any}	N_{any}	M1

Tx: Cannot assess
T0: No evidence of primary tumor
Tis: In situ
T1: ≤ 2 cm
  Tla: ≤ 0.5 cm
  T1b: > 0.5 cm, 1 cm
  Tlc: > 1 cm, ≤ 2 cm
T2: > 2 cm, < 5 cm
T3: > 5 cm
T4: Extension to chest wall or skin
  T4a: Extension to chest wall
  T4b: Edema or ulceration of the skin
  T4c: Both chest wall extension and skin involvement
  T4d: Inflammatory carcinoma
Nx: Cannot assess
N0: No regional nodal metastases
N1: Mobile ipsilateral axillary nodal metastases
N2: Fixed ipsilateral axillary nodal metastases
N3: Ipsilateral internal mammary nodal metastases
Mx: Cannot be assessed
M0: No distant metastases
M1: Distant metastases

APPROACH TO Breast Carcinoma

DEFINITIONS

DOMINANT BREAST MASS: A 3-dimensional breast mass that persists throughout the menstrual cycle is generally considered a "dominant breast mass."

FINE-NEEDLE ASPIRATION (FNA): A diagnostic procedure using a small-gauge needle and a syringe under vacuum for cytologic analysis, with or without image guidance. FNA can identify cancer cells but cannot differentiate invasive cancers from in situ cancers.

CORE NEEDLE BIOPSY: Large-bore (usually 10- to 14-gauge) needle biopsy that provides a histologic diagnosis. This procedure can be done with image guidance via stereotactic techniques (Figure 1–1).

NEOADJUVANT CHEMOTHERAPY: Chemotherapy given *prior* to surgery to shrink the tumor and provide a better cosmetic result. Adjuvant therapy is chemotherapy or radiotherapy following surgery.

BREAST CONSERVATION THERAPY: Partial mastectomy with axillary staging by sentinel lymph node biopsy or axillary dissection. Generally, radiation therapy (to the chest wall) is added to decrease local recurrence rate.

LEVEL 1, 2, AND 3 AXILLARY NODES: Level 1 nodes are lateral to the pectoral minor muscles; level 2 nodes are deep to the pectoral minor muscles; and level 3 nodes are medial to the pectoral minor muscles.

TRIPLE RECEPTIVE-NEGATIVE BREAST CANCER: A term describing breast cancers that are being increasingly identified in premenopausal women, particularly of African American descent. These tumors are typically biologically aggressive and are estrogen, progesterone, and HER2-neu receptors negative. Unfortunately, the prognosis of patients with these tumors is poor at this time. These tumors represent approximately 10% to 15% of all breast cancers.

CLINICAL APPROACH

The steps in the management of breast cancer include diagnosis, locoregional therapy, and systemic therapy. The history, clinical examination, imaging, and tissue biopsy are applied for diagnosis in most cases. Standard breast imaging includes mammography and ultrasound, and for selective patients, magnetic resonance imaging (MRI) is applied. A tissue diagnosis can be obtained with FNA, core needle biopsy, or excisional biopsy. Once the tissue diagnosis confirms cancer, the extent of disease and metastasis must be defined, including evaluation of the ipsilateral and contralateral breasts. Patients with suspected stage I or stage II tumor could be staged with a CBC, liver function tests, and CXR. Individuals with bone pain or abdominal symptoms should be evaluated with a bone scan or an abdominal computed tomography (CT) to rule out metastases. Stage III disease should be evaluated with a CBC, liver function tests, a CXR, a bone scan, an abdominal CT scan, and brain CT or MRI if the patient has headaches or neurologic complaints (Figure 1–2). Positron emission tomography (PET) is more sensitive than conventional imaging in identifying distant metastases, and in many institutions, PET + brain MRI are the modalities commonly used for disease staging.

The surgical options are individualized. If the patient desires breast conservation therapy, feasibility is based on the likely cosmetic outcome, the ability to obtain negative margins safely without a total mastectomy, and the patient's compliance with postoperative radiation therapy and follow-up breast cancer surveillance. The treatment of large lesions requiring partial mastectomy may cause significant cosmetic distortion; in such cases, patients

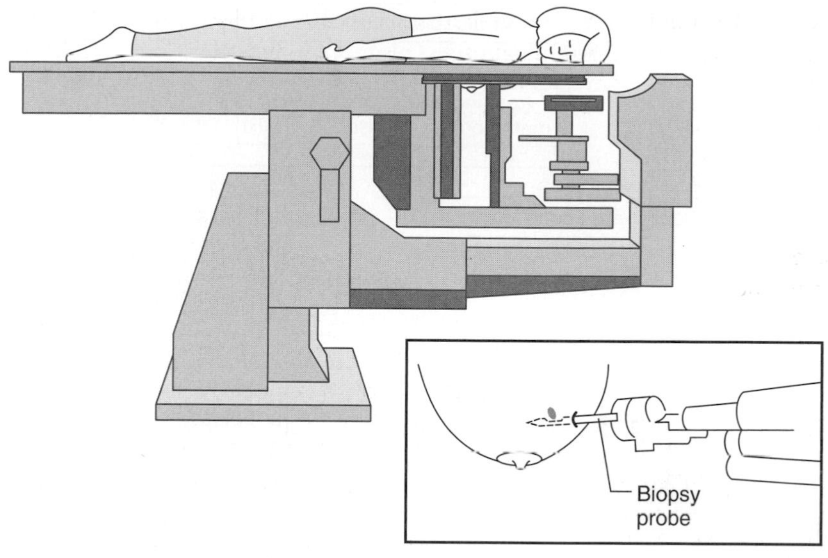

Figure 1–1. Stereotactic core breast biopsy. The patient is prone on a table undergoing a biopsy with image guidance.

commonly undergo neoadjuvant chemotherapy prior to surgery to shrink the tumor to obtain better cosmetic results. Alternatively, with a more favorable tumor/breast size ratio, it is often possible to perform a partial mastectomy and obtain a good cosmetic result without the use of neoadjuvant chemotherapy.

MANAGEMENT

1. The first step is obtaining a tissue diagnosis and staging the breast cancer.
2. **Locoregional therapy:** BCT and mastectomy offer equivalent survival benefits with proper patient selection and follow-up. In addition to resection of the primary tumor, assessment of the regional lymph node basin is important for local control, accurate staging, and determination of the appropriate adjuvant therapy (such as chemotherapy and/or radiation therapy) to be undertaken. **Options for nodal staging include levels 1 and 2 axillary lymph node dissection (ALND) versus sentinel lymph node biopsy (SLNB).** The rationale for sentinel node sampling is to identify tumor involvement in the primary lymphatic drainage area and perform biopsy on only these nodes. The sentinel lymph nodes are localized following radiotracers and blue dye injection at the site of the primary tumor. A small incision is then made in the axilla over the areas of increased radioactivity, followed by the removal of lymph nodes with high radioactive counts and/or stained with blue dye. SLNB has been shown to provide satisfactory staging of the axilla and produce less morbidity in comparison

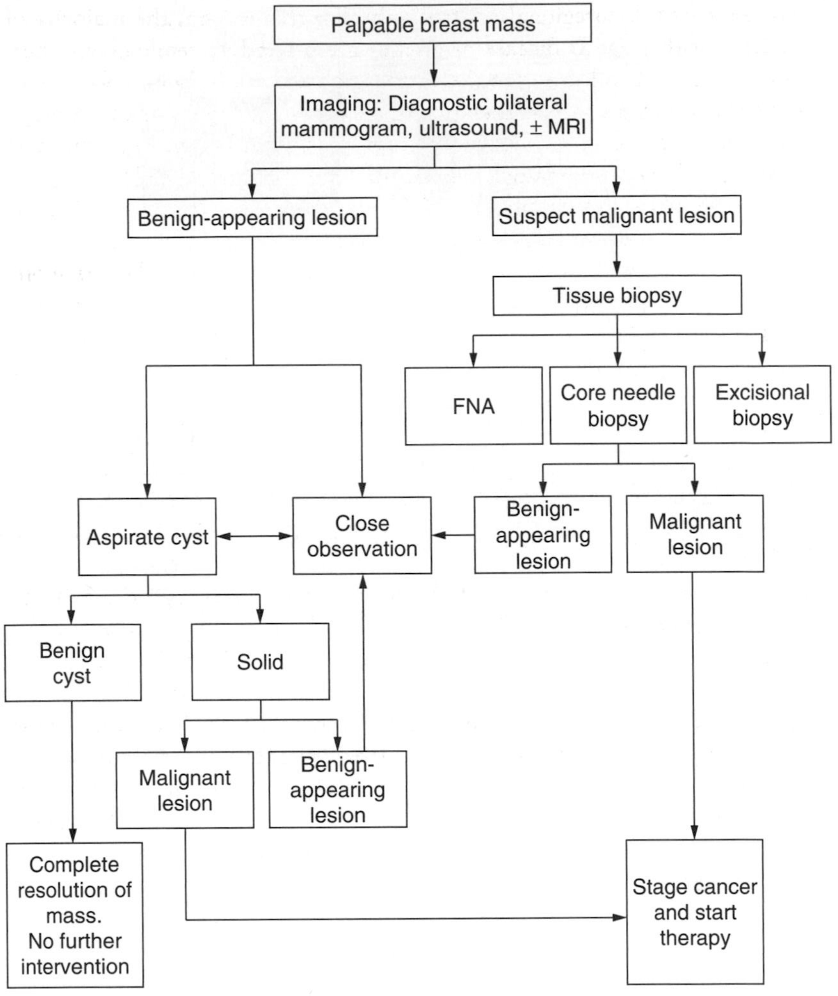

Figure 1–2. The evaluation of a palpable breast mass. MRI, magnetic resonance imaging; FNA, fine-needle aspiration.

to ALND. However, when the SLN is positive for metastasis, a complete dissection of the level 1 and 2 axilla is usually performed.

3. **Systemic therapy:** Systemic therapy is given to patients who are at risk for or who have known metastatic diseases (stages III and IV). The options for treatment include surgery followed by chemotherapy or preoperative (neoadjuvant) chemotherapy followed by surgery. **Patients with stage II breast cancer have a 33% to 44% risk of recurrence of the disease at**

20 years with locoregional control only. For this reason, the majority of patients with stage II disease or greater are offered systemic chemotherapy in addition to locoregional control, with radiation therapy for breast-conserving surgery. Chemotherapy practice has undergone many changes over the past few years. The most common chemotherapy regimens currently used in the United States include 5-fluorouracil/doxorubicin (Adriamycin)/cyclophosphamide (FAC) and Adriamycin/cyclophosphamide (AC). Recent data suggest that the addition of docetaxel (Taxotere) to AC produces additional survival benefits when compared to FAC. Furthermore, clinical evidence demonstrates that the addition of a HER2/neu–receptor antagonist (trastuzumab) may produce additional survival benefits in patients with tumors that overexpress HER2/neu. Another aspect of chemotherapy that shows some promise is "dose-dense" therapy in which the intervals between the cycles of AC is reduced from 3 to 4 weeks to 1 to 2 weeks; clinical trials involving dose-dense therapy has produced survival benefits from cancer-related death, but this approach is associated with an increase in chemotherapy-related complications and toxicities. **Generally, antiestrogen therapy is given for 5 years to patients with estrogen and/or progesterone receptor–positive tumors.** Antiestrogen therapy can be given alone or after the completion of adjuvant chemotherapy. Based on the demonstration of survival advantages and fewer side effects associated with aromatase inhibitors (AIs) in postmenopausal women with ER-positive tumors, **AIs have become the hormonal therapy of choice in these patients.**

The implied advantages of neoadjuvant chemotherapy include in vivo determination of tumor sensitivity to therapy and improved tumor response. Despite these theoretical benefits, **randomized controlled clinical trial evidence does not demonstrate a survival difference between patients treated with neoadjuvant versus adjuvant therapy. The proven advantage of neoadjuvant therapy includes** improvements in breast conservation rate and therefore likely improved cosmetic results.

Comprehension Questions

1.1 A 38-year-old woman is noted on routine physical examination to have a painless 1-cm right breast mass. There is no skin dimpling or adenopathy. An FNA is performed revealing malignant cells. Which of the following is the best next step?

A. Total mastectomy
B. Partial mastectomy and radiation therapy
C. PET scan and MRI of brain
D. Core needle biopsy of mass

1.2 A 54-year-old woman is noted to have a 1.5 breast mass, which on stereotactic core needle biopsy is diagnosed as intraductal carcinoma. The surgeon is planning on a local tumor resection and sentinel lymph node assessment. Which of the following most accurately describes a sentinel lymph node?

A. A lymph node containing cancer metastases
B. The lymph node that is most likely to become infected postoperatively
C. The first lymph node in the lymph node basin draining a tumor
D. The surgical margins of an axillary dissection

1.3 A 60-year-old woman undergoes breast-conserving surgery (a lumpectomy) for a 0.3-cm tumor. The axillary lymph nodes are negative. Which of the following is the best therapy?

A. Radiation therapy to the affected breast
B. No further therapy and observation
C. Combined chemotherapy such as the AC regimen
D. A radical mastectomy

1.4 A 62-year-old woman complains of painful enlargement of her right breast. She has no family history of breast cancer. The right breast reveals warmth, redness, and right axilla nontender adenopathy. Which of the following is the best next step?

A. Oral antibiotic therapy
B. IV antibiotic therapy
C. Biopsy
D. Observation

1.5 Which of the following is considered appropriate treatment option for a 53-year-old woman who develops 2 liver metastases 2 years following left modified radical mastectomy, chest wall radiation, systemic chemotherapy (A+C), and tamoxifen therapy for her T2N2, estrogen receptor positive, and HER/2neu negative invasive ductal carcinoma?

A. Aromatase inhibitor
B. Trastuzumab
C. Radiation therapy to the liver
D. Liver resection

ANSWERS

1.1 **D.** Even though FNA showed cancer cells, this diagnostic modality involves cytology (loose cells), and does not allow for the differentiation of invasive versus in situ breast cancer. A core needle biopsy should be performed to determine the histology of the tumor and assess receptor status and tumor biology of the cancer. PET scan+ brain MRI is systemic staging options that may be applied for patient with invasive cancer but is not needed if the tumor turns out to be in situ only. Mastectomy and segmental mastectomy are treatment options that should be withheld until the nature and stage of the tumor is fully determined.

1.2 **C.** The sentinel node is the first lymph node in the lymph node basin draining a tumor. The advantages are that the procedure determines whether axillary lymph nodes contain metastasis without the extensive surgery of complete lymph node dissection.

1.3 **A.** Radiation therapy is indicated for a patient with stage I disease treated by BCT. The addition of radiation therapy reduces the local recurrence rate from 30% to 9%, and it is an integral part of the treatment program. Chemotherapy may or may not be indicated in a postmenopausal patient with early breast cancer. Radical mastectomy is rarely indicated for breast cancer treatment.

1.4 **D.** A postmenopausal or nonlactating woman who presents with red and/or tender breasts should be assumed to have breast cancer until it is proven otherwise. Inflammatory breast cancer is characterized by edema, redness, and tenderness caused by tumor occlusion of the dermal lymphatic channels.

1.5 **A.** Aromatase inhibitor is an appropriate treatment option for this patient with ER-receptor positive tumor who develops systemic disease relapse. Tratuzamab provides only survival advantages for patients whose cancers over express HER2/neu. Radiation therapy to the liver is not an option because the liver is highly susceptible to radiation injury. Liver resection is not an option at this time, because the probability of other microscopic metastases in this scenario is high. Another possible treatment option for this patient that is not listed is the application of additional systemic chemotherapy with Taxotere.

Clinical Pearls

- Tamoxifen therapy is associated with the development of uterine cancer.
- Aromatase inhibitors are used for postmenopausal women who have ER positive tumors.
- The initial workup for a dominant breast mass generally involves obtaining tissue to identify the breast mass and mammography to assess for other occult abnormalities.
- A sentinel node biopsy can eliminate the need for axillary node dissection in selected patients.
- Patients with triple negative tumors (ER negative, PR negative, and HER2/neu negative) have a poor prognosis.
- Surgery and radiation therapy are locoregional treatment modalities, and chemotherapy and antiestrogen therapies are systemic treatment strategies.

REFERENCES

Bland KI, Beenken SW, Copeland EM III. The breast. In: Brunicardi FC, Andersen DK, Billiar TR, et al, eds. *Schwartz's Principles of Surgery*. 8th ed. New York, NY: McGraw-Hill, 2005:453-499.

Iglehart JD, Smith BL. Diseases of the breast. In: Townsend CM Jr, Beauchamp RD, Evers BM, et al, eds. *Sabiston Textbook of Surgery*. 17th ed. Philadelphia, PA: Saunders Elsevier, 2008:851-898.

Newman LA. Advances in adjuvant and neoadjuvant therapy for breast cancer. In: Cameron JL, ed. *Current Surgical Therapy*. 9th ed. Philadelphia, PA: Mosby Elsevier, 2008:662-670.

1. Tamoxifen (Tx of Breast Ca) → uterine ca

2. ER pos. tumor → Aromatase i

3 Chemoth. FAC 5Fluor Adriamycin Cyclophos
AC + Taxotere shows additional benefit.

Case 2

A 48-year-old man presents for evaluation of burning epigastric and substernal pain that has recurred almost daily for the past 4 months. He says that these symptoms seem to be worse when he lies down and after meals. He denies difficulty swallowing or weight loss. The patient has been taking a proton pump inhibitor (PPI) regularly over the past 12 weeks with partial resolution of his symptoms. His past medical history is significant for frequent early morning wheezing and hoarseness that have been present for the past few months. The patient has no other known medical problems, and he has had no prior surgeries. He consumes alcohol occasionally but does not use tobacco. On examination, he is moderately obese. No abnormalities are identified on the cardiopulmonary or abdominal examination.

- ➤ What is the most likely diagnosis?
- ➤ What are the mechanisms contributing to this disease process?
- ➤ What are the complications associated with this disease process?

ANSWERS TO CASE 2:

Gastroesophageal Reflux Disease

Summary: A 48-year-old man complains of a 4-month history of daily burning epigastric pain. It is worse after eating and lying down and minimally improved with the use of a PPI. He also has symptoms of reactive airway disease and hoarseness.

- **Most likely diagnosis:** Gastroesophageal reflux associated with silent aspiration and pharyngitis.
- **Mechanisms contributing to this disease process:** Diminished lower esophageal sphincter (LES) function, impaired esophageal clearance, excess gastric acidity, diminished gastric emptying, and abnormal esophageal barriers to acid exposure.
- **Complications associated with the disease process:** Peptic stricture, Barrett esophagus, and extraesophageal complications.

ANALYSIS

Objectives

1. Learn the physiologic mechanisms that prevent the pathologic processes that lead to gastroesophageal reflux disease (GERD).
2. Learn a rational diagnostic and therapeutic approach to suspected GERD.

Considerations

This patient's history of substernal chest pain associated with meals is typical for GERD. Hoarseness and wheezing are atypical symptoms that may be related to pharyngeal reflux with silent aspiration. Evaluation by an otolaryngologist may be needed to rule out oropharyngeal and vocal cord pathology.

One of the most alarming features in the history is the lack of response to the PPI, which produces symptoms relief in more than 95% of treated patients; therefore it is extremely important to confirm the diagnosis of GERD and to rule out other pathology. Endoscopy should be performed. A 24-hour pH monitoring while the patient is off medication is appropriate to correlate the symptoms with episodes of reflux and quantify the severity of the reflux. Pharyngeal pH monitoring, which measures proximal esophageal acid exposure, may help support a diagnosis of silent aspiration.

Although H_2 blockers can provide symptomatic relief for mild reflux, PPIs are far more effective for the relief of GERD symptoms. However, patients with extraesophageal symptoms and pharyngeal reflux may be less responsive to medical treatment. Surgical therapy is an alternative to medical therapy and may be considered if the patient does not respond to medical therapy, cannot tolerate the medications, or prefers surgical intervention.

APPROACH TO Gastroesophageal Reflux Disease

DEFINITIONS

GASTROESOPHAGEAL REFLUX DISEASE: Symptoms of heartburn caused by acid regurgitation from the stomach into the distal esophagus.

BARRETT ESOPHAGUS: Replacement of the normal squamous epithelium of the distal esophagus with columnar epithelium with intestinal metaplasia, which places the patient at risk for esophageal adenocarcinoma.

MANOMETRY AND PH MONITORING: Combined procedure in which a small electronic pressure transducer is swallowed by the patient to be positioned in the vicinity of the LES. The most commonly used pH monitor involves a 24-hour ambulatory device that measures pH at 5 cm above the LES.

CLINICAL APPROACH

Occasional gastroesophageal reflux, or heartburn, occurs in approximately 20% to 40% of the adult population. Not all patients with typical GERD-like symptoms have reflux (60%); therefore, it is important to look for alternative causes of symptoms in patients with atypical symptoms or inappropriate response to PPI. Patients with long-standing GERD may develop complications such as peptic strictures, Barrett esophagus, and extraesophageal complications. **Barrett esophagus** is associated with an **increased risk for esophageal adenocarcinoma. Extraesophageal complications,** postulated to be caused by pharyngeal reflux and silent aspiration, include **laryngitis, reactive airway disease, recurrent pneumonia, and pulmonary fibrosis.**

Pathophysiology

Normal physiologic mechanisms are important in preventing abnormal gastroesophageal reflux. For example, abnormalities in the resting pressure, intra-abdominal length, or number of relaxations of the LES can contribute to abnormal reflux. The LES normally serves as a zone of increased pressure between the positive pressure in the stomach and the negative pressure in the chest. A hypotensive or incompetent LES can result in increased reflux. The **crural diaphragm,** which is attached to the esophagus by the phrenoesophageal ligament, also contributes to the normal barrier against reflux. **When the LES**

is abnormally located in the chest, as with a hiatal hernia, the antireflux mechanism may be compromised at the gastroesophageal (GE) junction. Also, the esophagus normally undergoes transient relaxations, but patients with abnormal GERD experience an increased number and duration of relaxations. Other potential contributory factors include excess acid production, abnormal esophageal clearance of acid, delayed gastric emptying, and decreased mucosal resistance to acid injury.

Workup

Patients with self-limiting or mild GERD symptoms do not automatically require further workup. **Those with long-standing or atypical symptoms (wheezing, cough, hoarseness), recurrence of disease after the cessation of medical therapy, or unrelieved symptoms when taking maximal-dose PPIs should undergo diagnostic testing to confirm the diagnosis and to rule out complications of GERD.** Also, patients being considered for a surgical antireflux procedure should undergo further evaluation. Although not all surgeons routinely perform all four studies, a standard workup prior to a surgical antireflux procedure includes endoscopy, manometry, 24-hour pH probe testing, and barium esophagography (Table 2–1).

Treatment

The initial treatment of patients with GERD consists of lifestyle modifications (Table 2–2) and medications as needed. For patients with esophagitis or frequent symptoms, **the mainstay of treatment is acid suppression therapy with PPI.** High-dose PPI therapy is often required for severe symptoms or refractory esophagitis. Most patients with frequent severe GERD symptoms will likely need lifelong high-dose PPI therapy. A lack of any symptomatic relief with PPIs suggests the possibility of an alternative diagnosis.

Surgical therapy is an alternative to medical therapy and **indicated in patients with documented GERD who have persistent symptoms when taking maximal doses of PPI.** Although several antireflux operations are available, the standard operation is laparoscopic Nissen fundoplication, which involves performing a 360-degree wrap of the fundus of the stomach around the GE junction to create a valve effect (Figure 2-1). Long-term success with antireflux surgery exceeds 90%. Two newer endoscopic endoluminal techniques have been developed to treat reflux: delivery of radiofrequency energy to the GE junction and endoluminal suturing of the GE junction. Further prospective data are required for these newer procedures.

Table 2–1 DIAGNOSIS OF GASTROESOPHAGEAL REFLUX DISEASE

TEST	PURPOSE OF TEST
Endoscopy	Evaluates for erosive esophagitis or Barrett esophagus, or alternative pathology. Biopsy for suspected dysplasia or malignancy.
Barium esophagogram Identifies the GE jxn in relation to the Diaphragm	Identifies the location of the gastroesophageal junction in relation to the diaphragm. Identifies a hiatal hernia or shortened esophagus. Evaluates for gastric outlet obstruction (in which case fundoplication is contraindicated). Can demonstrate spontaneous reflux.
pH monitoring for 24 h	Correlates symptoms with episodes of reflux. Quantitates reflux severity.
Pharyngeal pH monitoring	Correlates respiratory symptoms with abnormal pharyngeal acid exposure.
Manometry Peristalsis Achalasia = Diffuse Esophageal Spasm	Evaluates the competency of the lower esophageal sphincter. Evaluates the adequacy of peristalsis prior to planned antireflux surgery. Partial fundoplication may be indicated if aperistalsis is noted. Can diagnose motility disorders such as achalasia or diffuse esophageal spasm.
Nuclear scintigraphy	May confirm reflux if pH monitoring cannot be performed. Evaluates gastric emptying.

Nisson Funduplication - 360° wrap of the stomach Fundus around the GE jxn

Table 2–2 TREATMENT OF GASTROESOPHAGEAL REFLUX DISEASE

Behavioral therapy	Avoidance of caffeine, alcohol, and high-fat metals Avoidance of meals within 2–3 h of bedtime Elevation of the head of the bed Weight loss in obese individuals Smoking cessation
Medical therapy	Antacids H_2 blockers Proton pump inhibitors Prokinetic agents
Surgical therapy	Laparoscopic or open antireflux procedure
Endoscopic therapy	Radiofrequency energy directed to the gastroesophageal junction Endoscopic endoluminal gastroplication

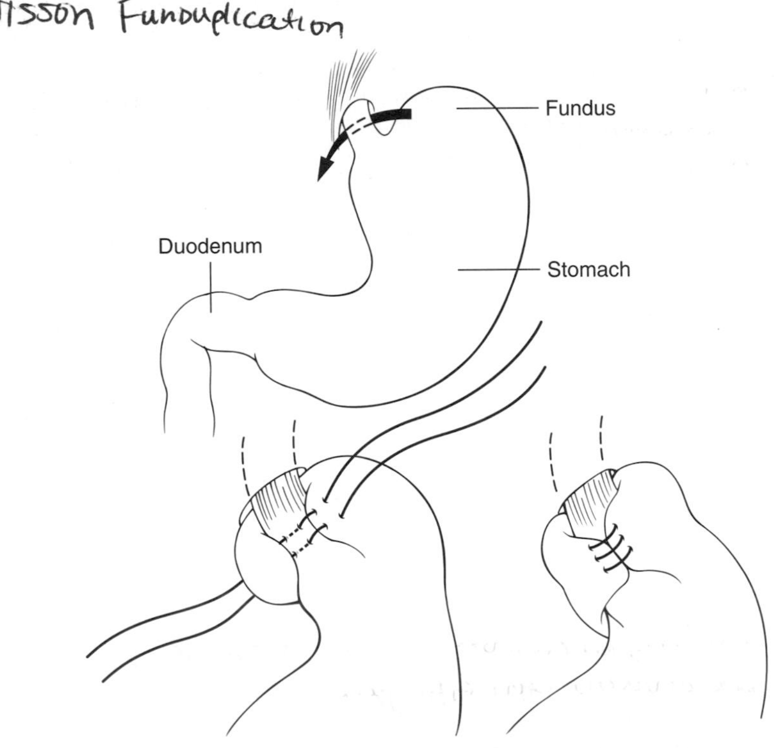

Figure 2–1. Nissen fundoplication. The fundus of the stomach is wrapped around the distal esophagus and sutured.

Comprehension Questions

2.1 A 62-year-old man with congestive heart failure (CHF) and emphysema has symptoms of substernal chest pain and regurgitation after meals and at bedtime. He obtains incomplete relief of his symptoms with ranitidine. An endoscopy confirms mild esophagitis. Which of the following is the most appropriate next step?

A. Reassure him that continued occurrence of symptoms while receiving therapy is normal.
B. Prescribe omeprazole 20 mg per day.
C. Schedule him for 24-hour pH monitoring, manometry, and a barium esophagogram for further evaluation.
D. Schedule him for a laparoscopic Nissen fundoplication.

2.2 A 51-year-old woman has a 6-month history of substernal chest pain and vague upper abdominal discomfort. She has been taking antacid therapy with minimal relief and has had a negative upper endoscopy. Which of the following is the best next step in her workup?

A. Barium esophagogram to evaluate for a hiatal hernia
B. Performing manometry to rule out a motility disorder such as diffuse esophageal spasm or achalasia
C. Referring the patient for cardiac workup as a potential cause of her chest pain
D. Referring to a psychiatrist for a possible conversion reaction

2.3 A 45-year-old man has had a diagnosis of GERD for 3 years with treatment with H_2 blocking agents. Recently, he has complained of epigastric pain. An upper endoscopy was performed showing Barrett's esophagus at the distal esophagus. Which of the following is the best next step in the treatment of this individual?

A. Initiate a PPI.
B. Advise the patient to continue to take the H_2 blocker.
C. Advise surgical therapy involving gastrectomy and esophageal bypass.
D. Discontinue the H_2 blocker and initiate antacids.

2.4 A 24-year-old man with long-standing GERD, currently taking PPIs, is being evaluated for possible surgical therapy. Which of the following is an indication for surgery?

A. Inability to tolerate PPIs
B. Incomplete relief of symptoms despite a maximum dosage of medical therapy
C. The patient's desire to discontinue medication
D. All of the above

ANSWERS

2.1 **B.** Given the patient's comorbidities (congestive heart failure and emphysema), he is not a good candidate for surgical therapy. Patient should be switched to a PPI because the relapse rate associated with H_2 blockers is much higher than those associated with PPI.

2.2 **C.** When chest or epigastric pain does not respond to antacid therapy, and especially with a negative upper endoscopy, etiologies other than GERD (such as cardiac pain) should be considered. Documentation of a hiatal hernia does not necessarily correlate causally to her symptoms. Cardiac disease would be the most concerning disease, and that is why this disorder should be ruled out first.

2.3 **A.** The next step in medical therapy for GERD is the addition of a PPI. The patient has been symptomatic and developed Barrett esophagitis on an H_2 blocker, and therefore additional therapy is needed for relief of symptoms and to decrease the progression of the Barrett esophagitis to adenocarcinoma. An antireflux surgery (such as the Nissen fundoplication) is an option but not gastrectomy and esophageal bypass. This patient also needs endoscopic surveillance of the Barrett esophagus.

2.4 **D.** The indications for surgery are relative and determined in part by the patient; thus, inability to tolerate or a desire to discontinue medical therapy is a consideration for operative management.

Clinical Pearls

- Diagnostic endoscopy should be performed when patients have long standing GERD symptoms and when patients' symptoms are refractory to medical treatment.
- The long-term efficacy of PPI and antireflux operations in reducing esophageal cancer development appears to be equivalent.
- Adenocarcinoma of the esophagus is a complication of long-standing GERD.
- Surgical therapy for GERD is indicated in patients with documented GERD who have persistent symptoms while taking maximal dose PPIs, cannot tolerate PPIs, or do not wish to take lifelong medications.
- The response to PPI is one of the most reliable clinical indicators of GERD.
- A 24-hour pH monitoring is the most reliable objective indicator of GERD.

REFERENCES

Bhanot P, Soper NJ. Gastroesophageal reflux disease. In: Cameron JL, ed. *Current Surgical Therapy*. 9th ed. Philadelphia, PA: Mosby Elsevier; 2008:34-41.

Peters JH, DeMeester TR. Esophagus and diaphragmatic hernia. In: Brunicardi FC, Andersen DK, Billiar TR, et al, eds. *Schwartz's Principles of Surgery*. 8th ed. New York, NY: McGraw-Hill; 2005:835-931.

Spechler SJ, Lee E, Ahnen D, et al. Long-term outcome of medical and surgical therapies for gastroesophageal reflux disease: Follow-up of a randomized controlled trial. *JAMA*. 2001;285:2331-2338.

rinantidine- H_2 → high rate of relapse

omeprazole - PPI

Case 3

A 43-year-old man presents to the emergency department with severe abdominal pain and substernal chest pain. The patient's symptoms began approximately 12 hours earlier after he returned from a party where he consumed a large amount of alcohol that made him ill. Subsequently, he vomited several times and then went to sleep. A short time thereafter, he was awakened with severe pain in the upper abdomen and substernal area. His past medical history is unremarkable, and he is currently taking no medications. The patient appears uncomfortable and anxious. His temperature is 38.8°C (101.8°F), pulse rate 120 beats/min, blood pressure 126/80 mm Hg, and respiratory rate 32 breaths/min. The findings from an examination of his head and neck are unremarkable. The lungs are clear bilaterally with decreased breath sounds on the left side. The cardiac examination reveals tachycardia and no murmurs, rubs, or gallops. The abdomen is tender to palpation in the epigastric region, with involuntary guarding. The results of a rectal examination are normal. Laboratory studies reveal that his white blood count is 26,000/mm^3 and that his hemoglobin, hematocrit, and electrolyte levels are normal. The serum amylase, bilirubin, aspartate transaminase (AST), alanine transaminase (ALT), and alkaline phosphatase values are within normal limits. A 12-lead electrocardiogram shows sinus tachycardia. His chest radiograph reveals moderate left pleural effusion, a left pneumothorax, and pneumomediastinum.

➤ What is the most likely diagnosis?

➤ What is your next step?

ANSWERS TO CASE 3:
Esophageal Perforation

Summary: A 43-year-old man presents with a spontaneous thoracic esophageal perforation (Boerhaave syndrome). The patient has a left pneumothorax and exhibits a septic process from the mediastinitis.

- **Most likely diagnosis:** A spontaneous esophageal rupture (Boerhaave syndrome).
- **Next step:** Management of the airway, breathing, and circulation (ABCs), including the placement of a left chest tube, fluid resuscitation, and the administration of broad-spectrum antibiotics, followed by a water-soluble contrast study of the esophagus.

ANALYSIS

Objectives

1. Recognize the clinical settings, early signs and symptoms, and complications of esophageal perforation.
2. Learn the diagnostic and therapeutic approach to a suspected esophageal perforation.

Considerations

This is a young patient with forceful retching followed by severe chest and abdominal pain, and now with fever. The chest radiograph reveals pneumomediastinum, with air entering from the esophagus into the mediastinum.

This patient's clinical presentation is classic for a spontaneous esophageal perforation; however, delay in diagnosis and treatment can still occur because many physicians do not have extensive experience in the evaluation and treatment of this problem. Maintaining a high index of suspicion and pursuing an early diagnosis and early treatment are essential.

APPROACH TO
Suspected Esophageal Perforation

DEFINITIONS

BOERHAAVE SYNDROME: Spontaneous esophageal syndrome.
PNEUMOMEDIASTINUM: Air within the mediastinal space.

Esophageal perforation remains a surgical emergency. A delay in diagnosis leads to increased morbidity and mortality; therefore, a high index of suspicion should be maintained. Most esophageal perforations are iatrogenic and occur during a diagnostic or therapeutic procedure. Spontaneous esophageal perforation, also referred to as Boerhaave syndrome, accounts for approximately 15% of all causes of esophageal perforation.

The development of an **acute onset of chest pain after an episode of vomiting** is typical of Boerhaave syndrome. Other symptoms that may be present include shoulder pain, dyspnea, and midepigastric pain. Findings from a physical examination, screening radiographs, and laboratory results depend on (1) the integrity of the mediastinum, (2) the location of the perforation, (3) and the time elapsed since the perforation. Seventy-five percent of patients present with a **pleural effusion** indicating disruption of the mediastinal pleura. Contamination of the mediastinum with esophageal luminal contents often leads to **mediastinitis and chest pain.** A delay in treatment leads to sepsis with signs of systemic infection (tachycardia, fever, and leukocytosis). Perforation into the mediastinum leads to pneumomediastinum that can be seen on a chest radiograph and subcutaneous emphysema that can be demonstrated by physical examination. Because **most spontaneous esophageal ruptures occur in the distal third of the esophagus** above the GE junction, **two-thirds of patients present with a left pleural effusion.** The time from perforation to the time of diagnosis is of paramount importance to the ultimate outcome (see Table 3–1).

Table 3–1 CLINICAL PROGRESSION OF SPONTANEOUS ESOPHAGEAL PERFORATION

SIGN OR SYMPTOM	TIME OF OCCURRENCE	COMMENTS
Chest pain	Immediate, persistent	Most common presenting symptom; less specific are shoulder and abdominal pain
Subcutaneous emphysema	1 h after perforation	Occurs more frequently with iatrogenic cervical perforation; perforation; may not be present with lower esophageal perforation
Pleural effusion on chest radiograph	May be immediate or late (> 6 h)	Occurs in 75% of cases; most often on left side (66%) but may occur on right side (20%)
Fever, leukocytosis	> 4 h	Sepsis from mediastinitis
Death	Diagnosis made < 24 h, 15% Diagnosis made > 24 h, > 40%	Outcome is dependent on early diagnosis and treatment

DIAGNOSIS

The best initial diagnostic test to confirm an esophageal rupture is a water-soluble contrast esophagogram, which identifies perforation in 90% of cases. Water-soluble contrast is preferred during the initial examination because it causes less mediastinal irritation than barium if a large leak is discovered. Water-soluble contrast (Gastrografin) esophagram should be obtained with the patient in the right lateral decubitus position to improve its diagnostic sensitivity, and

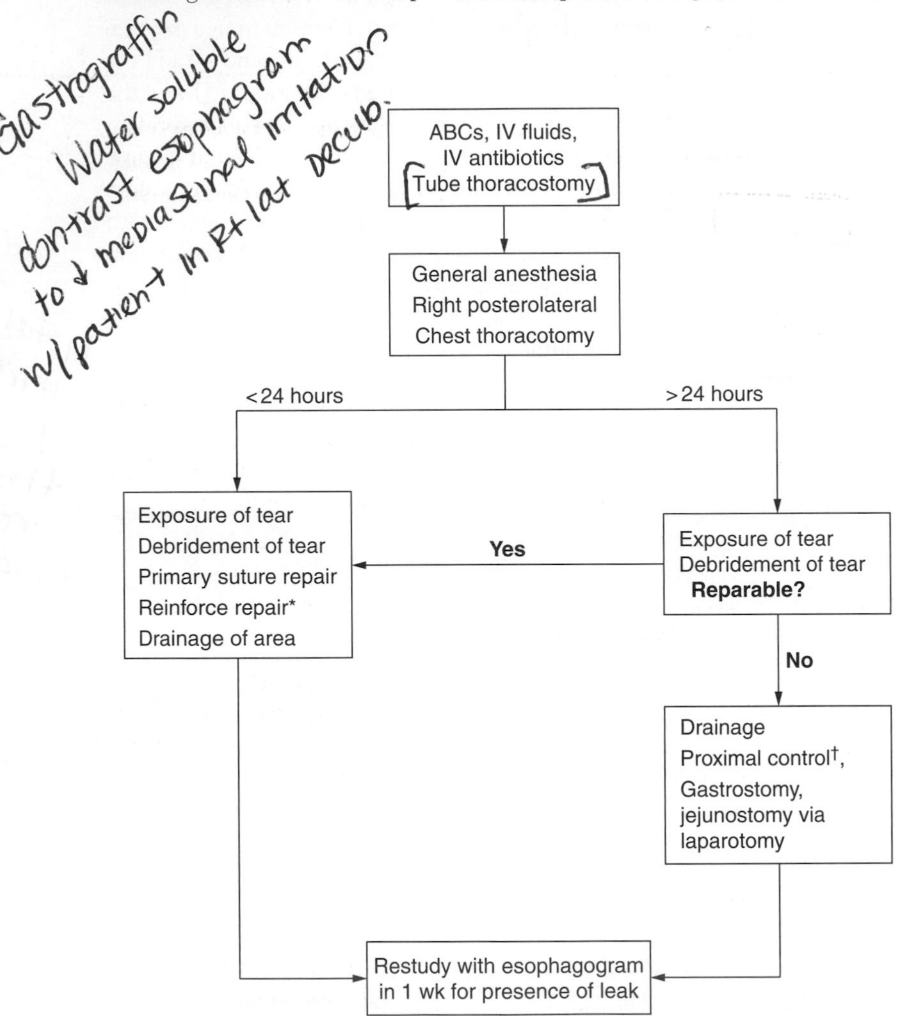

*Reinforce with flap (eg, intercostal, pleural).

†Proximal control refers to diversion (eg, nasogastric tube drainage, cervical stoma).

Figure 3–1. Algorithm for managing esophageal perforation. ABCs, airway, breathing, circulation; IV, intravenous.

if no leak is visualized, barium contrast may be given to confirm the absence of a leak. Once perforation is diagnosed, the initial treatments include prompt resuscitation (directed toward airway, breathing, and circulation—the ABCs), antibiotics therapy, and preparation for operative therapy. **The treatment principles for spontaneous esophageal perforation include surgical drainage, debridement, repair, and diversion** (Figure 3–1).

Comprehension Questions

3.1 A 26-year-old male is brought into the emergency center for severe chest pain and upper abdominal pain. He is diagnosed with esophageal perforation. Which of the following is the most likely etiology of his condition?

A. Trauma
B. Iatrogenic (endoscopy)
C. Spontaneous rupture (Boerhaave syndrome)
D. Caustic injury

3.2 A 60-year-old man has a 10-year history of achalasia. His dysphagia has been worsening, and he underwent an esophageal dilation; shortly after this procedure, he develops acute chest pain, tachycardia, and fever 6-hour after esophageal dilatation for achalasia. Which of the following diagnostic procedures is most appropriate for this patient?

A. A barium esophagogram
B. A Gastrografin esophagogram
C. Esophagoscopy
D. Computed tomography

3.3 The family member of the patient in 3.2 is very concerned about the prognosis. Which of the following is the most important factor that determines the outcome in esophageal perforation?

A. The size of the perforation
B. Whether a meal has been ingested recently
C. The duration between the event and the corrective surgery
D. Leukocytosis

3.4 After eating some stale pizza, a 21-year-old college student presents to the emergency department with a 24-hour history of nausea, vomiting, and severe chest pain. An esophageal perforation is diagnosed by a contrast study, with the best clinical impression of its onset occurring approximately 12 hours previously. Which of the following is the best treatment?

A. Primary surgical repair
B. Endoscopic repair
C. Gastrostomy tube and observation
D. Continued observation for spontaneous healing

ANSWERS

3.1 **B.** Diagnostic endoscopy is associated with the risk of cervical esophageal perforation and therapeutic endoscopy (pneumatic dilatation) is most commonly associated with perforation of the distal esophagus.

3.2 **B.** Barium study is the most sensitive diagnostic method; however, barium leak is associated mediastinitis and peritonitis. A Gastrografin (water-soluble) esophagogram is the most appropriate initial diagnostic study that is more than 90% accurate in identifying a perforation.

3.3 **C.** The outcome to an esophageal perforation is directly related to the elapsed time between the perforation and the treatment. Although the other answer choices are also potential factors in outcome, the time delay is most important as it is associated with infection and sepsis.

3.4 **A.** Primary esophageal repair is generally performed when the perforation is less than 24 hours in duration. In patients in good physiologic condition, surgical repair is generally used regardless of the duration of perforation.

Clinical Pearls

- Spontaneous esophageal perforation should be suspected in a patient with chest pain after vomiting, subcutaneous emphysema found on physical examination, and left-sided effusion demonstrated on a chest radiograph.
- A high index of suspicion is needed because a delay in diagnosis directly compromises patient outcome.
- Most spontaneous esophageal ruptures occur in the distal third of the esophagus.
- Most iatrogenic esophageal perforations are associated with endoscopy.

REFERENCES

DeMeester SR. Esophageal perforation. In: Cameron JL, ed. *Current Surgical Therapy*. 8th ed. Philadelphia, PA: Mosby Elsevier, 2008:16-20.

Peters JH, DeMeester TR. Esophagus and diaphragmatic hernia. In: Brunicardi FC, Andersen DK, Billiar TR, et al, eds. *Schwartz's Principles of Surgery*. 8th ed. New York, NY: McGraw-Hill, 2005:835-831.

Case 4

During the routine physical examination of a 30-year-old, fair-complexioned white man, you discover a 1.5-cm pigmented skin lesion on the posterior aspect of his left shoulder. This lesion is nonindurated, has ill-defined borders, and is without surrounding erythema. Examination of the patient's left axilla and neck reveals no identifiable abnormalities. No other pigmented skin lesions are observed during your thorough physical examination. According to the patient's wife, this skin lesion has been present for the past several months, and she believes it has increased in size and become darker during this time. The patient is otherwise healthy.

- ➤ What is your next step?
- ➤ What is the most likely diagnosis?
- ➤ What is the best treatment for this problem?

ANSWERS TO CASE 4: Malignant Melanoma

Summary: A 30-year-old man has a suspicious pigmented skin lesion on his left shoulder.

- **Next step:** Perform an excisional biopsy.
- **Most likely diagnosis:** Malignant melanoma.
- **Best treatment for this problem:** If this proves to be melanoma, wide local excision with an appropriate clear margin is the best initial treatment. Additionally, evaluation and excision of the regional lymph nodes may be appropriate depending on the depth of invasion of the tumor.

ANALYSIS

Objectives

1. Learn to recognize the clinical presentation of malignant melanomas.
2. Learn the principles involved in performing biopsies of suspected melanomas.
3. Learn about the treatment and prognosis associated with melanomas.

Considerations

Melanoma should be considered whenever a patient presents with a pigmented skin lesion, and lesions should be assessed with the following ABCDE approach. **A: asymmetry; B: border irregularity; C: color change; D: diameter increase; E: enlargement or elevation.**

All suspicious lesions should undergo a diagnostic biopsy and be assessed for depth of tumor invasion. A simple excision can be used to perform a biopsy on small lesions on the extremities. Lesions that are large or involve cosmetically important areas require an incisional biopsy. During the initial biopsy, no attempts are made to achieve a wide margin. Once the melanoma is confirmed and microstaged via biopsy, the patient will require a thorough examination for locoregional metastases and distant metastasis before treatment of the primary melanoma.

APPROACH TO
Pigmented Skin Lesions

DEFINITIONS

MALIGNANT MELANOMA: Cancer of the pigmented cells of the skin.

MALIGNANT MELANOMA STAGING: Surgical staging procedure that depends on the depth of invasion, ulceration, and lymph node status.

CLINICAL APPROACH

The **incidence of cutaneous melanoma is increasing at an alarming rate.** In the year 2000, there were 60,000 new cases and 7700 deaths. Melanoma accounts for 4% of all newly diagnosed cancers in the United States and for 1% of all cancer deaths. It is responsible for six out of seven deaths caused by skin cancer. Melanoma is now the fifth most common cancer in men and the seventh most common cancer in women in the United States. The site of occurrence is evenly distributed among the head and neck, trunk, and upper and lower extremities. Risk factors can be divided into environmental, genetic, and other (Table 4–1), with an associated increase in the overall relative risk.

Melanocytes, dendritic cells found at the dermal/epidermal junction, are found in the skin, choroids of the eye, mucosa of the respiratory and gastrointestinal tracts, lymph node capsules, and substantia nigra in the brain.

Table 4–1 RISK FACTORS FOR MELANOMA

GENETIC*	ENVIRONMENTAL FACTORS	OTHER
Fair skin (2.1) Red hair (3) White (5-10) More than 20 nevi on body (3.4) Blue eyes (4.5) Easily burned and unable to tan (4.5) Familial cases (4-10) Prior history of melanoma (900)	Sunlight (especially ultraviolet B) Areas near the equator First sunburn at young age	Age Gender Tanning lamps Ultraviolet A Higher socioeconomic class Immunosuppression Halogenated compounds Alcohol/tobacco Coffee/tea

*Relative risk is shown in parentheses.

The **four types of melanoma are (1) superficial spreading, (2) nodular sclerosis, (3) lentigo maligna, and (4) acral lentiginous.** By far the most common is **superficial spreading,** which accounts for 70% of all cases. It has a slight female predominance and typically has a prolonged radial growth phase (1-10 years) and a late vertical growth phase. In comparison to that for the other types of melanoma, the prognosis is favorable. **Nodular sclerosis** is the second most common form, accounting for 15% to 30% of all cases. It has no radial growth phase but has an aggressive vertical growth phase that spreads quickly, partially explaining its poorer prognosis. **Lentigo maligna** occurs in approximately 4% to 10% of patients and has a relatively long radial growth phase (5-15 years) and a good prognosis. **Acral lentiginous** melanoma represents 35% to 60% of cases occurring in **African Americans, Asians, and Hispanics** and appears primarily on the palms and soles of the hands and feet and in the nail beds. Similar to nodular sclerosis, it has a very aggressive vertical growth phase and is associated with a poor prognosis.

The incidence of melanoma is directly related to sun exposure. To reduce sun damage, patients should be advised to avoid exposure during the hours of 10 AM to 4 PM, seek shade at all times, and apply sunscreen liberally to protect against ultraviolet (UV) radiation, primarily ultraviolet B (UVB). Other measures include the use of titanium dioxide or zinc oxide for ultraviolet A (UVA) protection, a wide-brimmed hat, sunglasses, darker clothes, and the avoidance of tanning booths and sunlamps.

The treatment and prognosis are determined by the microstage and the pathologic stage of the tumor. The American Joint Committee on Cancer (AJCC) revised staging system for melanoma from 2002, introduced some important changes, and included the following: (1) Thickness and ulceration continue to be used for the T classification; however, the level of invasion is no longer used except for T1 lesions. (2) The number of metastatic lesions (rather than the largest dimension) is now used for the N classification as well as whether the nodes are microscopic versus macroscopic. (3) The site of distant metastases and the serum lactate dehydrogenase levels are used for the M classification. (4) All patients with stage I, II, or III disease with an associated primary lesion that is **ulcerated should be upstaged.** (5) Satellite and in-transit metastases are all combined under stage III disease. (6) The information gained from a sentinel lymph node (SLN) biopsy for staging is used in making clinical management decisions. Table 4–2 lists the new melanoma TNM classification and AJCC stage grouping.

Two methods of microstaging for melanomas have been described by Clark and Breslow. The Clark method is based on the level of invasion of the dermal layers (ie, intraepithelial, into or filling the papillary dermis, into the reticular dermis). The Breslow method of microstaging level is based on the depth of invasion, which is the vertical height of the melanoma from the granular layer to the area of deepest penetration. Most studies have shown that in comparison to the Clark method, Breslow depths of invasion are more accurate prognostic indicators; the overall 5-year survival correlates with tumor thickness. **The 5-year survival rate for stage I melanoma with a thickness of less than 0.75 mm is more than 96%.**

Table 4–2 TNM CLASSIFICATION

T CLASSIFICATION	
Thickness	Ulceration status
T1: 1.0 mm	a: level II/III and without; b: level IV/V or with
T2: 1.01-2 mm	a: without; b: with ulceration
T3: 2.01-4 mm	a: without; b: with ulceration
T4: > 4.0 mm	a: without; b: with ulceration
N CLASSIFICATION	
Metastatic nodes	Nodal metastatic mass
N1: 1 node	a: micro; b: macro
N2: 2-3 nodes	a: micro; b: macro; c: in-transit or satellite lesions
N3: > 4 nodes or in-transit lesions	
M CLASSIFICATION	
Site	
M1: Distant skin, subcutaneous, or nodal	Normal lactate dehydrogenase level
M2: Lung metastsis	Normal lactate dehydrogenase level
M3: Any other distant site	Elevated lactate dehydrogenase level

Revised American Joint Committee on Cancer classification, 2002.

TREATMENT

Primary Tumor

The surgical treatment of melanoma begins with proper management of the primary lesion. Table 4–3 summarizes a treatment plan. Because wide local excision is necessary for treatment of the primary tumor, reexcision of the previous biopsy scar is generally needed. Therefore, orientation of the initial biopsy is extremely important in avoiding unnecessary tissue loss and morbidity. In general, biopsy incisions on the extremities should be oriented longitudinally.

Table 4–3 SUGGESTED SURGICAL MARGINS

MINIMUM MARGIN WIDTH	CLINICAL SITUATION
0.5 cm	Melanoma in situ
1.0 cm	Lesions < 1.5 mm in thickness
2 cm	Lesions 1.5-4 mm in thickness
At least 2 cm	Lesions > 4 mm in thickness

Lymph Nodes

When palpable adenopathy is present, complete lymphadenectomy of the involved lymph node basin should be performed. However, an attempt should be made to obtain a tissue diagnosis (either with fine-needle aspiration or excisional biopsy) before this procedure. Patients with **intermediate-depth melanoma (0.76-4 mm) seem to have a longer survival after prophylactic lymph node dissection,** suggesting that a subset of patients without clinically evident lymph node involvement may also benefit from regional lymphadenectomy. Because of the morbidity associated with lymphadenectomy, prophylactic dissection is not done routinely, but instead the lymph node basins are generally assessed by SLN biopsy. The SLN is the first node in the lymphatic channel through which the primary melanoma drains and can be identified with greater than 90% accuracy by using the combined technique of vital blue dye and radiolymphoscintigraphy. This approach offers the advantages of identifying patients with regional nodal metastases who may potentially benefit from therapeutic lymph node dissection and avoids exposing patients without regional lymph node metastases to the morbidity associated with a lymphadenectomy. Additionally, the histologic analysis results from an SLN biopsy can be used to stage the disease process more accurately.

All patients with confirmed lymph node metastases should undergo a thorough workup to exclude or identify extranodal spread. **Surgery is the primary therapy for patients with nodal** involvement, and adjuvant therapy provides minimal benefits for stage I and II disease and only limited benefits for stage III disease. Currently, **interferon-2A** (Intron-A) is the treatment offered for stage III disease and provides marginal improvements in overall and disease-free survival. However, because of side effects, Intron-A therapy is generally poorly tolerated.

The prognosis for patients with stage IV disease remains dismal, with a median survival of 6 to 9 months. Again, it is essential that a thorough workup be performed to develop a therapeutic plan for all sites of disease involvement. Therapeutic options for patients with stage IV disease are limited. The most promising treatment, now approved by the Food and Drug Administration **(FDA) for stage IV melanoma patients, is high-dose interleukin-2,** which has a known complete, durable response rate of 9% and a partial response rate of 8%.

Comprehension Questions

4.1 A 50-year-old man is noted to have a growing pigmented lesion of the right forearm. On biopsy, it is noted to be malignant melanoma. Which of the following is the most likely type of melanoma?

A. Superficial spreading
B. Nodular sclerosis
C. Acral lentiginous
D. Lentigo maligna

4.2 Which of the following is the most accurate predictor of clinical prognosis during microstaging of a melanoma?
A. Breslow depth of invasion
B. Clark level of invasion
C. T-cell infiltration
D. Size of the primary tumor

4.3 Based on the current consensus, which of the following is the most appropriate surgical margin for a 2.0-mm-depth melanoma?
A. 0.5 cm
B. 1 cm
C. 2 cm
D. 4 cm

4.4 A 30-year-old man had a melanoma biopsied from his left forearm. The initial pathology finding revealed this lesion with a maximal depth of 1.5 mm and microscopically uninvolved margins. Which of these is the most appropriate treatment?
A. Thorough skin examination, wide local excision with 2-cm margin, and interferon therapy
B. Thorough skin examination, wide local excision with 2-cm margin, and PET scan
C. Thorough skin examination, wide local excision with 1-cm margin, PET scan, and interferon therapy
D. Thorough skin examination, wide local excision with 2-cm margin, lymphoscintigraphy, and sentinel lymph node biopsy

4.5 Which of the following is the most appropriate strategy for a 33-year-old man with a 1.2-mm-thick melanoma on the left shoulder?
A. Wide local excision of the melanoma followed by alpha interferon therapy
B. Lymphoscintigraphy, sentinel lymph node biopsy, and wide local excision of the melanoma, and alpha interferon therapy
C. Lymphoscintigraphy, sentinel lymph node biopsy, and wide local excision of the melanoma.
D. Wide local excision of the melanoma and radiation therapy

ANSWERS

4.1 **A.** Superficial spreading is the most common form of melanoma and consists of 70% of all cases. It has a slight female predominance and typically has a prolonged radial growth phase and a late vertical growth phase. In comparison to that for the other types of melanoma, the prognosis is favorable.

4.2 **A.** Although Breslow and Clark staging both use depth of invasion, the Breslow criterion is considered to reflect the prognosis more accurately.

4.3 **C.** Margins of 2 cm are considered adequate for a tumor with a depth between 1.5 mm and 4 mm.

4.4 **D**. Thorough skin examination is important for all patients with skin cancers. Wide local excision with adequate margins (2-cm) in this case is the mainstay of treatment for this intermediate depth melanoma, and in this patient without obvious regional and distant metatstases, lymphoscintigraphy and SLNB may be beneficial for regional lymph node staging and treatment.

4.5 **C.** Lymphoscintigraphy is needed to identify the appropriate lymphatic drainage basins and the sentinel lymph nodes. Sentinel lymph node biopsy is beneficial in identifying the subset of patients with intermediate depth melanoma who may potentially benefit from identification and resection of involved regional lymph nodes. Radiation therapy is usually reserved for the treatment of symptomatic recurrences and selective patients with close resection margins. Alpha-interferon treatment is not indicated in patients without documented lymph node involvement.

Clinical Pearls

- A full-thickness biopsy should be performed on all suspicious pigmented skin lesions.
- **A**symmetry, **B**order irregularity, **C**olor change, **D**iameter increase, and **E**nlargement or **E**levation is more suspicious for malignant melanoma.
- The Breslow system is more accurate than the Clark system for microstaging.
- Excision of the melanoma with adequate skin margins remains the mainstay of therapy, and in patients with prior excisions, the margins are measured in a radial fashion from the edge of the biopsy scar or edge of the melanoma, therefore planning of the initial skin biopsy incision is important.

REFERENCES

Faries MB, Morton DL. Cutaneous melanoma. In: Cameron JL, ed. *Current Surgical Therapy*. 9th ed. Philadelphia, PA: Mosby Elsevier, 2008:1096-1101.

Hansen SL, Mathes SJ, Young DM. Skin and subcutaneous tissue. In: Brunicardi FC, Andersen DK, Billiar TR, et al, eds. *Schwartz's Principles of Surgery*. 8th ed. New York, NY: McGraw-Hill, 2005:429-452.

Case 5

A 63-year-old man complains of a 6-month history of difficulty voiding and feeling as though he cannot empty his bladder completely. After voiding, he often feels as though he needs to urinate again. He denies a urethral discharge. He has mild hypertension and takes hydrochlorothiazide. His only other medication is ampicillin prescribed for two urinary tract infections during the past year. On examination, his blood pressure is 130/84 mm Hg and his pulse rate 80 beats/min; he is afebrile. Findings from examinations of the heart and lungs are normal, and the abdomen reveals no masses.

- ➤ What is the most likely diagnosis?
- ➤ What is the best therapy for this patient?

ANSWERS TO CASE 5: Benign Prostatic Hyperplasia

Summary: A 63-year-old hypertensive man complains of a 6-month history of difficulty voiding and feeling as though he cannot empty his bladder completely. He has experienced two episodes of cystitis. He denies dysuria or urgency and does not have a urethral discharge.

➤ **Most likely diagnosis:** Benign prostatic hyperplasia (BPH).

➤ **Best therapy:** Transurethral prostatectomy (TURP).

ANALYSIS

Objectives

1. Learn the clinical presentation of BPH.
2. Learn the differential diagnosis for urinary outlet obstruction in males and when a biopsy is appropriate.

Considerations

The prostate gland is the male reproductive organ positioned at the base of the bladder that completely encircles the urethra as it exits the bladder and before it becomes part of the penile urethra. The physiologic function of the prostate is to produce the ejaculate, which serves as a vehicle for spermatozoa. As the man ages, the prostate increases in size. This increase in size can have consequences because the human prostate is the only mammalian prostate with a capsule. The capsule restricts expansion of the prostate gland as BPH progresses. The bladder neck and prostatic urethra become compromised in their function, leading to a condition known as bladder outlet obstruction.

Symptoms of BPH, known as **prostatism,** include irritative and obstructive symptoms. They can **include frequent urination of small amounts,** a feeling of **incomplete voiding** with subsequent attempts to urinate to achieve the feeling of bladder emptying, **slow urinary flow, voiding at night** after sleep (nocturia), **hesitancy** at the beginning of urinary flow, and, in its extreme form, **complete urinary retention.** Several conditions that produce similar symptoms mimic BPH. Urethral stricture disease (a narrowing of the urethra with scarring), urinary tract infection, including infection of the prostate (prostatitis), prostate cancer, and neurologic conditions affecting the control and strength of bladder contraction all mimic and may be indistinguishable from BPH. When there is **nodularity or an elevation in the prostate-specific antigen (PSA), biopsy of the prostate is generally indicated.**

APPROACH TO
Urinary Outlet Obstruction

DEFINITIONS

MICTURITION: The physiologic act of voiding. This involves contraction of the detrusor (bladder muscle) followed by relaxation of the bladder neck and other urinary sphincters to allow unrestricted, complete emptying of the bladder in a single setting.

DIGITAL RECTAL EXAMINATION (DRE): The prostate is palpated with a gloved examining finger inserted into the rectum. The normal prostate has the "feel" of the thenar eminence of the thumb (Figure 5–1).

PROSTATE-SPECIFIC ANTIGEN: A blood protein normally produced by the prostate. PSA is specific to the prostate but not to a particular condition of the prostate because age, size, infection, and cancer are among the several reasons why PSA values can be elevated.

URODYNAMICS: Testing performed on the function of the bladder in both its filling and emptying phases, which may be as simple as voiding into a specially developed toilet to measure the voiding flow rate to as complicated as the placement of a catheter into the urinary bladder to measure pressures and volumes during filling and emptying.

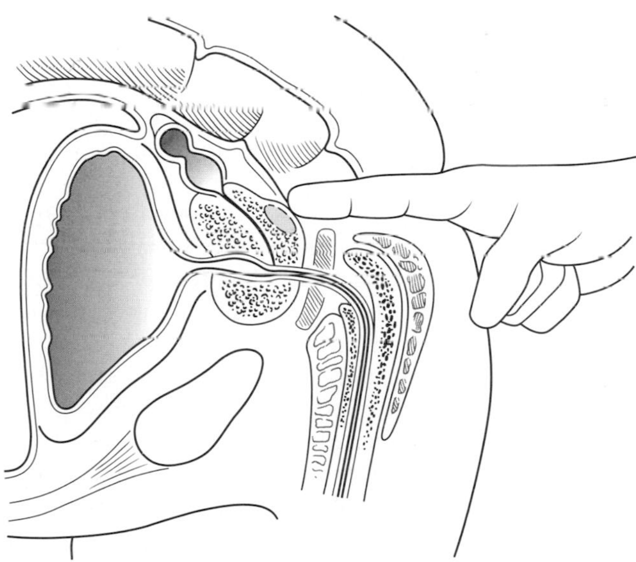

Figure 5–1. A digital rectal examination is performed to detect nodularity in the prostate gland.

CLINICAL APPROACH

When faced with the vague symptomatology of prostatism, the initial duty of the physician is to exclude other etiologies because the treatment would differ. This exclusion process begins with obtaining a history and looking for associated signs and symptoms of other disease processes. A **review of systems** should entail a search for **neurologic abnormalities.** A **urinalysis** is the cornerstone of laboratory testing to exclude the presence of a **urinary tract infection or microscopic hematuria** that might indicate a **bladder tumor. PSA blood testing** should be performed as well as determination of the **serum creatinine** level to rule out severe prostatism with renal compromise. A **DRE** not only characterizes the **size of the prostate** but also is performed to exclude the **presence of a palpable nodule suggestive of prostate cancer** (Figure 5–1). Even the best history and physical and laboratory testing may not discriminate between bladder outlet obstruction secondary to BPH and a urethral stricture because both of these pathologic entities are secondary to restriction of the urethra. If a patient requires urodynamic testing in cases in which the diagnosis is not clear, consultation with a urologist is generally helpful. Making matters more difficult, prostatism may coexist with a urinary tract infection and/or a neurologic disease such as Parkinson disease. Evidence of **renal compromise,** an **elevated serum creatinine value** and/or **urinary retention,** multiple small voids with incomplete emptying, and/or a **palpable bladder** on physical examination call for **urgent urologic intervention.**

Once the correct diagnosis of BPH is made, **initial treatment is often medical.** Two classes of medication are available for the management of prostatism. The first class are α_1-antagonist agents, which cause relaxation of the prostate smooth muscle, thereby increasing the functional diameter of the urethra (common agents include terazosin, doxazosin, and tamsulosin). Another class of medication used in the management of prostatism causes a reduction in prostate size by blocking a metabolite of testosterone (5-alpha reductase inhibitor, most commonly used is finasteride), thus leading to the involution of prostate glandular tissue and shrinkage of the overall prostate size. When medical therapy fails, surgical intervention, which serves to destroy prostate obstructing tissue, is used. The **standard operative procedure** is known as transurethral resection of the prostate, or **TURP.** This procedure is carried out transurethrally using a specially developed scope that has attached to it a cutting element with water irrigation. "Chips" of the prostate are carved out from within the prostate urethra and removed via the scope. Alternative methods to destroy prostate tissue include the use of a laser, radiofrequency waves, or microwaves. Rarely, the prostate enlarges to such a size that open surgical removal known as a suprapubic prostatectomy is required. Regardless of the method of therapy chosen to manage BPH, the patient needs to be monitored thereafter for response to therapy because residual glandular tissue will continue to grow.

Comprehension Questions

5.1 A 57-year-old asymptomatic man is noted to have a prostate that is normal in shape and size on rectal examination. His PSA level is 18 ng/mL (normal, 2.5 ng/mL). Which of the following is the best next step for this patient?

A. Observation
B. Transrectal ultrasound examination with a prostate biopsy
C. Repeated PSA testing in 6 months
D. Initiation of finasteride therapy

5.2 A 72-year-old man has a lower abdominal mass and constantly dribbles urine. Which of the following is the best next step in management?

A. Computed tomography scan of the pelvis
B. Enema
C. Placement of a Foley catheter
D. Referral to a general surgeon and a neurologist

5.3 A 58-year-old commercial airline pilot has confirmed prostatism. He is being treated by a doctor but seeks treatment in the emergency department for dizziness, which precludes his flying. Which of the following is the most likely problem?

A. Unrecognized Parkinson disease
B. Undiagnosed metastatic prostate cancer
C. Drug side effect
D. Silent renal failure

5.4 A 42-year-old man requests prostate "testing" because his father has recently been given a diagnosis of prostate cancer. You perform a DRE, which reveals a normal-sized, smooth prostate gland. A PSA test is then performed and is run immediately because the patient insists on knowing the results before leaving the office. The PSA result is 3.2 ng/mL (normal, 2.5 ng/mL). Which of the following is the best next step?

A. CT scan of the abdomen and pelvis for a workup for prostatic cancer
B. Sonographically directed prostate biopsy
C. Repeated PSA test
D. Prostatectomy with possible lymphadenectomy

ANSWERS

5.1 **B.** A substantially elevated PSA value in this patient generally requires a prostate biopsy to assess for prostate cancer. Transrectal sonography is performed to help determine the location of the biopsy.

5.2 **C.** Overflow incontinence occurs when the urinary bladder is filled to capacity. As the pressure rises, with standing and coughing, a small amount of urine leaks out of the bladder through the restricted bladder outlet in a dribbling fashion. A small amount of urine is seen to squirt from the penis as the Valsalva maneuver pushes on the massively distended bladder. Immediate urinary drainage and hospitalization are in order.

5.3 **C.** The α_1-antagonist class of medications, originally developed for blood pressure control, relax the smooth muscle within the arterial wall, leading to a decrease in blood pressure that may result in dizziness and/or syncope (fainting). Patients must be warned of this side effect. Titration and nighttime dosing are often required.

5.4 **C.** Mild elevations of the PSA value may be seen immediately after a DRE. The best course in this case is to repeat the PSA test several days to 1 week later. The PSA is most useful for patients who have had treatment for prostate cancer to detect recurrence. PSA screening has not be shown definitively to impact mortality due to prostate cancer. Nevertheless, many practitioners advocate screening after the age of 50.

Clinical Pearls

- Patients with symptoms suggestive of BPH should undergo a renal function test (creatinine), a PSA test, urinalysis, and a digital rectal examination.
- The International Prostate Symptom Score can characterize voiding symptoms based on a patient's report of incomplete emptying, frequency, intermittency, urgency, weak stream, straining, and nocturia.
- Although there is no physiologic relationship between BPH and prostate malignancy, the age of onset of these two clinical entities overlaps.
- Distinguishing characteristics of prostate cancer include a firm, hard, and/or misshapen prostate gland on examination and/or an elevated or elevating PSA value. Both BPH and prostate malignancy can coexist in the same patient.
- The diagnosis of prostate cancer is made with transrectal biopsy of the prostate.

REFERENCES

Tanagho EA, McAninch JW, eds. *Smith's General Urology*. 17th ed. New York, NY: McGraw-Hill; 2007.

Walsh PC, Wein AJ, Dorracott E, et al, eds. *Campbell's Urology*. 9th ed. Philadelphia, PA: Saunders; 2006.

Case 6

A 43-year-old man presents with a 16-hour history of intermittent, crampy abdominal pain and bilious vomiting. He states that the symptoms began approximately 3 hours after lunch on the previous day, improved after vomiting, but returned after 1 to 2 hours. He had a bowel movement shortly after the onset of the pain, but there has been no passage of flatus or stool since then. The patient denies any similar episodes previously and has no current medical problems. He underwent exploratory laparotomy for trauma to the abdomen 3 years previously. On examination, his temperature is 38°C (100.5°F), pulse rate 105 beats/min, blood pressure 140/80 mm Hg, and respiratory rate 24 breaths/min. The abdomen is distended, with a well-healed midline surgical scar. The abdomen is tender throughout with no masses or peritonitis. The bowel sounds are hypoactive with occasional high-pitched rushes. No hernias are identified. A rectal examination reveals no masses and no stool in the rectal vault. Laboratory studies reveal normal electrolyte levels. His white blood cell (WBC) count is 16,000/mm^2 with 85% neutrophils, 4% bands, 10% lymphocytes, and 1% monocytes; the hemoglobin and hematocrit values are 18 g/dL and 48%, respectively. The serum amylase value is 135 IU/L. An abdominal radiograph was obtained (see Figure 6–1 on the following page).

- What is your next step in management?
- What are the complications associated with this disease process?
- What is the probable therapy?

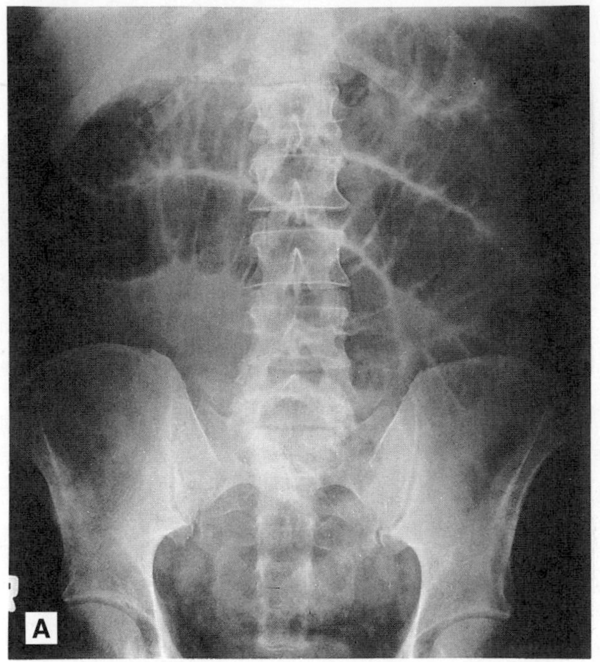

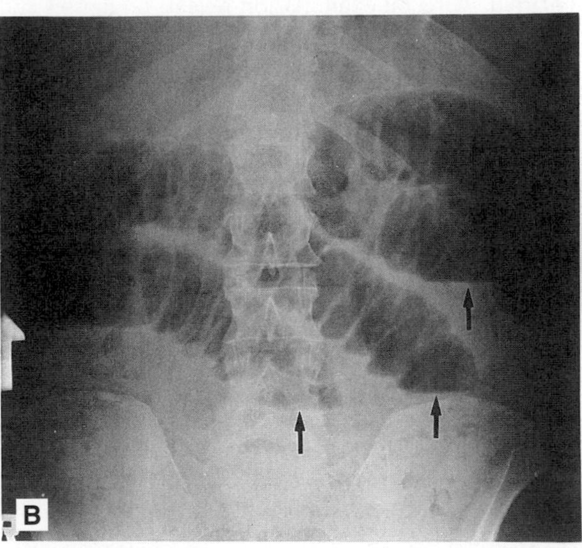

Figure 6–1. Abdominal radiographs in the supine (**A**) and upright (**B**) positions show a dilated small bowel with air-fluid levels. *Reproduced, with permission, from Kadell BM, Zimmerman P, Lu DSK. Radiology of the abdomen. In: Zinner MJ, Schwarz SI, Ellis H, et al., eds.* Maingot's Abdominal Operations. *10th ed. New York, NY: McGraw-Hill; 1997:24.*

ANSWERS TO CASE 6:
Small Bowel Obstruction

Summary: A 43 year old patient has signs, symptoms, and radiographic evidence of a high-grade mechanical small bowel obstruction.

- **Next step in management:** Place a nasogastric (NG) tube to decompress the stomach, begin fluid resuscitation, and place a Foley catheter to monitor urine output and assess his response to the fluid resuscitation.
- **Complications associated with this disease process:** Mechanical small bowel obstruction may lead to strangulation, bowel necrosis, and sepsis. Vomiting may result in aspiration pneumonitis. When unrecognized or untreated, intravascular fluid loss (from third-space fluid loss and vomiting) can lead to prerenal azotemia and acute renal insufficiency.
- **Probable therapy:** Exploratory laparotomy after fluid resuscitation.

ANALYSIS

Objectives

1. Learn the clinical and radiographic features associated with mechanical small bowel obstruction and strangulating or complicated disease processes.
2. Learn the management strategy for mechanical small bowel obstruction.

Considerations

An otherwise healthy 43-year-old man presents with typical signs and symptoms associated with mechanical small bowel obstruction, presumably secondary to intra-abdominal adhesions. The change in pain pattern from intermittent to persistent is a concern. **Persistent pain** in this setting can be produced by severe bowel distension (which may produce venous congestion, decreased bowel perfusion, and necrosis) or **bowel ischemia secondary to strangulation.** Other features of this patient's presentation suggesting the presence of a complicated bowel obstruction include **fever, tachycardia, leukocytosis, an elevated serum amylase level, and radiographic signs of a high-grade small bowel obstruction.** Mechanical obstruction of the bowel results in the accumulation of fluid in the bowel lumen and bowel wall, in addition to extravasation of fluid into the peritoneal cavity. The net result of these fluid shifts is a depletion of intravascular volume and decreased perfusion of all organs. Therefore, **one of the most vital aspects of treatment is early recognition of the problem and restoration of the intravascular**

volume to reestablish organ perfusion. Restoration of intravascular volume is critical in this patient prior to operative therapy because the induction of general anesthesia in a volume-depleted individual may lead to profound hypotension. Nonoperative therapy is frequently successful for mechanical small bowel obstruction caused by adhesions; however, this approach is inappropriate in a patient exhibiting signs and symptoms suggestive of existing or impending bowel ischemia and/or necrosis. The most appropriate management in this case consists of NG tube placement to prevent further vomiting and potential aspiration, fluid resuscitation, administration of broad-spectrum antibiotics, and urgent laparotomy.

APPROACH TO Small Bowel Obstruction

DEFINITIONS

CLOSED-LOOP OBSTRUCTION: This can develop when intestinal blockage occurs at both the proximal and distal ends of a bowel segment. Examples include small bowel incarcerated in a tight hernia defect and intestinal volvulus. This situation is associated with more rapid progression to strangulation, and it is unlikely to resolve without operative therapy.

ILEUS: Distension of the small bowel and/or colon from nonobstructive causes. Common causes include local or systemic inflammatory or infectious processes, a variety of metabolic derangements, recent abdominal surgery, and adverse effects of medications.

INTERNAL HERNIA: A congenital or acquired defect within the peritoneal cavity that can lead to small bowel obstruction.

GALLSTONE ILEUS: Mechanical obstruction of the small bowel due to large gallstone(s) in the bowel lumen. This condition generally occurs when a stone or stones in the gallbladder enter the adjacent duodenum. The typical clinical presentation is characterized by intermittent bowel obstruction for several days until the stone lodges in the distal small bowel and causes complete obstruction.

CLINICAL APPROACH

Mechanical small bowel obstruction is a common clinical problem. The cause of the obstruction, treatment considerations, and the approach to the disease differ based on the patient's age, the duration of symptoms, and whether or not the patient has a history of abdominal operation or trauma. An obstruction in a neonate, an infant, or a young **child** is most likely the result of a **hernia, malrotation, meconium ileus, Meckel diverticulum, intussusception, or intestinal**

atresia. In contrast, small bowel obstruction in an **adult** is most commonly caused by **adhesions, a hernia, Crohn disease, gallstone ileus, or a tumor.** Because a mechanical small bowel obstruction prevents the passage of intestinal luminal contents, the patient develops cramplike abdominal pain, nausea, and bilious vomiting. It is not uncommon for patients to describe the occurrence of a bowel movement at the onset of an acute obstruction, which generally is because of the stimulation of peristalsis leading to evacuation of the distal gastrointestinal tract contents. **The presence of a bowel movement thus does not rule out bowel obstruction.** Whenever the small bowel obstruction is nearly complete or complete (high grade), there may be a cessation of flatus and stool passage following the initial bowel movement. Figure 6–2 outlines the recommended approach to patient evaluation and treatment.

Physical Examination

The physical examination of a patient with small bowel obstruction may initially reveal a low-grade fever and tachycardia as a result of dehydration and inflammatory changes. The persistence of tachycardia after the restoration of intravascular volume may suggest unresolved inflammation from small bowel ischemia and/or necrosis. Similarly, the presence of fever should raise the suspicion for bowel ischemia and/or pulmonary complications due to aspiration of gastric contents. In most patients, abdominal examinations reveal mild, diffuse tenderness. Nonspecific tenderness that improves following successful decompression by the placement of an NG tube is observed commonly in patients with an uncomplicated obstruction. Localized tenderness directly over distended bowel loops suggests the presence of severe distension or bowel ischemia; although a worrisome finding, this localized tenderness is not specific for ischemia. A digital rectal examination (DRE) of patients with small bowel obstruction often reveals little or no stool in the rectal vault, which is because of continued peristalsis and evacuation of stool from the distal bowel. The finding of a large amount of stool in the rectum is unusual and may suggest ileus rather than mechanical obstruction as the cause of distension.

Pathophysiology

Mechanical obstruction of the small bowel reduces bowel absorptive function and causes luminal fluid accumulation. Additionally, there is a fluid shift into the extravascular space because of local inflammatory stimulation and venous congestion. As the obstruction continues, transudative fluid loss into the peritoneal cavity occurs. These losses, along with vomiting, generally produce tremendous intravascular volume depletion and place untreated patients at risk for the development of remote organ dysfunction caused by hypoperfusion. Generally, patients with **proximal small bowel obstruction have more frequent vomiting, and those with more distal obstruction have more distension and**

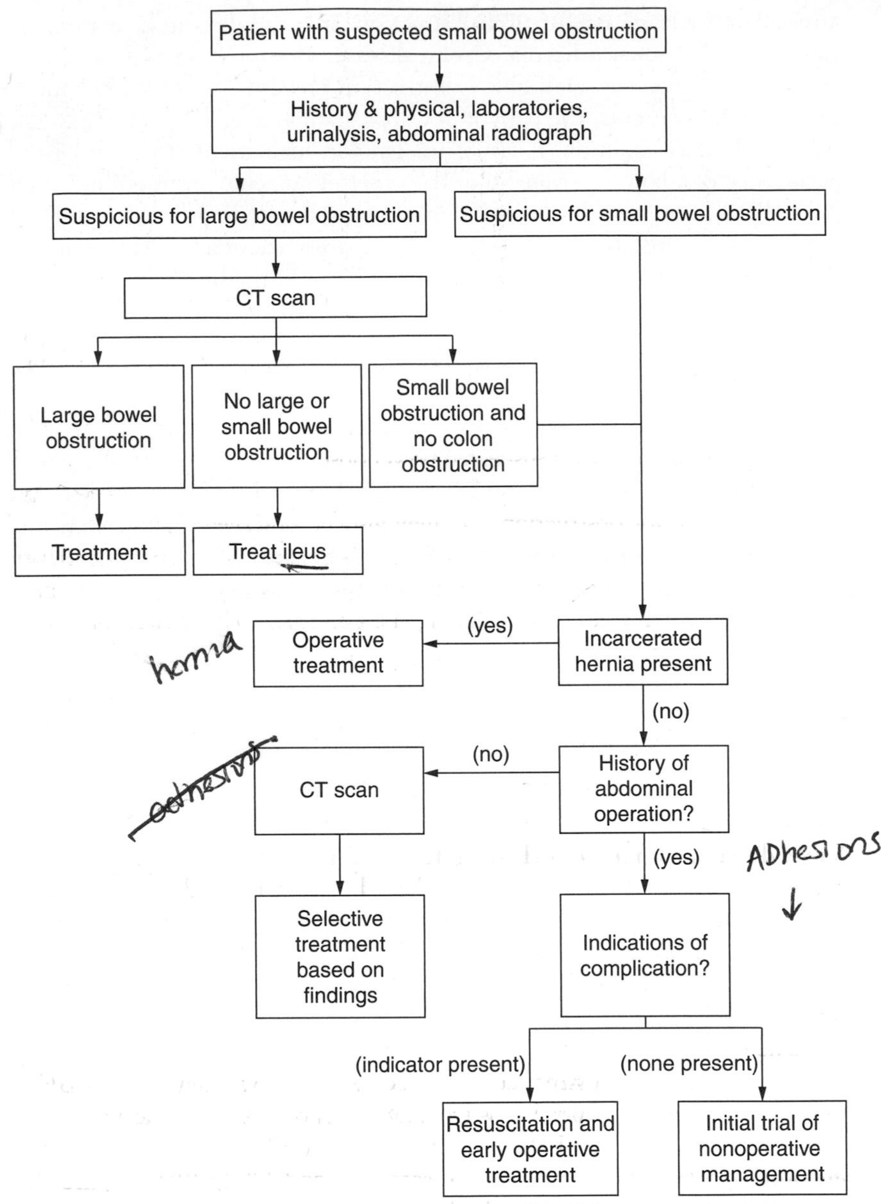

Figure 6–2. Algorithm for the management of small bowel obstruction. CT, computed tomography.

less vomiting. With long-standing distal small bowel obstruction, bacterial overgrowth can develop and lead to feculent vomitus. Prolonged distal small bowel obstruction can lead to further intra-abdominal and pulmonary (aspiration) infectious complications.

Laboratory and Radiographic Evaluations

The initial laboratory evaluation should include a complete blood count with a differential count, serum electrolyte and amylase determinations, urinalysis, and arterial blood gas studies (for selected patients). With dehydration and a physiologic response to bowel obstruction, patients with uncomplicated small bowel obstruction may initially present with mild leukocytosis (WBC count, 10,000-14,000/mm^3) and a left-shifted differential. Generally, the leukocytosis resolves with therapy. **Persistent leukocytosis after hydration should raise a suspicion of complications** and may mandate early surgical intervention or an additional diagnostic evaluation. An elevation in the serum amylase level is most commonly associated with pancreatitis but may also develop with complicated small bowel obstruction.

Plain radiographs of the abdomen are generally obtained during the initial evaluation of patients with suspected bowel obstruction. These usually reveal dilated small bowel with or without colonic air. These findings are not pathognomonic for obstruction and may also be observed in the setting of ileus. Not uncommonly, radiographs of an advanced obstruction demonstrate a fluid-filled bowel with a paucity of air rather than a dilated bowel. Similarly, patients with an obstruction involving the proximal small bowel may have radiographs showing little or no air-filled bowel.

Additional Radiographic Studies

A **CT scan provides additional information** for patients in whom the **etiology is obscure, such as those with a functional obstruction (ileus), inflammatory bowel disease, a tumor, or gallstone ileus.** CTs are also being utilized increasingly to determine the severity of small bowel obstruction and for localization of the obstructive site. CT scans can reliably identify the transition from dilated to decompressed bowel, which is diagnostic for mechanical obstruction. In addition, CT imaging may be useful in visualizing peritoneal tumor spread (carcinomatosis), primary small bowel tumors, Crohn disease, gallstone ileus, and clinically obscure hernias. Alternatively, contrast radiography such as **upper gastrointestinal and small bowel follow-through (UGI/SBFT) can be used to differentiate between mechanical obstruction and ileus** or to assist in determining the location and severity of a bowel obstruction. It is important to bear in mind that CT scanning and UGI/SBFT require the administration of contrast into the bowel lumen and can aggravate patient vomiting and contribute to aspiration. **The goals in patient evaluation are to diagnose the bowel obstruction and identify patients with complicated small bowel obstruction, who may benefit from early operative interventions.** Table 6–1 lists some of the more commonly used indicators to identify bowel strangulation.

Table 6–1 INDICATORS SUGGESTIVE OF STRANGULATED SMALL BOWEL OBSTRUCTION

HISTORY	PHYSICAL EXAMINATION	LABORATORY FINDINGS	RADIOGRAPHY†
Constant pain* Constipation*	Localized tenderness* Fever*,† Tachycardia*,† Peritonitis† Tender mass*,†	Leukocytosis* Elevated amylase level† Elevated lactate level†	Complete obstruction*,† Fluid-filled bowel* Thickened bowel wall* Mesentery edema (CT)* Free-fluid (CT)*

Abbreviation: CT, computed tomography.
*Nonspecific (ie, may occur without strangulation).
†Not sensitive (ie, may not occur with strangulation).

Treatment

Patients with **uncomplicated partial small bowel obstruction** from adhesions can be initially treated with a trial of **nonoperative therapy** consisting of nothing by mouth (NPO), placement of an NG tube, close monitoring of fluid status, serial clinical examinations, and laboratory and radiographic follow-up. Most patients who are successfully treated nonoperatively demonstrate improvement within 6 to 24 hours after the initiation of treatment. These improvements include a decrease in abdominal discomfort and distension, a decrease in the volume of NG aspirate, and radiographic resolution of bowel distension. The absence of early improvement with nonoperative treatment should prompt further evaluation with a CT scan or UGI/SBFT to confirm the diagnosis and/or further define the obstruction for possible surgical therapy. When operative treatment is determined to be necessary, perioperative broad-spectrum antibiotics are administered to prevent wound and intra-abdominal infectious complications. Operative therapy for adhesive small bowel obstruction consists of careful exploration and identification of the obstruction source. Adhesive bands responsible for the obstruction are divided, and ischemic or necrotic bowel is resected.

Early Postoperative Small Bowel Obstruction

Early postoperative small bowel obstruction is characterized by symptoms developing within 30 days following an abdominal operation. This condition can result from narrowing of the lumen because of mechanical causes or ileus. An exact determination of the cause is generally not necessary because nonoperative observation is the usual treatment for both. A CT scan may be useful in some patients to identify or rule out an intra-abdominal infection as the cause.

Outcome

The mortality associated with small bowel obstruction has improved over the past 50 years with improved medical technology and supportive care. Despite this overall improvement in patient outcome, a significant increase in morbidity and mortality continues to be associated with complicated small bowel obstruction. Therefore, one of the major goals in patient treatment is early diagnosis and treatment of uncomplicated small bowel obstruction to prevent a progression to strangulation and bowel necrosis. Patients with a **high-grade bowel obstruction or suspected of having a strangulated bowel should undergo prompt resuscitation and early operative therapy,** which may prevent the development and/or progression of bowel necrosis.

Comprehension Questions

6.1 A 79-year-old woman who has had no previous abdominal surgery presents with intermittent abdominal distension and pain of 1 week's duration and persistent vomiting for the past 1 day. Her physical examination does not reveal any hernias and is consistent with that of distal small bowel obstruction. She is afebrile. Her WBC count is 4000/mm^2. Which of the following is the most appropriate next step?

A. Attempt nonoperative treatment for 48 hours.
B. Perform upper gastrointestinal tract endoscopy.
C. Proceed with an immediate exploration laparotomy.
D. Perform a CT scan.

6.2 Which of the following situations is most likely to respond to nonsurgical management?

A. A 72-year-old woman with a bowel obstruction because of midgut volvulus
B. Small bowel obstruction caused by gallstone ileus
C. A 45-year-old woman who has small bowel obstruction after open gallbladder surgery 20 days previously
D. A 2-day-old male infant who has small bowel obstruction because of jejunal atresia

6.3 A 72-year-old white man arrives in the emergency department with nausea and vomiting following an appendectomy performed 25 days previously. He is afebrile. The abdomen is slightly tender and distended. The WBC count is $18,000/\text{mm}^2$. Electrolyte studies reveal a sodium level of 140 mEq/L, potassium 4.2 mEq/L, chloride 105 mEq/L, and bicarbonate 14 mEq/L. Which of the following is the best therapy for this patient?

A. Placement of an NG tube and observation
B. Colonoscopy for possible intussusception
C. A barium enema to relieve a volvulus
D. Surgical therapy

6.4 A 33-year-old woman with a history of 3 previous C-sections presents to the hospital with her third bout of small bowel obstruction over the past 2 years. She has been managed with nonoperative treatment consisting of NG suction, NPO, and IV fluid for the past 4 days. With her course of management, the patient has had a decrease in abdominal distension but her NG-tube output has diminished but continues to be bilious and voluminous (currently 600 mL/24 hours). Which of the following is the most appropriate management option?

A. Place a central venous catheter for TPN administration and continue her nonoperative treatment for an additional 2 weeks.
B. Obtain a CT scan.
C. Perform a laparotomy.
D. Remove her NG tube and initiate PO feedings.

ANSWERS

6.1 **D.** Patients without previous abdominal surgery or hernias who present with symptoms and signs of bowel obstruction may benefit from CT imaging (to identify possible malignancy, gallstone ileus, or internal hernia), and most patients with this presentation would ultimately require exploratory laparotomy to diagnose and correct the cause of obstruction. CT in these patients may also help differentiate mechanical obstruction from an ileus.

6.2 **C.** Early small bowel obstruction (within 30 days) following abdominal surgery is generally caused by early adhesions or persistent inflammation that frequently resolves with NG decompression and supportive care.

6.3 **D.** The patient has anion gap acidosis as evidenced by the low bicarbonate level, which is probably caused by lactic acid, reflecting ischemic bowel or severe fluid depletion. Elderly patients, age 65 or older often have a minimum of symptoms and are afebrile. Surgical therapy may be indicated if CT imaging confirms intra-abdominal sepsis or high-grade obstruction.

6.4 **B.** This patient is a difficult patient from the management standpoint because though she is demonstrating some signs of improvement, such as decreased distension and decreasing NG output, she continues to have a fairly high NG output that is bilious. A CT scan may be highly appropriate to look for signs of continued mechanical obstruction and it also may be useful to quantify the degree of obstruction and plan the next step in treatment. Laparotomy is a reasonable option, if the patient has not made any progress with conservative management. NG removal and PO feeding could be attempted but may not be successful given the volume and quality of the patient's NG output. Continued nonoperative treatment without further assessment is not appropriate in this patient who is without any prohibitive risks or contraindications for surgery.

Clinical Pearls

- A significant proportion of patients with small bowel obstruction can be treated conservatively (NPO, placement of an NG tube, close monitoring of fluid status, serial clinical examinations, and laboratory and radiographic follow-up) while constantly being assessed for bowel ischemia or strangulation.
- Persistent pain, fever, tachycardia, leukocytosis, an elevated serum amylase level, and radiographic signs of high-grade small bowel obstruction are often signs of complicated bowel obstruction and the need for surgical therapy.
- CT imaging plays an important role in patient evaluation. The exceptions to this rule include patients with simple adhesive obstruction and an absence of indicators of complicated small bowel obstruction (Table 6–1), as well as patients in whom early operative intervention is clinically indicated.
- Patients with closed-loop obstruction require early operative treatment.

REFERENCES

Evers BM. Small intestine. In: Townsend CM Jr, Beauchamp RD, Evers BM, et al, eds. *Sabiston Textbook of Surgery*. 18th ed. Philadelphia, PA: Saunders Elsevier; 2008:1278-1332.

Whang EE, Ashley SW, Zinner MJ. Small intestine. In: Brunicardi FC, Andersen DK, Billiar TR, et al, eds. *Schwartz's Principles of Surgery*. 8th ed. New York, NY: McGraw-Hill; 2005:1017-1054.

Case 7

A 34-year-old diabetic woman complains of a 6-month history of progressive numbness and pain in her right hand that wakes her up at night. She states that her thumb is especially affected. She says that she is beginning to drop objects she is carrying in her right hand. She denies a history of trauma, exposure to heavy metals, or a family history of multiple sclerosis. The only medication she takes is an oral hypoglycemic agent.

- ➤ What is the most likely diagnosis?
- ➤ What is the mechanism of the disorder?
- ➤ What is your next step?

ANSWERS TO CASE 7:
Carpal Tunnel Syndrome

Summary: A 34-year-old diabetic woman complains of a 6-month history of progressive numbness and pain in her right hand occurring especially at nighttime and affecting her thumb. She states that she is beginning to drop objects she carries in her right hand.

- ➤ **Most likely diagnosis:** Carpal tunnel syndrome.
- ➤ **Mechanism of the disorder:** Median nerve compression.
- ➤ **Next step in therapy:** Nighttime splint and nonsteroidal anti-inflammatory drugs (NSAIDs).

ANALYSIS

Objectives

1. Learn the clinical presentation, pathophysiology, and risk factors for carpal tunnel syndrome.
2. Learn the medical and surgical options for treating carpal tunnel syndrome.

Considerations

The distribution of the progressive numbness and pain is suggestive of median nerve compression. In addition, exacerbation of the patient's symptoms at night is typical of carpal tunnel syndrome. The mechanism of this disorder is compression of the median nerve as it passes within the carpal tunnel. This causes axonal damage and narrowing of the nerve. Median nerve compression causes numbness and pain in the thumb, index finger, and middle and lateral aspects of the ring finger. The median nerve may be compressed anywhere along its length from the brachial plexus down to the hand, but the most common site of compression is within the carpal tunnel, where it is dorsal to the transverse carpal ligament. The carpal canal is a rigid structure that causes physiologic dysfunction by producing median nerve ischemia. The best initial management is a nighttime splint for the wrist and avoidance of excess activity with the hand.

APPROACH TO
Carpal Tunnel Syndrome

DEFINITIONS

CARPAL TUNNEL SYNDROME: Median nerve compression at the wrist leading to paresthesias of the radial three fingers and sometimes hand weakness.

TINEL SIGN: Reproduction of the patient's symptoms by percussion of the median nerve at the wrist.

ELECTROPHYSIOLOGIC STUDIES: Investigation of nerve conduction and muscle innervation.

CLINICAL APPROACH

The carpal canal serves as a mechanical conduit for the digital flexor tendons. The walls and floor on the dorsal surface of the canal are formed by the carpal bones, and the ventral aspect is confined by the strong, inelastic, transverse carpal ligament. The smallest cross-sectional area of the canal is created by extremes of flexion and extension of the wrist (Figure 7–1). Exacerbation of symptoms at night is thought to be caused by edema; tenosynovitis may also be present. Carpal tunnel syndrome is associated with endocrine conditions, diabetes, myxedema, hyperthyroidism, acromegaly, and pregnancy. Other causes are autoimmune disorders, lipomas of the canal, bone abnormalities, and

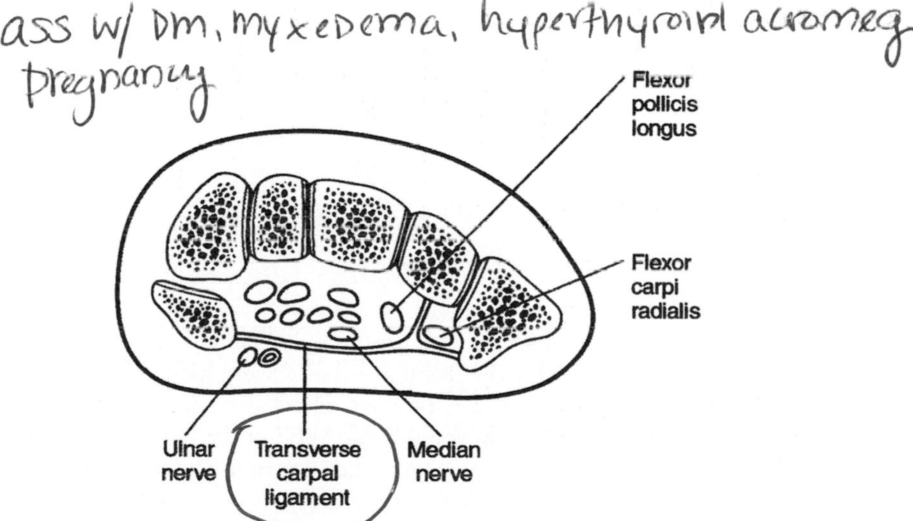

Figure 7–1. The carpal tunnel. The wrist in cross section reveals that the median nerve is susceptible to impingement.

hematomas. The etiology is often multifactorial. Women are more commonly affected in a ratio of approximately 3:1.

Diagnosis

The diagnosis of carpal tunnel syndrome is clinical, and the symptoms are typical. The exertion of direct digital pressure by the examiner over the median nerve at the carpal tunnel frequently reproduces the symptoms in approximately 30 seconds. In the Phalen maneuver, gravity-induced wrist flexion also produces the classic symptoms of this condition. A positive Tinel sign is present when direct percussion over the nerve reproduces paresthesia. Sensory loss, particularly vibration sense, and motor loss may be present with thenar muscle wasting and decreased abductor muscle resistance. Because CTS is found bilaterally in up to half of patients, comparison to the contralateral hand can be misleading. Electrophysiologic studies may be helpful. A comparison of median and ulnar or median and radial sensory stimulation values at the wrist is useful in confirming the diagnosis. Radiographs, including a "carpal tunnel view," are recommended to detect arthritis or fractures. Computed tomography and magnetic resonance imaging are rarely needed; however, in the case with a symptomatic patient with equivocal EMG findings, imaging can be helpful. MR imaging has the greatest sensitivity and specificity in the evaluation of CTS.

Treatment

Conservative therapy consists of the use of splints and nonsteroidal anti-inflammatory agents. Splints should be light and hold the wrist in a neutral or slightly extended position. Local steroid injections are effective in 80% to 90% of patients, but symptoms tend to return after months or sometimes years. Injections should not be given more frequently than on two or three occasions per year. Care must be taken not to inject directly into the median nerve. Diuretics have not been shown to be efficacious. **Surgery is indicated for intractable symptoms that are refractory to medical management.** It consists of complete division of the transverse carpal ligament extending distally from the ulnar side of the median nerve. The results of surgery are generally good. Poor results are usually associated with either a misdiagnosis or failure to divide the ligament completely. The surgery can be performed with an open or an endoscopic approach. A tourniquet is used to exsanguinate the limb, and the operative field is infiltrated with a local anesthetic agent such as Xylocaine; in addition, intravenous sedation can be used. The Palmer fascia and the ligament are divided vertically from the proximal end of the carpal tunnel to its most distal point, and a wide separation of the ends of the ligament is observed (Figure 7–2). The underlying median nerve is carefully protected. A small tissue flap is left attached to the hook of the hamate, and the skin is closed. Postoperatively, the wrist is splinted in slight extension for approximately 2 weeks.

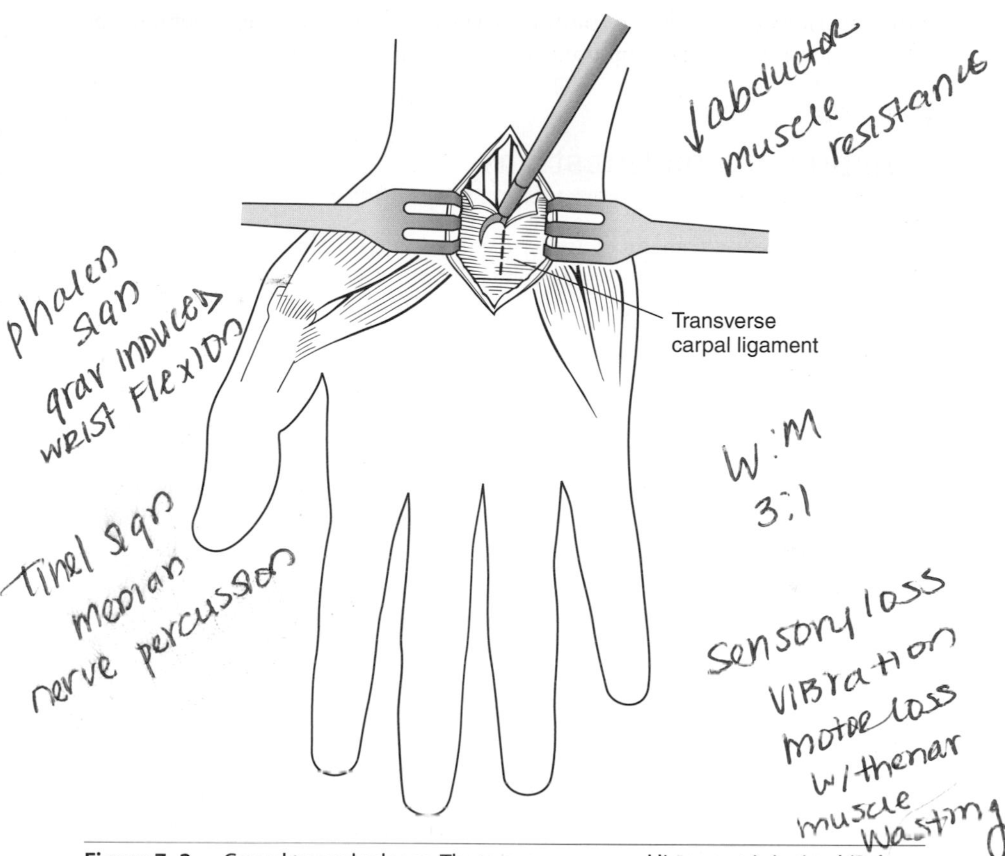

Figure 7–2. Carpal tunnel release. The transverse carpal ligament is incised (Palmar view of the wrist).

The potential advantages of the endoscopic approach are less discomfort, minimal scarring, a shorter period of immobilization, and a more rapid recovery. Persistent or recurrent symptoms should be investigated by repeated electrophysiologic studies and by exclusion of other causes of nerve compression. Occasionally, the ulnar nerve is compressed at the wrist, but more commonly, compression of this nerve occurs in the fibromuscular groove posterior to the medial epicondyle.

Prognosis

In general, conservative treatment of mild CTS is effective. In conditions that are temporary such as pregnancy, temporizing measures are common. Overall surgery is approximately 85% effective in alleviating symptoms; however, some patients may have residual numbness of the fingers even after carpal tunnel release. Additionally, patients with advanced disease (significant motor deficits or muscular atrophy, concomitant neuropathy or diabetes, longer duration of condition, or older age group have a poorer prognosis.

Comprehension Questions

7.1 A 24-year-old medical student notes some numbness and tingling of her right hand. She states that primarily her little finger is affected. Which of the following is the most likely etiology?

A. Median nerve
B. Radial nerve
C. Ulnar nerve
D. Long thoracic nerve

7.2 Which of the following patients is most likely to develop carpal tunnel syndrome?

A. A 45-year-old woman with diabetes insipidus
B. A 32-year-old woman with hypothyroidism
C. An 18-year-old man with addisonian syndrome
D. A 51-year-old woman with fibromyalgia

7.3 A 30-year-old man complains of numbness and tingling of his right thumb and index finger. He also has pain at night on the same hand. The Tinel sign is positive. He is diagnosed with CTS and given a nighttime splint. After 3 months, the symptoms have worsened. An electrophysiologic study is performed, and the results are equivocal. Which of the following is the best next step for this patient?

A. Refer to psychiatrist
B. Question about drug-seeking behavior
C. Refer for cervical spine surgery
D. MRI of the wrist

ANSWERS

7.1 **C.** The sensory innervation of the little finger and the ulnar side of the ring finger is achieved with the ulnar nerve. Median nerve distribution is to the sensory aspect of the thumb, index and middle fingers on the palmar aspect.

7.2 **B.** Hypothyroidism (as well as diabetes mellitus, hyperthyroidism, pregnancy, and acromegaly) is associated with carpal tunnel syndrome. Diabetes insipidus is associated with loss of dilute urine and not associated with CTS.

7.3 **D.** When the clinical findings are present, but the EMG studies are equivocal, MR imaging can be helpful in assisting with the diagnosis. No imaging test is considered to be routinely needed in the evaluation of CTS, but in selected circumstances, it may be helpful. In mild cases of CTS, clinical examination is sufficient.

Clinical Pearls

- Carpal tunnel syndrome usually involves pain to the radial three fingers, especially at night.
- The initial treatment of carpal tunnel syndrome includes administration of NSAIDs and the use of a wrist splint.
- Surgery is indicated when severe pain or progressive motor weakness occurs despite conservative measures.

REFERENCE

Peimer CA. Surgery of the hand and wrist. In: Brunicardi FC, Andersen DK, Billiar TR, et al, eds. *Schwartz's Principles of Surgery*. 8th ed. New York, NY: McGraw-Hill; 2005:1721-1787.

Case 8

A 46-year-old woman presents with a 24-hour history of abdominal pain that began approximately 1 hour after a large dinner. The pain initially began as a dull ache in the epigastrium but then localized in the right upper quadrant (RUQ). She describes some nausea but no vomiting. Since her presentation to the emergency department, the pain has improved significantly to the point of her being nearly pain free. She describes having had similar pain in the past with all previous episodes being self-limited. Her past medical history is significant for type II diabetes mellitus. On physical examination, her temperature is 38.1°C (99°F), and the rest of her vital signs are normal. The abdomen is nondistended with minimal tenderness in the RUQ. Findings from the liver examination appear normal. The rectal and pelvic examinations reveal no abnormalities. Her complete blood count reveals a white blood cell (WBC) count of 13,000/mm^3. Serum chemistry studies demonstrate total bilirubin 0.8 mg/dL, direct bilirubin 0.6 mg/dL, alkaline phosphatase 100 U/L, aspartate transaminase (AST) 45 U/L, and alanine transaminase (ALT) 30 U/L. Ultrasonography of the RUQ demonstrates stones in the gallbladder, a thickened gallbladder wall, and a common bile duct diameter of 4.0 mm.

- ➤ What is the most likely diagnosis?
- ➤ What is the best therapy?
- ➤ What are the complications associated with this disease process?

ANSWERS TO CASE 8: Gallstone Disease

Summary: A 46-year-old woman presents with a 1-day history of RUQ abdominal pain and a physical examination and laboratory findings suggestive of gallstone disease.

- **Diagnosis:** Cholecystitis, likely acute and chronic.
- **Best therapy:** Laparoscopic cholecystectomy is the preferred treatment for all patients with a reasonable life expectancy and no prohibitive risks for general anesthesia and abdominal surgery.
- **Complications:** Complications from gallstone disease include complications involving the gallbladder (acute and chronic cholecystitis) and complications involving the passage of stones from the gallbladder (including pancreatitis, choledocholithiasis, cholangitis, and gallstone ileus.

ANALYSIS

Objectives

1. Know the etiology of gallstone disease and learn the differences among biliary colic, acute cholecystitis, and chronic cholecystitis.
2. Know the basic diagnostic and therapeutic plans for patients with gallstone disease.
3. Learn the complications that can develop from gallstone disease.

Considerations

This patient provides a good history of recurrent upper abdominal pain episodes following meals, consistent with biliary colic. Although she demonstrates minimal tenderness to palpation in her right upper abdomen on physical examination, the **elevated leukocyte count and ultrasound findings of gallbladder wall thickening are consistent with acute or chronic cholecystitis**. If this patient had a normal WBC count and an ultrasound examination demonstrating stones in the gallbladder and no other abnormalities, the presentation would be consistent with biliary colic, which can be treated by elective cholecystectomy. Since findings in this patient are consistent with cholecystitis; the treatment consists of hospital admission, administration of intravenous antibiotics, and laparoscopic cholecystectomy prior to discharge from the hospital.

APPROACH TO
Gallstone Disease

DEFINITIONS

BILIARY COLIC: Characterized by waxing and waning, poorly localized postprandial upper abdominal pain radiating to the back and normal laboratory evaluations of liver functions. It is caused by cholecystokinin-stimulated gallbladder contraction, following food ingestion. The condition is generally produced by gallstone obstruction at the gallbladder neck or, less commonly, by gallbladder dysfunction.

ACUTE CHOLECYSTITIS: In 95% of patients, acute cholecystitis results from a stone or stones obstructing the cystic duct. Bacterial infection is thought to occur via the lymphatics, with the most commonly found organisms being *Escherichia coli, Klebsiella, Proteus,* and *Streptococcus faecalis.* Patients generally present with persistent RUQ pain, with or without fever, gallbladder tenderness, leukocytosis, and often mild, nonspecific elevated liver enzyme levels, which may or may not indicate common bile duct stones. Treatment includes hospital admission, administration of intravenous fluids, nothing by mouth, antibiotics directed at the organisms just listed, and cholecystectomy during the hospitalization.

ACALCULOUS CHOLECYSTITIS: Gallbladder inflammation caused by biliary stasis (in 5% of patients with acute cholecystitis) leading to gallbladder distension, venous congestion, and decreased perfusion; it nearly always occurs in patients hospitalized with a critical illness.

CHRONIC CHOLECYSTITIS: Results from repeated bouts of biliary colic and/or acute cholecystitis leading to gallbladder wall inflammation and fibrosis. The patient may present with persistent or recurrent localized RUQ pain without fever or leukocytosis. Sonography may demonstrate a thickened gallbladder wall or a contracted gallbladder.

CHOLANGITIS: Infection within the bile ducts, most commonly because of complete or partial obstruction of the bile ducts by gallstones or strictures. The classic **Charcot triad (RUQ pain, jaundice, and fever)** is seen in only 70% of patients. This condition may lead to life-threatening sepsis and multiple-organ failure. Treatment consists of antibiotic therapy and supportive care; in cases of severe cholangitis, endoscopic decompression of the bile duct by endoscopic retrograde cholangiopancreatography (ERCP) or surgery is indicated.

RIGHT UPPER QUADRANT ULTRASONOGRAPHY: Ninety-eight to ninety-nine percent sensitivity in identifying gallstones in the gallbladder. The examination is also useful for measuring the diameter of the common bile duct, which can indicate the possible presence of stones in the common bile duct (choledocholithiasis). When present, common bile duct stones are visualized less than 50% of the time with this imaging modality.

BILIARY SCINTIGRAPHY: The study of gallbladder function and biliary patency using an intravenous radiotracer. Normally the liver is visualized, followed by the gallbladder, followed by emptying of the radiotracer into the duodenum. Nonvisualization of the gallbladder in a patient with RUQ pain indicates gallbladder dysfunction caused by acute or chronic cholecystitis.

ENDOSCOPIC RETROGRADE CHOLANGIOPANCREATOGRAPHY: Endoscopic common bile duct cannulation and direct injection of contrast material to visualize the duct. An endoscopic sphincterotomy in the duodenum during the procedure may facilitate bile drainage and the clearance of bile duct stones, which is especially useful in treating cholangitis and choledocholithiasis. The procedure requires sedation and may be associated with complication rates of 8% to 10%.

CLINICAL APPROACH

Pathophysiology

At least 16 million Americans have gallstones, and 800,000 new cases occur each year. Gallstones are categorized as either cholesterol stones or pigmented stones. Cholesterol stones are most common and form as the result of the combined effects of cholesterol supersaturation in the bile and gallbladder dysfunction. Only a small fraction (15%-20%) of patients with gallstones develop symptoms. Although it is unknown why some patients with gallstones develop symptoms whereas others do not, it is clear that those who develop symptoms are at risk for the subsequent development of complications, including acute and chronic cholecystitis, choledocholithiasis, pancreatitis, and cholangitis.

Patient Evaluation and Treatment

The evaluation in every patient should consist of a history, a physical examination, a complete blood count, liver function studies, a serum amylase determination, and RUQ ultrasonography (Table 8–1). It is important to differentiate biliary colic from complicated gallstone disease, such as acute or chronic cholecystitis, choledocholithiasis, cholangitis, and biliary pancreatitis, because the management varies for these conditions. For example, a patient with **choledocholithiasis (common bile duct stone) may present with symptoms identical to those of biliary colic, but the condition may be differentiated on the basis of an elevation in serum liver enzyme levels and dilation of the common bile duct by ultrasound.** In contrast to patients with biliary colic, who are treated by elective cholecystectomy, patients with choledocholithiasis require in-hospital observation for the development of cholangitis and early endoscopic clearance of common bile duct stones, in addition to cholecystectomy. A major goal in

Table 8–1 GALLSTONE DISEASE PRESENTATIONS

DISEASE	SYMPTOMS	PHYSICAL EXAMINATION	ULTRASONOGRAPHY	LABORATORY STUDIES
Biliary colic	Postprandial pain, usually < 6 h in duration	Afebrile, mild tenderness over gallbladder	Gallstones in gallbladder but no wall thickening, no CBD dilation	Normal WBC count, normal LFT values, normal serum amylase level
Acute cholecystitis	Persistent epigastric or RUQ pain lasting > 8 h	May be febrile or afebrile; usually localized gallbladder tenderness	Gallstones in gallbladder; may have pericholecystic fluid; may or may not have CBD dilation	Normal or elevated WBC count; may have normal or mildly elevated LFT values
Chronic cholecystitis	Persistent recurrent RUQ pain	Afebrile; may have localized tenderness over a palpable gallbladder	Stones in gallbladder, thickened gallbladder wall; in advanced cases contracted gallbladder	Normal WBC count; may have mild elevation in LFT values
Choledocholithiasis	Postprandial abdominal pain that improves with fasting	May or may not be clinically jaundiced; nonspecific RUQ abdominal tenderness	Gallstones in gallbladder; CBD usually dilated	Elevation in LFT values; the pattern of elevation is dependent on the chronicity and partial versus complete obstruction
Biliary pancreatitis	Persistent epigastric and back pain	Epigastric tenderness to deep palpation is present	Gallstones in gallbladder; CBD dilation may occur because of pancreatitis (does not always indicate CBD stones)	Leukocytosis, serum amylase level frequently > 1000 U/L, LFT values may be transiently elevated, but persistence may indicate CBD stones

Abbreviations: CBD, common bile duct; LFT, liver function test; RUQ, right upper quadrant; WBC, white blood cell.

patient evaluation is to make an accurate diagnosis without using unnecessary imaging and invasive diagnostic studies. **Choledocholithiasis should be suspected** if the RUQ ultrasound findings include a **common bile duct diameter greater than 5 mm in the presence of elevated liver enzyme levels. Gallstone pancreatitis** should be considered in the presence of **significantly elevated amylase and lipase values.**

Sometimes, acute and chronic cholecystitis may be difficult to differentiate clinically because in both cases patients may have localized tenderness over the gallbladder. When this situation arises, patients should be treated as if they had acute cholecystitis. The treatment for both acute and chronic cholecystitis is cholecystectomy. The operation of choice is a laparoscopic cholecystectomy with or without cholangiography (radiopaque dye injected into the common bile duct and a radiograph taken). Some surgeons selectively perform cholangiograms if the common bile duct is dilated and liver enzyme levels are elevated. Other surgeons obtain cholangiograms with every laparoscopic cholecystectomy performed. Patients with gallstone pancreatitis are treated with bowel rest and intravenous hydration. When the pancreatitis resolves clinically, a laparoscopic cholecystectomy can be done. Generally, patients with **uncomplicated biliary pancreatitis should undergo cholecystectomy** during the same hospitalization. When cholecystectomy is delayed, 25% to 30% of patients may develop recurrent bouts of pancreatitis within a 6-week period.

Comprehension Questions

8.1 A 65-year-old woman presents to the emergency department with postprandial RUQ pain, nausea, and emesis over the last 12 hours. The pain is persistent and radiates to her back. She is afebrile, and her abdomen is tender to palpation in the RUQ. Sonography demonstrates cholelithiasis, gallbladder wall thickening, and a dilated common bile duct measuring 12 mm. Laboratory studies reveal the following values: WBC count 13,000/mm^3, AST 220 U/L, ALT 240 U/L, alkaline phosphatase 385 U/L, and direct bilirubin 4.0 mg/dL. Which of the following is the most appropriate treatment at this time?

A. Admit the patient to the hospital, provide intravenous hydration, and check hepatitis serology values.

B. Admit the patient to the hospital and perform a laparoscopic cholecystectomy.

C. Admit the patient to the hospital, provide intravenous hydration, begin antibiotic therapy, and recommend ERCP.

D. Provide pain medication in the emergency department and ask the patient to follow up in the clinic.

8.2 A 28-year-old woman undergoing an obstetric ultrasound during the second trimester of pregnancy is found to have gallstones in her gallbladder. She claims to have had indigestion with frequent belching throughout her pregnancy. Which of the following is the most appropriate treatment?

A. A low-fat diet until the end of her pregnancy and then a postpartum laparoscopic cholecystectomy
B. Elective laparoscopic cholecystectomy during the second trimester
C. Follow-up after completion of her pregnancy
D. Open cholecystectomy during the second trimester

8.3 A 45-year-old man is seen in the emergency center for abdominal pain. A presumptive diagnosis of acute cholecystitis is made. Which of the following findings is most consistent with this diagnosis?

A. Fever, intermittent RUQ pain, and jaundice
B. Persistent abdominal pain, RUQ tenderness, and leukocytosis
C. Intermittent abdominal pain and minimal tenderness over the gallbladder
D. Epigastric and back pain

8.4 A 69-year-old man presents with confusion, abdominal pain, shaking chills, a rectal temperature of 34°C (94°F), and jaundice. An abdominal radiograph shows air in the biliary tree. Which of the following is the most likely diagnosis?

A. Acute cholangitis
B. Acute pancreatitis
C. Acute cholecystitis
D. Acute appendicitis

8.5 A 33-year-old otherwise healthy woman presents to the hospital with localized right upper quadrant pain. Her temperature is 38.2°C. Her abdomen is tender locally in the right upper quadrant. Her WBC is 12,000/mm^3 and her liver function tests are all within normal limits. An ultrasound of the right upper quadrant revealed gallstones with the gall bladder, pericholecystic fluid, and a common bile duct measuring 4.5 mm in diameter. What is the most appropriate management for this patient?

A. NPO, antibiotics, followed by cholecystecomy in 6-8 weeks
B. NPO, antibiotics, and ERCP with endoscopic drainage of the biliary tract
C. NPO, antibiotics
D. NPO, antibiotics, and laparoscopic cholecystectomy

8.6 A 30-year-old woman presents with postprandial upper abdominal pain that has been recurrent over the past several months. She has undergone ultrasound evaluation of the gallbladder that has not demonstrated gallstones. Her liver function studies have been normal. Which of the following is the most appropriate next step for this patient?

A. Obtain a CCK-stimulated HIDA scan.
B. Cholecystectomy.
C. Refer patient to a gastroenterologist for treatment of irritable bowel syndrome.
D. Repeat the gallbladder ultrasound.

ANSWERS

8.1 **C.** Admission to the hospital, administration of intravenous fluids and antibiotics, and ERCP are appropriate in managing this patient. This patient's presentation is highly suggestive of cholangitis, with the presence of a significant elevation in her liver enzyme levels, common bile duct dilation, and tenderness in the RUQ.

8.2 **C.** Reevaluation after the completion of pregnancy is appropriate for this patient, who has stones in her gallbladder and symptoms of belching and indigestion that are most likely unrelated to gallstones and may be pregnancy induced. Indications for cholecystectomy in pregnancy include cholecystitis, intractable pain, and cholangitis.

8.3 **B.** Persistent abdominal pain, RUQ tenderness, and leukocytosis indicate acute cholecystitis. Choice A is most consistent with cholangitis; choice C is typical of biliary colic, and choice D is consistent with acute pancreatitis.

8.4 **A.** Elderly patients older than 65 years of age who present with fever (or hypothermia), jaundice, abdominal pain, and shaking chills often have acute cholangitis (purulent infection of the biliary tract). The presence of air in the biliary tree is consistent with this illness. This is a life-threatening condition and often requires urgent surgical or endoscopic decompression of the biliary system, in addition to aggressive supportive care and broad-spectrum antibiotic therapy.

8.5 **D.** This patient has signs, symptoms, and finding compatible with acute cholecystitis. The treatment of acute cholecystitis consists of antibiotics and early cholecystectomy. Early cholecystectomy has been compared to delayed cholecystectomy and the investigations have shown that early operative treatment did not contribute to increase in operative complications and that early surgery resulted in the reduction in length of stay and readmissions to the hospital.

8.6 **A.** This patient has fairly typical signs and symptoms of biliary colic. Biliary colic is most commonly produced by the mechanical obstruction of gallbladder drainage by a gallstone; however, in a small subset of patients, these symptoms can be produced by primary gallbladder dysfunction that is not related to gallstones. This condition is referred to as *biliary dyskenesia*, and its presumptive diagnosis is based on classic biliary colic symptoms, absence of gallstones, and evidence of gallbladder dysfunction. Gallbladder dysfunction could be demonstrated in these patients with a HIDA scan following CCK administration. Normal gallbladders generally will demonstrate ejection fraction of more than 50% following CCK injection, and biliary dyskenesia patients may have lower ejection fraction and reproduction of symptoms with CCK injections.

Clinical Pearls

- Cholecystectomy is generally not indicated unless there is a clear link between the patient's symptoms and gallstones or if there is objective evidence of gallbladder dysfunction (eg, a thickened gallbladder wall on ultrasonography, nonvisualization of the gallbladder on biliary scintigraphy) or gallstone-related complications.
- In general, the treatment of cholecystitis is hospitalization, administration of intravenous antibiotics, and a laparoscopic cholecystectomy prior to discharge from the hospital.
- **Cholangitis, which can be diagnosed with Charcot triad—RUQ pain, jaundice, and fever** is life threatening. Treatment consists of antibiotics therapy, supportive care, and, in cases of severe cholangitis biliary duct, decompression via ERCP.
- Choledocholithiasis should be suspected if the RUQ ultrasound findings include a common bile duct diameter > 5 mm in the presence of elevated liver enzyme levels.

REFERENCES

Chari RS, Shah SA. Biliary system. In: Townsend CM Jr, Beauchamp RD, Evers BM, et al, eds. *Sabiston Textbook of Surgery*. 18th ed. Philadelphia, PA: Suanders Elsevier; 2008:1547-1588.

Kao LS, Liu TH. Calculous disease of the gallbladder and biliary tract. In: Miller T, Bass BL, Fabri PJ, et al, eds. *Modern Surgical Care: Physiological Foundations and Clinical Applications*. 3rd ed. New York, NY: Informa Healthcare; 2007: 455-468.

Oddsdottir M, Hunter JG. Gallbladder and the extrahepatic biliary system. In: Brunicardi FC, Andersen DK, Billiar TR, et al, eds. *Schwartz's Principles of Surgery*. 8th ed. New York, NY: McGraw-Hill; 2005:1187-1219.

Acute Cholecystitis

Pain

RUQ tenderness

Leukocytosis

Cholangitis (Virchow)

Fever

Pain

Jaundice

Case 9

A 38-year-old man presents at the emergency department with tarry stools and a feeling of light-headedness. The patient indicates that over the past 24 hours he has had several bowel movements containing tarry-colored stools and for the past 12 hours has felt light-headed. His past medical and surgical history is unremarkable. The patient complains of frequent headaches caused by work-related stress for which he has been self-medicating with 6-8 tablets of ibuprofen a day for the past 2 weeks. He consumes two to three martinis per day and denies tobacco or illicit drug use. On examination, his temperature is 37.0°C (98.6°F), pulse rate 105 beats/min (supine), blood pressure 104/80 mm Hg, and respiratory rate 22 breaths/min. His vital signs upright are pulse 120 beats/min and blood pressure 90/76 mm Hg. He is awake, cooperative, and pale. The cardiopulmonary examinations are unremarkable. His abdomen is mildly distended and mildly tender in the epigastrium. The rectal examination reveals melanotic stools but no masses in the vault.

- What is your next step?
- What is the best initial treatment?

ANSWERS TO CASE 9: Upper Gastrointestinal Tract Hemorrhage

Summary: A 38-year-old man presents with signs and symptoms of acute upper gastrointestinal (GI) tract hemorrhage. The patient's presentation suggests that he may have had significant blood loss leading to class III hemorrhagic shock.

- **Next step:** The first step in the treatment of patients with upper GI hemorrhage is intravenous fluid resuscitation. The etiology and severity of the bleeding dictate the intensity of therapy and predict the risk of further bleeding and/or death.

- **Best initial treatment:** Prompt attention to the patient's airway, breathing, and circulation (ABCs) is mandatory for patients with acute upper GI hemorrhage. After attention to the ABCs, the patient is prepared for endoscopy to identify the etiology or source of the bleeding and possible endoscopic therapy to control hemorrhage.

ANALYSIS

Objectives

1. Be able to outline resuscitation and treatment strategies for patients presenting with acute upper GI tract hemorrhage and hemorrhagic shock.
2. Learn the common causes of upper GI tract hemorrhage and their therapies.
3. Know the adverse prognostic factors associated with continued bleeding and increased mortality.

Considerations

The treatment of patients with suspected upper GI tract hemorrhage begins with an initial assessment to determine if the bleeding is acute or occult. Acute bleeding is recognized by a history of hematemesis, coffee-ground emesis, melena, or bleeding per rectum, whereas patients with occult bleeding may present with signs and symptoms associated with anemia and no clear history of blood loss. **A critical part of the initial evaluation is assessment of the patient's physiologic status to gauge the severity of blood loss. The sequence in the management** of acute upper GI tract hemorrhage consists of **(1) resuscitation, (2) diagnosis, and (3) treatment,** in that order. In this patient's case, his symptoms and physiologic parameters suggest severe, acute blood loss (class III hemorrhagic shock with up to 35% total blood volume loss) and should prompt immediate resuscitation with close monitoring of patient response (urine output, clinical appearance, blood pressure, heart rate, serial hemoglobin and hematocrit values, and consideration of central venous pressure [CVP] monitoring). A nasogastric tube should be inserted following resuscitation to determine whether bleeding is active. The stomach should be irrigated with room-temperature water or saline until gastric aspirates are clear. For patients with **massive upper GI tract bleeding, agitation, or impaired respiratory status, endotracheal intubation is recommended prior to endoscopy.** Laboratory studies to be obtained include a complete blood count (CBC), liver function studies, prothrombin time (PT), and partial thromboplastin time (PTT). A type and cross-match should be ordered. Platelets or fresh-frozen plasma should be administered when thrombocytopenia or coagulopathy is identified, respectively. Early endoscopy identifies the bleeding source in patients with active ongoing bleeding and may achieve early control of bleeding. Given the history of nonsteroidal anti-inflammatory drug (NSAID) use, it would be appropriate to begin empirical therapy for a presumed gastric ulcer and gastric erosions with a proton pump inhibitor prior to endoscopic confirmation.

APPROACH TO Upper Gi Bleeding

DEFINITIONS

MALLORY-WEISS TEAR: A proximal gastric mucosa tear following vigorous coughing, retching, or vomiting. The bleeding is generally self-limiting, mild, and amenable to supportive care and endoscopic management.

DIEULAFOY EROSION: Infrequently encountered, this problem describes bleeding from an aberrant submucosal artery located in the stomach. This bleeding is frequently significant and requires prompt diagnosis by endoscopy, followed by endoscopic or operative therapy.

ARTERIOVENOUS (AV) MALFORMATION: A small mucosal lesion located along the GI tract. Bleeding is usually abrupt, but the rate of bleeding is usually slow and self-limiting.

ESOPHAGITIS: Mucosal erosions frequently resulting from gastroesophageal (GE) reflux, infections, or medications. Patients most frequently present with occult bleeding, and treatment consists of correction or avoidance of the underlying causes.

ESOPHAGEAL VARICEAL BLEEDING: Engorged veins of the GE region, which may ulcerate and lead to massive hemorrhage; related to portal hypertension and cirrhosis.

SHOCK: Insufficient physiologic mechanism to adequately supply substrate to tissue. The American Trauma Life Support (ATLS) system grades shock from stage I to IV.

Stage I: Less than 750 mL blood loss, well compensated
Stage II: 750-1500 mL blood loss, slight tachycardia, normal blood pressure
Stage III: 1500-2000 mL blood loss, moderate tachycardia, hypotension
Stage IV: Less than 2000 mL blood loss, marked tachycardia, prominent hypotension

CLINICAL APPROACH

Upper GI bleeding describes bleeding from a location proximal to the ligament of Trietz and accounts for 80% of all significant GI bleeding. The sources of upper GI tract bleeding can be categorized as variceal (20%) versus nonvariceal (80%). Common nonvariceal bleeding sources include duodenal ulcers (25%), gastric erosions (20%), gastric ulcers (20%), and Mallory-Weiss tears (15%). Up to 30% of patients have multiple etiologies of bleeding identified during endoscopy. In addition, all studies indicate that a proportion of cases have no endoscopically discernible cause, and these cases are associated with an excellent outcome. Rare causes of upper GI tract bleeding include neoplasms (both benign and malignant), AV malformations, and Dieulafoy erosions. **Bleeding tends to be self-limited in approximately 80% of all patients with acute upper GI tract bleeding.** Continuing or recurrent bleeding occurs in 20% of patients and is the major contributor to mortality. The **overall mortality associated with upper GI tract bleeding is 8% to 10%** and has not changed over the last several decades. There are striking differences in the rates of rebleeding and mortality depending on the diagnosis at endoscopy (Table 9–1). **Patient mortality with acute upper GI tract bleeding increases with rebleeding, increased age, and in patients who develop bleeding in the hospital.** A number of clinical predictors and endoscopic stigmata

Table 9–1 RISK OF REBLEEDING BASED ON SOURCE

SOURCE	REBLEEDING (%)
Esophageal varices	60
Gastric cancer	50
Gastric ulcer	28
Duodenal ulcer	24
Gastric erosion (gastritis)	15
Mallory-Weiss tear	7
No identified source	2.5

Data from Silverstein FE, Gilbert DA, Tedesco FJ, et al. The national ASGE survey on upper gastrointestinal bleeding, Part I, II, and III. *Gastrointest Endosc.* 1981;27:73-101.

Table 9–2 FACTORS ASSOCIATED WITH INCREASED REBLEEDING AND MORTALITY

Clinical
- Shock on admission
- Prior history of bleeding requiring transfusion
- Admission hemoglobin < 8 g/dL
- Transfusion requirement ≥5 U of packed red blood cells
- Continued bleeding noted in nasogastric aspirate
- Age > 60 y (increased mortality but no increase in rebleeding)

Endoscopic
- Visible vessel in ulcer base (50% rebleeding risk)
- Oozing of bright blood from ulcer base
- Adherent clot at ulcer base
- Location of ulcer (worse prognosis when located near large arteries, eg, posterior duodenal bulb or lesser curve or stomach)

Data from Silverstein FE, Gilbert DA, Tedesco FJ, et al. The national ASGE survey on upper gastrointestinal bleeding, Parts I, II, and III. *Gastrointest Endosc.* 1981;27:73-101.

are associated with the increased risk of recurrent bleeding (Table 9–2). The use of NSAIDs contributes to the development of NSAID-induced gastric ulcers. All NSAIDs produce mucosal damage. The risk of developing an ulcer is dose related. Roughly 2% to 4% of NSAID users have GI tract complications each year. Approximately 10% **of patients taking NSAIDs daily develop an acute ulcer.**

Upper GI tract endoscopy establishes a diagnosis in more than 90% of cases and assesses the current activity of bleeding. It aids in directing therapy and predicts the risk of rebleeding. Furthermore, it allows for endoscopic therapy. Endoscopic hemostasis can be achieved through a variety of ways, including thermotherapy with a heater probe, multipolar or bipolar electrocoagulation, and ethanol or epinephrine injections. As shown in Figure 9–1, endoscopy can demonstrate bleeding, esophageal varices, gastroduodenal bleeding, or no bleeding. For nonvariceal bleeding, endoscopic hemostasis is usually achieved with the use of epinephrine injections followed by thermal therapy. Permanent hemostasis occurs in roughly 80% to 90% of patients. Once bleeding is controlled, long-term medical therapy with antisecretory agents such as histamine-2 blockers or proton pump inhibitors is used to treat the underlying disease. Testing for *Helicobacter pylori* should be performed, and if this organism is present, treatment should be initiated. Any NSAID use should be discontinued. If this is not possible, a prostaglandin analogue (such as misoprostol) should be used or, alternatively, one of the selective COX-2 inhibitors should be used to replace nonselective COX inhibitors.

If bleeding continues or recurs, surgery may be necessary. **Surgery is indicated for complicated peptic ulcer disease with massive, persistent, or**

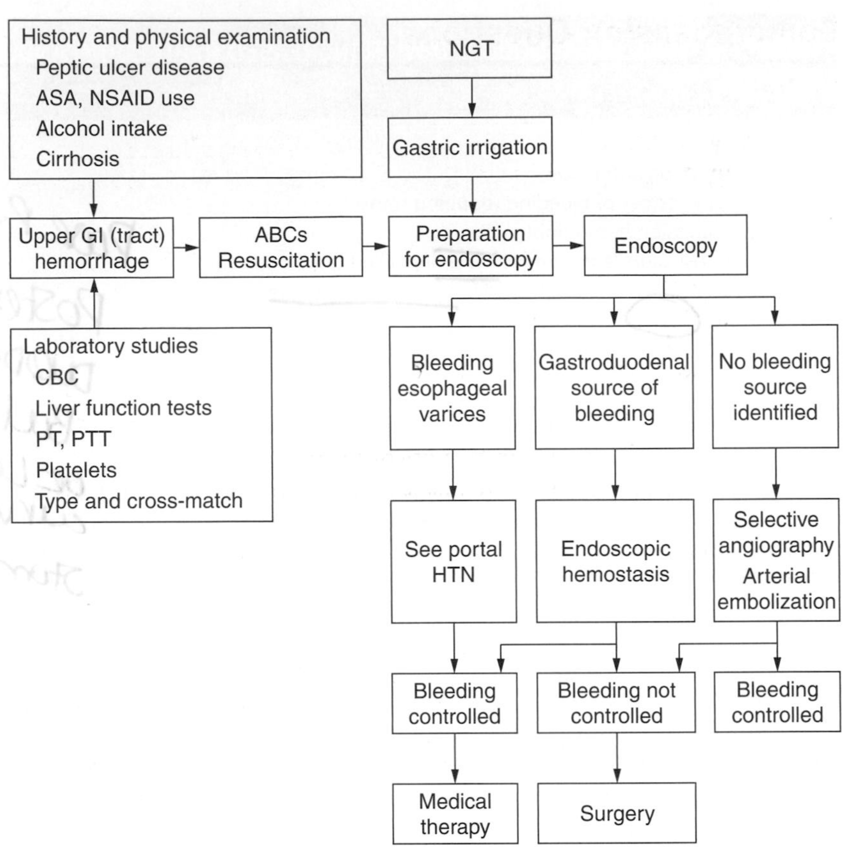

Figure 9–1. Algorithm for the treatment of patients with hematochezia or melena without hematemesis. ASA, aminosalicylate; NSAID, nonsteroidal anti-inflammatory drug; NGT, nasogastric tube; HTN, hypertension; GI, gastrointestinal; ABCs, airway, breathing, circulation; CBC, complete blood count; PT, prothrombin time; PTT, partial thromboplastin time.

recurrent upper GI tract hemorrhage or in association with nonhealing or giant ulcers (≥ 3 cm). For a bleeding gastric ulcer where there is a concern for possible malignancy either gastrectomy or excision of the ulcer is indicated. For other types of ulcers, the vessel may require ligation followed by a vagotomy procedure and pyloroplasty. If the bleeding source cannot be identified but active bleeding is clearly occurring, patients may undergo selective angiography. This treatment strategy can diagnose and treat bleeding in roughly 70% of patients; arterial embolization with gel foam, metal coil springs, or a clot can be used to control bleeding. In addition, arterial vasopressin can cause bleeding to stop in some patients with peptic ulcer disease.

Comprehension Questions

9.1 A 55-year-old man has undergone upper endoscopy. He is told by his gastroenterologist that although this disorder may cause anemia, it is unlikely to cause acute GI hemorrhage. Which of the following is the most likely diagnosis?
A. Gastric ulcer
B. Duodenal ulcer
C. Gastric erosions
D. Esophageal varices
E. Gastric cancer

9.2 A 32-year-old man comes to the emergency department with a history of vomiting "large amounts of bright red blood." Which of the following is the most appropriate first step in the treatment of this patient?
A. Obtaining a history and performing a physical examination
B. Determining hemoglobin and hematocrit levels
C. Fluid resuscitation
D. Inserting a nasogastric tube
E. Performing urgent endoscopy

9.3 A 65-year-old man is brought into the emergency department with acute upper GI hemorrhage. A nasogastric tube is placed with bright red fluid aspirated. After 30 minutes of saline flushes, the aspirate is clear. Which of the following is the most accurate statement regarding this patient's condition?
A. He has approximately 20% chance of rebleed.
B. The mortality for his condition is much lower today than 20 years ago.
C. His age is a poor prognostic factor for rebleeding.
D. Mesenteric ischemia is a likely cause of his condition.

9.4 A 52-year-old man with alcoholism and known cirrhosis comes into the emergency department with acute hematemesis. Bleeding esophageal varices are found during upper GI endoscopy. Which of the following is most likely to be effective treatment for this patient?
A. Balloon tamponade of the esophagus
B. Proton pump inhibitor
C. Triple antibiotic therapy
D. Misoprostol oral therapy
E. Endoscopic sclerotherapy

ANSWERS

9.1 **E.** Gastric cancer is relatively asymptomatic until late in its course. Weight loss and anorexia are the most common symptoms with this condition. Hematemesis is unusual, but anemia from chronic occult blood loss is common.

9.2 **C.** Fluid resuscitation is the first priority to maintain sufficient intravascular volume to perfuse vital organs. Assessment of volume status is best accomplished clinically; acutely the hemoglobin and hematocrit levels do not fall and do not reflect volume depletion.

9.3 **A.** Approximately 20% of patients with acute upper GI hemorrhage have continued or rebleeding episodes. The mortality has remained the same (approximately 8%-10%) over the past 20 years.

9.4 **E.** Endoscopic injection of sclerosing agents directly into the varix is effective in controlling acute hemorrhage caused by variceal bleeding in approximately 90% of cases. Balloon tamponade is a therapy used infrequently for acute esophageal variceal bleeding because of its limited effectiveness in achieving sustained control of bleeding. Other therapies include vasopressin or octreotide to decrease portal pressure.

Clinical Pearls

- Early endoscopy is useful in identifying the bleeding sources, and in patients with active ongoing bleeding it may help in achieving early control of bleeding.
- Approximately 10% of patients who take daily NSAIDs develop an acute ulcer.
- Surgery is indicated for complicated peptic ulcer disease with massive, persistent, or recurrent upper GI tract hemorrhage or in association with nonhealing or giant ulcers (> 3 cm).
- Acute GI tract hemorrhage should be treated with aggressive fluid resuscitation, close monitoring of patient response, nasogastric tube insertion following resuscitation to determine whether bleeding is active, and gastric irrigation with room-temperature water or saline until gastric aspirates are clear.
- The most common cause of upper GI tract hemorrhage in a patient with cirrhosis and portal hypertension is variceal bleeding, which carries a high rate of mortality and risk of rebleeding.
- The most common cause of pediatric significant upper GI tract hemorrhage is variceal bleeding from extrahepatic portal venous obstruction.

REFERENCES

Mercer DW, Robinson EK. Stomach. In: Townsend CM, Beauchamp RD, Evers BM, et al, eds. *Sabiston Textbook of Surgery*. 18th ed. Philadelphia, PA: Saunders Elsevier; 2008: 1223-1277.

Tavakkalizadeh A, Goldberg JE, Ashley SW. Acute gastrointestinal hemorrhage. In: Townsend CM, Beauchamp RD, Evers BM, et al, eds. *Sabiston Textbook of Surgery*. 18th ed. Philadelphia, PA: Saunders Elsevier; 2008:1199-1222.

Case 10

A 67-year-old man presented to the emergency department with a 6-hour history of bleeding per rectum. The patient's symptoms began after he developed an urge to defecate that was followed by several voluminous bowel movements containing maroon-colored stool mixed with blood clots. The patient complains of feeling light-headed just prior to arriving at the hospital but denies any abdominal pain. His past medical history is significant for borderline hypertension managed with diet control. His surgical history is significant for a right inguinal hernia repair 2 years ago. His blood pressure is 100/80 mm Hg, pulse rate 110 beats/min, and respiratory rate 20 breaths/min. The results of an examination of his abdomen are unremarkable. The rectal examination revealed no masses and a large amount of maroon-colored stool in the rectal vault.

- What should be your next step?
- What is the most likely diagnosis?
- How would you confirm this diagnosis?

ANSWERS TO CASE 10:
Lower Gastrointestinal Tract Hemorrhage

Summary: A 67-year-old man presents with acute lower gastrointestinal tract hemorrhage. The patient's symptoms and vital signs indicate a significant acute hemorrhage, likely class II hemorrhagic shock.

- **Next step:** The patient's presentation is highly suggestive of hypovolemic shock; therefore, the initial treatment should consist of volume resuscitation with isotonic crystalloid solution and close monitoring of his response to resuscitation.
- **Most likely diagnosis:** Acute lower GI tract hemorrhage.
- **How to confirm the diagnosis:** Place a nasogastric (NG) tube to sample the upper GI tract contents; the possibility of gastric bleeding can be eliminated if nonbloody, bilious material is recovered. Esophagogastroduodenoscopy (EGD) is the definitive method of evaluation to rule out a duodenal source of bleeding.

ANALYSIS

Objectives

1. Learn to differentiate the clinical presentations of occult and acute anorectal, nonanorectal lower GI tract, and upper GI tract bleeding.
2. Learn a rational diagnostic and therapeutic approach to lower GI tract bleeding.

Considerations

The passage of maroon-colored stool and blood clots generally indicates acute bleeding from a lower GI tract source (distal to the ligament of Treitz). Maroon-colored stool represents a mixture of fecal material and blood, indicating that the bleeding source is located proximal to the lower rectal segment and anus. **The passage of blood clots can occur with brisk bleeding from an upper GI tract source. Placement of an NG tube is useful during the initial evaluation for possible upper GI tract bleeding,** although up to 16% of patients may have nonbloody NG aspirate with upper GI tract bleeding originating from the duodenum. In patients older than 40 years, the **most likely causes of acute lower GI tract bleeding are diverticulosis, angiodysplasia, and neoplasm,** and these lesions are generally painless. When lower GI tract bleeding occurs in the presence of **abdominal pain,** the possibility of **an ischemic bowel, inflammatory bowel disease, intussusception, and a ruptured**

abdominal aneurysm should be entertained. Following resuscitation, the **primary goal in the treatment of a patient with acute and continued lower GI tract bleeding is localization of the bleeding site** (colonoscopy, mesenteric angiography, and/or an isotope-labeled red blood cell [RBC] scan).

mesenteric angiography.

APPROACH TO Lower GI Tract Bleeding

DEFINITIONS

OCCULT GI TRACT BLEEDING: Slow bleeding originating anywhere along the upper aerodigestive or lower GI tract, most commonly associated with neoplasm, gastritis, and esophagitis. Patients generally do not report bleeding and commonly present with iron deficiency anemia, fatigue, and Hemoccult-positive stool.

OVERT LOWER GI TRACT BLEEDING: Hematochezia or melena. The **most common causes in children and adolescents are Meckel diverticulum, inflammatory bowel disease, and polyps.** In adults aged 20 to 60 years, the most common causes are diverticulosis, neoplasm, and inflammatory bowel disease. In **older adults (> 60 years), the most common causes are diverticulosis, angiodysplasia, and neoplasm.**

TAGGED RBC SCAN: Nuclear medicine imaging using RBCs labeled with technetium 99m. This technique is highly sensitive in identifying active bleeding at a rate of 0.1 mL/min or greater; however, the images obtained may not localize the GI tract bleeding site accurately. Some recommend this imaging modality as an initial screening study before performing mesenteric angiography.

MESENTERIC ANGIOGRAPHY: Selective angiography of the superior and inferior mesentery arteries can localize bleeding from the midgut and hindgut. This procedure has greater specificity for bleeding localization than a tagged-RBC scan. Selective injection of vasopressin or gel foam can be applied to during angiography to treat active bleeding in patients who are not suitable surgical candidates. The bleeding generally has to be 0.5-1.0 mL/min to be visualized by angiography.

VIDEO CAPSULE ENDOSCOPY: A small capsular video camera can be swallowed to provide visualization of the entire GI tract lumen. This study is time consuming and does not offer therapeutic options for patients with acute bleeding.

RIGID PROCTOSIGMOIDOSCOPY: A simple bedside procedure in which a nonflexible endoscope is used to visualize the most distal 25-cm segment of the lower GI tract.

DIAGNOSTIC COLONOSCOPY: Flexible fiberoptic endoscopy that evaluates the entire colon and rectum and is reserved for hemodynamically stable patients. The reported success rate in identifying the bleeding source and site is as high as 75%, but this figure is highly variable depending on the operator and the timing. The advantages of this procedure are that it can rule out the possibility of a colorectal bleeding source and that identified bleeding angiodysplasia can be treated with epinephrine injection or coagulation.

ANGIODYSPLASIA: A common acquired degenerative vascular condition producing small, dilated, thin-walled veins in the submucosa of the GI tract. It occurs most commonly in the cecum and ascending colon of people older than 50 years. Approximately 50% of patients have associated cardiac disease. Up to 25% of patients with angiodysplasia have aortic stenosis. Most patients with angiodysplasia have chronic low-grade, self-limiting bleeding, although approximately 15% present with acute massive bleeding.

CLINICAL APPROACH

A patient presenting with overt lower GI tract bleeding should be quickly assessed for intravascular volume status and hemodynamic stability. A detailed history is important. The identification of coexisting medical problems may help identify patients whose bleeding is the result of coagulopathy, thrombocytopenia, or platelet dysfunction (medical causes of bleeding). **If the patient has had a previous abdominal vascular reconstruction, the possibility of an aortoenteric fistula must be strongly considered and ruled out.** The history elicited should include details regarding the quality and appearance of the bleeding. Melena (tarry stool) indicates the degradation of hemoglobin by bacteria and forms after blood has remained in the GI tract for more than 14 hours. **Melena is usually associated with upper GI tract or small bowel bleeding but can occur with bleeding from the ascending colon.** The passage of **maroon-colored stools** generally excludes a possible bleeding source in the rectum and anus. Bleeding from the rectum is usually characterized by the passage of formed stools streaked with blood or the passage of fresh blood at the end of a normal bowel movement. Most episodes of overt lower GI tract bleeding resolve spontaneously without specific therapy. It is important to rule out GI tract neoplasm as the source of bleeding in patients whose bleeding resolves. Patients whose bleeding creates adverse hemodynamic consequences or necessitates blood transfusion should undergo prompt evaluation to localize the source of bleeding so that operative excision can be accomplished. See Figure 10–1 for management strategy.

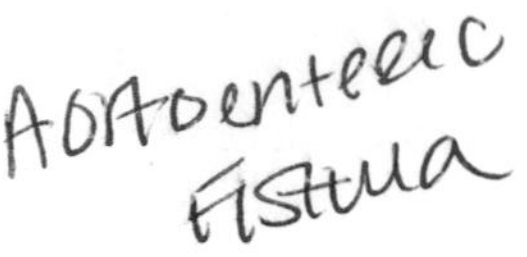

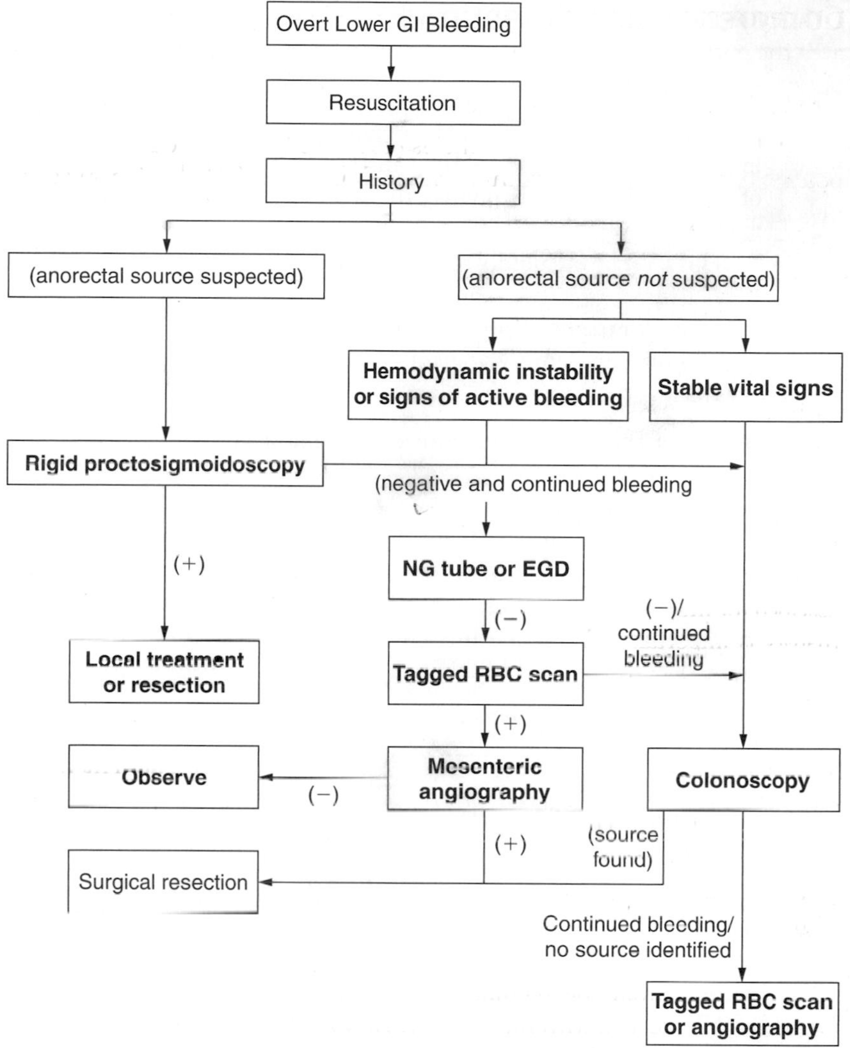

Figure 10–1. Algorithm for the management of hematochezia. Esophagogastroduodenoscopy (EGD), colonoscopy, and small bowel contrast radiography should be performed in patients whose gastrointestinal (GI) tract bleeding has resolved to eliminate the possibility of GI tract bleeding as the cause of bleeding. NG, nasogastric; RBC, red blood cell.

Comprehension Questions

10.1 A 75-year-old man develops hematochezia and presents with blood pressure of 90/60 mm Hg, and heart rate of 120 beats/min. His vital signs improve slightly with crystalloid and packed red cells infusion. Which of the following is considered the most appropriate next step(s) in management?

A. EGD, proctosigmoidoscopy, and a barium enema
B. NG tube, proctosigmoidoscopy, and a tagged RBC scan with or without mesentery angiography
C. NG tube, mesentery angiography, and colonoscopy
D. EGD and colonoscopy

10.2 Which of the following conditions is almost always associated with painless hematochezia?

A. Aortoenteric fistula developing 1 year after an abdominal aortic aneurysm repair
B. Ischemic colitis involving the descending colon
C. Bleeding duodenal ulcer
D. Superior mesentery artery embolus

10.3 Which of the following diagnostic modalities has the greatest specificity in identifying the source of lower GI tract bleeding?

A. Tagged RBC scan
B. Barium enema
C. Colonoscopy
D. Surgical exploration

10.4 A 66-year-old woman presents to the emergency center with a history of having passage of several maroon-colored stools earlier in the day. She complains of feeling light-headed following these episodes. The patient has a history of hypertension and osteoarthritis. She takes metoprolol and NSAIDs daily. Her initial blood pressure is 100/85 mm Hg, and heart rate is 90 beats/min. Her initial hematocrit is 34%. The patient's blood pressure improves with initial IV fluid resuscitation. An NG tube was placed and gastric lavage reveals only bilious fluid. During a 4-hour period of observation in the emergency center, the patient remains stable without further passage of bloody stools. Which of the following is the most appropriate next step?

A. EGD
B. Mesenteric angiography
C. Abdominal CT scan
D. Colonoscopy

10.5 A 72-year-old man presents to the emergency center with abdominal pain and the passage of bloody stools. His past medical history is significant for hypertension, noninsulin-dependent diabetes, and coronary artery disease. His blood pressure is 90/60 mm Hg, with a pulse rate of 120 beats/min. His temperature is 38.8°C. Palpation of his abdomen reveals tenderness in the left upper and lower quadrants. There is no evidence of peritonitis. Which of the following is the most appropriate next step?

A. EGD
B. Abdominal CT scan
C. Colonoscopy
D. Tag RBC scan

ANSWERS

10.1 **B.** In an initially unstable patient with overt GI bleeding, who has only partial response to initial resuscitation, it is critical to rapidly differentiate between upper and lower GI bleeding sources, and this is most rapidly accomplished with NG placement and gastric lavage. A proctosigmoidoscopy could be performed at the bedside to evaluate the anorectal segment of the GI tract. If no bleeding sources are identified with these initial bedside evaluations, a tag RBC scan and mesenteric angiography may be most appropriate to localize the site of bleeding.

10.2 **A.** Aortoenteric fistula following aortic reconstruction is nearly always associated with painless hematochezia while all the other conditions are likely to have pain and bleeding.

10.3 **C.** Colonoscopy has the highest specificity in identifying the source of lower GI tract bleeding (ie, the lowest false-positive rate for bleeding source identification).

10.4 **D.** This patient appears to have had a significant lower GI bleeding episode, which has either stopped or slowed. At this time, colonoscopy may be the best initial diagnostic modality to evaluate and potentially treat the cause of her bleeding. Because the bleeding has apparently stopped or slowed, a tagged RBC scan which is sensitive in localizing bleeding that is more than 0.1mL/min may not be helpful. Similarly, mesentery angiography that is sensitive in localizing bleeding sources that is more than 0.5-1.0 mL/min is not likely to be helpful. An abdominal CT is helpful in identifying overt anatomic changes would not be helpful for the identification of lower GI bleeding sources, which are most commonly colonic diverticulosis and angiodyplasia.

10.5 **B.** This patient's clinical presentation is atypical for lower hemorrhage, because the most common causes of lower GI hemorrhage are angiodysplasia and diverticulosis that do not produce pain. Given his picture of lower GI bleeding, fever, left-sided abdominal pain, and a history of atherosclerotic cardiac disease, the possibility of ischemic colitis needs to be entertained. Another diagnosis to consider is intestinal intussusception, which is uncommon in adults but would produce pain and mucosal sloughing that manifest as bloody mucous in the stool. CT scan in this setting may be useful to help identify the source of inflammatory changes that is producing the patient's abdominal pain, bleeding, and septic picture. With acute inflammatory process, colonoscopy is associated with an increased risk of perforation and is a less ideal diagnostic tool in this setting.

Clinical Pearls

- The primary goal in the treatment of a patient with acute and continued lower GI tract bleeding is localization of the bleeding site.
- The ability to localize the bleeding during an abdominal exploration is greatly compromised. Exploratory laparotomy thus should be avoided prior to precise localization of the bleeding site.
- Tagged RBC scan results should be interpreted with great caution because localization of bleeding to a region of the abdomen does not necessarily localize bleeding from a specific segment of the GI tract.
- Colonoscopy should be reserved for stable patients with lower GI tract bleeding.

REFERENCES

Lucas CE, Ledgerwood AM, Sugawa C. Approach to lower gastrointestinal bleeding. In: Cameron JL, ed. *Current Surgical Therapy*. 9th ed. Philadelphia, PA: Mosby Elsevier; 2008:306-310.

Tavakkalizadeh A, Goldberg JE, Ashley SW. Acute gastrointestinal hemorrhage. In: Townsend CM, Beauchamp RD, Evers BM, et al, eds. *Sabiston Textbook of Surgery*. 18th ed. Philadelphia, PA: Saunders Elsevier; 2008:1199-1222.

Case 11

A 38-year-old woman underwent initial screening mammography that revealed bilateral dense breast tissue shown in Figure 11–1. According to an evaluation by the radiologist, these abnormalities are probably benign (American College of Radiology category 3). The patient's past medical history is unremarkable. She has never had any previous breast mass or undergone mammography in the past. Her family history is significant in that her mother died of breast cancer at 45 years of age. On examination, extensive fibrocystic changes are found to be present in both breasts, and no dominant mass is identified. The examination results for both axillary areas are unremarkable.

➤ What is the most likely diagnosis?

➤ What complications are associated with these changes?

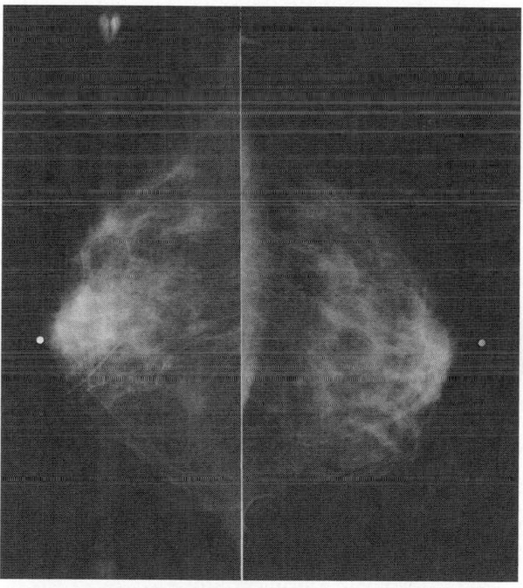

Figure 11–1. Bilateral mammogram showing dense fibrocystic changes in the breasts. *Courtesy of Dr. B. Steinbach.*

ANSWERS TO CASE 11: Breast Cancer Risk and Surveillance

Summary: The patient is a 38-year-old woman with a high-risk profile for breast cancer based on the maternal premenopausal breast cancer history, an unreliable breast examination because of dense fibrocystic changes, and a mammogram that is somewhat difficult to interpret due to increased density.

- **Diagnosis:** Benign fibrocystic changes
- **Complications:** These changes can lead to difficulty in detecting breast carcinoma by physical examination and mammography (Figure 11–1).

ANALYSIS

Objectives

1. Learn the relationship between benign breast changes and borderline malignant changes in breast cancer development (Table 11–1).
2. Understand the management principles for patients at risk for breast cancer development.
3. Learn the management options for patients with benign breast lesions, borderline malignancies, and high-risk profiles.

Considerations

For this patient, whose mother developed premenopausal breast cancer and who has clinically benign, dense fibrocystic changes in both breasts and a

Table 11–1 BENIGN BREAST LESIONS AND RELATIVE RISK OF BREAST CANCER

Benign breast histology not associated with an increased risk for breast cancer:
- Adenosis, apocrine metaplasia, cysts, ductal ectasia, fibroadenoma, fibrosis, mild hyperplasia, mastitis, squamous metaplasia

Risk increased 1.5- to 2.0- fold:
- Moderate or severe hyperplasia, papillomatosis

Risk increased 5-fold:
- Atypical hyperplasia

Risk increased 10-fold:
- Lobular carcinoma in situ
- Atypical hyperplasia with family history of breast cancer

screening mammogram showing no abnormalities, there is no uniform approach to treatment. The **ultimate decision** regarding **therapy or surveillance** is based on patient **risk factors,** her concerns about the threat of breast cancer, the **effectiveness of surveillance,** and the **anticipated cosmetic results** of a biopsy and/or treatment. These factors must be explored with the patient during the initial consultation. In this case, **breast ultrasonography** may provide additional information and should be done to establish a baseline evaluation. For an intermediate-risk patient, it may be worthwhile to consider chemoprevention strategies ranging from dietary supplements to the administration of antiestrogens.

APPROACH TO Surveillance and Management of High-Risk Patients

DEFINITIONS

INVASIVE LOBULAR CARCINOMA: Make up only 10% to 15% of all breast cancers. These frequently do not appear as dominant breast masses but instead as focal thickening (resembling fibrocystic changes). Mammography of these lesions has a tendency to be **negative**. Detection is by physical examination, magnetic resonance imaging (MRI), and ultrasonography.

ATYPICAL DUCTAL HYPERPLASIA: When this condition is diagnosed during core needle biopsy, 25% to 40% of patients have ductal carcinoma in situ diagnosed on excisional biopsy.

SCREENING MAMMOGRAPHY: Radiologic procedure for the examination of breast tissue with approximately 10% to 15% false-negative and 10% false-positive rates. The false-negative rate in younger patients (40 to 49 years) is higher and may approach 25%; consequently, the cost-benefit of screening mammography for 40- to 49-year-old women has been hotly debated. Roughly 20% of patients undergoing biopsies for mammographic abnormalities are found to have carcinoma.

ULTRASONOGRAPHY: Imaging using sound waves that can visualize small solid and cystic lesions (2-5 mm). It may be useful for the evaluation of cystic lesions and evaluating a low-risk patient with a palpable abnormality and a negative mammogram. When identified by ultrasound, a benign-appearing cyst characterized by the absence of septation and a solid component has a 99.5% negative predictive value for cancer; additional application of breast ultrasound is to differentiate benign and malignant characteristics of solid breast masses.

CHEMOPREVENTION: Tamoxifen (20 mg/day for 5 years) has been approved for chemoprevention in high-risk patients and has been reported to reduce the occurrence of subsequent cancer among high-risk patients. Chemoprevention must be weighed against the risks of thromboembolic complications, endometrial cancer, and the side effects of tamoxifen.

MRI: A useful technique for defining the local extent of breast cancers. It is sensitive in identifying small cancers in the breast, but it lacks specificity in that lesions identified as abnormal may not be cancerous (sensitivity, 90%-95%; specificity, ~45%). For premenopausal patients, MRI is even less useful in differentiating hormone-induced changes caused by cancers.

CLINICAL APPROACH

Familial Risk Factors

The risk of developing breast cancer increases **1.8-fold** in a woman whose **mother or sister has had breast cancer diagnosed.** This risk is further increased if the disease was diagnosed in the first-degree relative at a **premenopausal age (3.0-fold risk)** or if it was **bilateral breast cancer (4.0- to 5.4-fold if postmenopausal and 9.0-fold if premenopausal).** In addition, some families carry a genetic predisposition for breast cancer in the *BRCA1* or *BRCA2* gene. Whereas only 5% to 10% of cancers are attributed to mutations of the *BRCA* genes, the diagnosis of a *BRCA1* or *BRCA2* gene carrier significantly increases the lifetime risk of developing breast cancer by 3- to 17-fold.

Approach to Patient Treatment

Treatment options for benign breast lesions vary from patient to patient depending on each patient's **risk factors,** personal concerns regarding **cancer risk versus breast cosmesis,** and the **ability to continue close breast surveillance.** Low-risk benign lesions can be observed or excised based on the patient's clinical presentation and/or preference. A high-risk lesion or a patient with a high-risk history may opt for excision with observation and/or chemoprevention with antiestrogen therapy and close observation. Selective patients with a strong family history or known *BRCA* gene mutation may be treated with prophylactic mastectomy and/or bilateral oophorectomy. Regardless of the treatment selected, all high-risk patients should be followed with annual mammography and a physical examination and instructed on performing monthly breast self-examination (Table 11–2).

Screening ductal lavage: A new technology useful in the surveillance of patients with high-risk lesions or high-risk profiles. It involves aspiration of the areola to induce nipple discharge. The effluent produced is analyzed by **cytology.** Screening duct lavage may identify patients with early lesions who should be screened with more aggressive techniques including ductography, ductoscopy, or MRI, but it currently **remains an investigational tool.**

Table 11–2 NATIONAL COMPREHENSIVE CANCER NETWORK HIGH-RISK SCREENING ALGORITHM (> 25 Y OF AGE)

Prior thoracic chest radiograph: Annual mammogram and physical examination every 6 mo beginning 10 y after the XRT.

GAIL* model risk > 1.67% (> 35 y of age): Annual mammogram and physical examination; consider risk reduction strategies.

Family history or genetic predisposition (mutations of BRCA1 or BRCA2): Annual mammogram and physical examination every 6 mo starting at age 25 or 5-10 y prior to the earliest familial case; consider risk-reduction strategies.

Lobular carcinoma in situ: Annual mammogram and physical examination every 6-12 mo; consider risk-reduction strategies.

*GAIL, mathematical model risk factors: age, menarche, age at first live birth, number of first-degree relatives with breast cancer, number of previous benign breast biopsies, atypical hyperplasia in previous biopsy, race. The percent estimation refers to the annual probability of cancer development.

Comprehension Questions

11.1 A 44-year-old woman underwent a streotactic core biopsy of a suspicious mammographic lesion in the left breast. The biopsy revealed lobular carcinoma in situ. Which of the following is the most appropriate management recommendation for this patient?

A. Left mastectomy
B. Left partial mastectomy and radiation therapy
C. Tamoxifen, clinical examination, and mammography every 2 years
D. Tamoxifen, clinical examination, and mammography every 6 months

11.2 Which of the following factors is associated with the highest risk of developing breast cancer?

A. < 25 years of age
B. First-degree relative with breast cancer
C. Previous breast biopsy
D. Mutation of the *BRCA1* gene

11.3 A 37-year-old woman, who has multiple family members with breast cancer, is noted to have a BRCA-1 mutation. She is counseled about her 50-70% lifetime risk of breast cancer. She asks whether mastectomy would be advisable. Which of the following states regarding prophylactic mastectomy is most accurate?

A. Prophylactic mastectomy is an acceptable treatment option.
B. Prophylactic mastectomy is rarely if ever indicated.
C. Unilateral prophylactic mastectomy is the preferred method.
D. Prophylactic mastectomy is an acceptable treatment option only when the patient agrees to undergo immediate breast reconstruction.

11.4 Which of the following statements is most accurate regarding mammography?

A. The radiation has led to pulmonary malignancies.
B. Its primary role is to determine a malignant versus a benign condition of masses found on physical examination.
C. Its main role is to detect nonpalpable breast masses.
D. It is more accurate in younger patients.

11.5 A 41-year-old woman with a significant family history of breast cancer, including her mother who developed breast cancer at the age 62, underwent a stereotactic core biopsy of a suspicious left breast mammographic abnormality. The biopsy revealed the presence of atypical ductal hyperplasia (ADH). Which of the following is the most appropriate treatment option?

A. Tamoxifen chemoprevention
B. Left breast biopsy with needle localization
C. Left modified radical mastectomy
D. Tamoxifen chemoprevention and surveillance mammography every 6 months

11.6 A 33-year-old woman has a strong family history of breast cancer, including breast cancer occurrence in her mother at age 44 and history of breast cancer in a sister at age 40. She is concerned about her risk of cancer development but does not wish to have prophylactic mastectomies performed. Which of the following management options is considered most acceptable?

A. Prophylactic breast radiation and tamoxifen.
B. Begin annual screening mammography and clinical breast examinations.
C. Recommend counseling and genetic testing, initiate annual mammography and clinical breast examinations, and tamoxifen therapy.
D. Recommend counseling and genetic testing, if no abnormalities identified then begin surveillance mammography and clinical breast examinations at age 40.

ANSWERS

11.1 **D.** The findings of lobular carcinoma in situ (LCIS) carry a 10-fold increased risk of subsequent breast cancer, and this increased risk is bilateral. LCIS is considered a marker for subsequent breast cancer and not an early stage of existing breast cancer; the subsequent breast cancer development can be in the form of invasive ductal cancer or invasive lobular cancer. Left mastectomy and left partial mastectomy are not acceptable options given the nature of LCIS and the distribution of potential future breast cancers in this patient. Based on the increased risk of future breast cancers, intensified surveillance and chemoprevention with tamoxifen are justifiable.

11.2 **D.** *BRCA1* gene carriers have a 3- to 17-fold increased risk for breast cancer development. Female carriers of the *BRCA1* gene have a 56% to 85% lifetime risk of developing breast cancer and a 15% to 45% risk of developing ovarian cancer. Breast cancer history in a female first-degree relative is associated with 1.8-fold increase in cancer risk.

11.3 **A.** Prophylactic mastectomy is an acceptable management option for some patients with high risk profile, who has received sufficient counseling regarding risks and benefits of all options. When performed, prophylactic mastectomy is often bilateral and reconstruction following prophylactic mastectomy is individualized based on patient's desires. A patient with a BRCA-1 mutation has a very high lifetime risk for breast cancer, and discussion about risk reducing therapies, including prophylactic mastectomy.

11.4 **C.** The main purpose of mammography is to detect nonpalpable breast cancers. Surveillance mammograms have not been shown to increase the risk of other malignancies.

11.5 **B.** The diagnosis of atypical ductal hyperplasia (ADH) by core needle biopsy has been demonstrated to be associated with the findings of invasive or in situ ductal carcinoma during subsequent excisional biopsies. ADH is believed to represent a carcinogenic progression of the ductal epithelial cells. Even if the subsequent excisional biopsy demonstrates no evidence of cancer, the patient should be advised of her increased cancer risk and the need for clinical follow-up and surveillance mammography.

11.6 **C.** This patient's family history of premenopausal breast cancers is quite suspicious for familial breast cancer syndromes produced by BRCA mutations. Genetic testing is a reasonable recommendation after appropriate counseling regarding the implications, consequences, and management option for individuals and family members with BRCA mutations. For the very high risk patients such as this, annual surveillance mammography and clinical breast examinations should begin at age 25 or 5-10 years prior to the earliest familial case. Chemoprevention with Tamoxifen has been demonstrated to reduce the risk of subsequent breast cancer in high-risk patients, however its application may be associated with significant side effects that include hot flashes and uterine carcinoma. Prophylactic breast radiation has not been shown to reduce subsequent breast cancer risks and is not an option.

Clinical Pearls

- The primary role of mammography is the detection of nonpalpable breast masses.
- Having a first-degree relative with breast cancer, especially if this individual is premenopausal and the disease is bilateral, represents a risk factor for developing mammary cancer.
- Mammography in younger women under 30 years tends to be less sensitive because of the possibility of dense fibrocystic changes.

REFERENCES

Igelhart JD, Smith BL. Diseases of the breast. In: Townsend CM, Beauchamp RD, Evers BM, et al, eds. *Sabiston Textbook of Surgery*. 18th ed. Philadelphia, PA: Saunders Elsevier; 2008:851-914.

Kinsinger LS, Harris R, Woolf SH, et al. Chemoprevention of breast cancer: a summary of the evidence from the U.S. Preventative Services Task Force. *Ann Intern Med*. 2002;137(1):E59-E69.

Qaseem A, et al. Screening mammography for women 40 to 49 years of age: a clinical practice guideline from the American College of Physicians. *Ann Intern Med* 2007;146:511-515.

Vogel VC. Management of the high-risk patient. *Surg Clin N Am*. 2003;83:733-751.

Case 12

A 22-year-old man was walking past a construction site when a brick fell off the scaffold and struck him in the head. Witnesses noted that the patient was unconscious immediately after the incident and did not regain consciousness for approximately 10 minutes. The paramedics placed the patient in cervical-spine precautions and brought him to the emergency department. During the primary survey at the emergency department, the patient has apparently normal air exchange, a respiratory rate of 18 breaths/min, blood pressure of 138/78 mm Hg, and a pulse of 80 beats/min. The patient does not open his eyes in response to voice commands but has eye opening in response to painful stimuli. He withdraws from painful stimuli. His only verbal responses are incomprehensible sounds. The secondary survey demonstrates a 3-cm scalp laceration and a contusion over the right temporal region. The right pupil is dilated 6 mm and sluggishly reactive to light; the left pupil is 4 mm in diameter and reacts normally to light. No blood is visualized behind the tympanic membranes. The results from an examination of the truncal region and extremities are within normal limits.

- What is the most likely diagnosis?
- What should be your next step?

ANSWERS TO CASE 12:

Closed Head Injury

Summary: A 22-year-old man has an injury mechanism and presentation indicating an isolated severe closed head injury. He has an initial Glasgow Coma Scale (GCS) aggregate score of 8 (see Table 12–1).

➤ **Most likely diagnosis:** Severe closed head injury with possible mass effect.

➤ **Next step:** Immediate endotracheal intubation to control ventilation and oxygenation.

ANALYSIS

Objectives

1. Be able to calculate and know the significance of the GCS score.
2. Learn the causes and preventive measures for secondary brain injury.
3. Learn the emergent management for patients with intracranial mass lesions.

Table 12–1 GLASGOW COMA SCALE

ASSESSMENT AREA	SCORE
EYE OPENING	
Spontaneous	4
To speech	3
To pain	2
None	1
BEST MOTOR RESPONSE	
Obeys commands	6
Localizes pain	5
Withdraws to pain	4
Decorticate posture (abnormal flexion)	3
Decerebrate posture (extension)	2
No response	1
VERBAL RESPONSE	
Oriented	5
Confused conversation	4
Inappropriate words	3
Incomprehensible sounds	2
None	1

GCS is the aggregate score of all three components

Considerations

This patient may have an epidural hematoma, subdural hematoma, intraparenchymal injury, subarachnoid hemorrhage, diffuse axonal injury, or any combination of these injuries. The anatomic classification of the injury is **not important** in the initial treatment of this patient. **For a patient with a severe head injury, the most important management principle is avoidance of secondary brain injury.** The injured brain is much more susceptible to hypoxia and hypotension; **in brain injury patients with both hypoxia and hypotension, mortality is approximately 75%, and hypotension alone doubles the mortality risk compared to that for normotensive patients with a severe head injury.** Definitive **airway management by endotracheal intubation** is vital in the initial treatment of this patient.

This patient also has evidence of increased intracranial pressure with localizing signs, **unequal pupils, and hemiparesis.** The Monro-Kellie doctrine governs intracranial pressure and expanding mass lesions. This equation states that the volume of blood, brain, and cerebrospinal fluid within the nonexpansile cranium must remain constant for intracranial pressure to remain constant. If an additional substance, such as an expanding hematoma is added, the intracranial pressure will increase unless a compensatory amount of blood, brain, or cerebrospinal fluid is removed. Once the patient has been intubated and appropriately resuscitated with crystalloids and blood, the **emergent treatment of a patient with localizing signs includes controlled hyperventilation and administration of mannitol.** Hyperventilation causes cerebral vasoconstriction, reducing the volume of blood in the cranium and allowing room for the intracranial mass lesion. It must be used cautiously; however, because prolonged use can cause cerebral ischemia secondary to reduced blood flow. Intravenous mannitol, at a dose of 1 g/kg, is also used to decrease the volume of blood in the brain and to decrease brain volume related to edema. **Mannitol should not be used unless the patient is adequately resuscitated because it can aggravate hypovolemia and cause uncompensated shock.**

APPROACH TO
Closed Head Injury

DEFINITIONS

EPIDURAL HEMATOMA: The collection of blood outside the dura but beneath the skull, most often in the temporal region (middle meningeal artery laceration). These hematomas are uncommon, occurring in 0.5% of all head injuries and 9% of severe head injuries, and they have a better prognosis than other types of cerebral hematomas. They appear classically biconvex or lens shaped on a CT scan.

SUBDURAL HEMATOMA: The collection of blood between the brain surface and the dura, commonly as a result of the tearing of bridging veins. They are much more common than epidural hematomas, and their prognosis is worse than that for epidural hematomas because of coexisting brain injury.

CONCUSSION: Transient loss of consciousness associated with no CT scan abnormalities.

MILD HEAD INJURY: GCS of 13 to 15.

MODERATE HEAD INJURY: GCS of 9 to 12.

SEVERE HEAD INJURY: GCS of 8 or less.

COMA: Severe head injury generally with a GCS of 8 or less.

BURR HOLE: A hole drilled through the skull, usually on the side of the larger pupil to decompress an intracranial mass lesion. The procedure should only be performed by a physician with adequate training by neurosurgeons, and the procedure should only be done as a lifesaving maneuver when timely transfer to a neurosurgeon is not possible.

CLINICAL APPROACH

As in any trauma patient, airway, breathing, and circulation concerns should be addressed first. The goals include avoidance of hypoxia and hypotension that can exacerbate head injury, and stabilization of associated spine, chest, abdomen, pelvic, and extremity injuries. A neurologic assessment should then be performed and include a pupillary examination and calculation of the GCS. The pupillary examination determines pupil size and reactivity to light. **Dilation of a pupil with a sluggish response to light is an early sign of temporal lobe herniation.** The third nerve becomes compressed against the tentorium with herniation of the temporal lobe. **Ninety percent of the time this herniation and pupillary abnormality** occur on **the same side of the intracranial lesion.** This can direct the placement of emergency burr holes should they become necessary. The **GCS** evaluates **eye opening, motor response, and verbal response.** The best motor response is a better indicator of prognosis than the worst response. The **trend** observed in a patient's examination is **much more important than a single examination.** The diagnostic test of choice for all patients with a head injury is CT imaging. This scan should *not* be obtained at a facility that is not able to treat the head-injured patient definitively if it will delay transfer to a qualified neurosurgeon or trauma surgeon.

Comprehension Questions

12.1 A 46-year-old intoxicated man was driving down the highway in the wrong direction when his vehicle struck a pickup truck head-on. He presents with pulse rate of 130 beats/min, blood pressure of 90/62 mm Hg, and respiratory rate of 30 breaths/min. His pupils are 5 mm and are equally round and reactive bilaterally, he does not open his eyes to painful stimulus, he moans with painful stimulus, and he withdraws from painful stimulus. His oxygen saturation with oxygen by facemask is 91%. In addition to the possibility of closed head injury, what other factor most likely is a contributing factor for his low GCS?

A. Hypoxia
B. History of seizure disorder
C. Alcohol intoxication
D. Chronic syphilis infection

12.2 A short time after arrival to the ED, the patient described in 12.1 underwent intubation, mechanical ventilation, and placement of bilateral chest tubes for bilateral pneumothoraces. After an additional infusion of 1000 mL of Lactated Ringer solution, the patient's blood pressure improves to 120/80 mm Hg, heart rate decreased to 100 beats/min. With painful stimuli, the patient does not open his eyes and he withdraws to painful stimulation. A CT scan of the brain demonstrates bilateral frontal contusions, subarachnoid hemorrhage, and diffuse brain edema bilaterally. Which of the following is the most appropriate next step?

A. Craniectomy for the evacuation of subarachnoid hemorrhage.
B. Continue mechanical ventilation, IV fluids, and monitoring.
C. Place bilateral burr holes in the ED.
D. Administer IV corticosteroids.

12.3 An 18-year-old skier who was not wearing a helmet runs into a tree during a downhill run. He is brought to the emergency department where he is noted to be screaming random words and phrases, localizing to pain, opening his eyes to his name. Following your initial evaluation, you contact the neurosurgeon for consultation. How would you classify the severity of his closed head injury?

A. Mild
B. Moderate
C. Severe
D. Poor prognosis

12.4 An 18-year-old man presents with the injury mechanism described in 12.3, with normal blood pressure, does not open eyes to painful stimuli, has abnormal flexion of the upper extremities with pain, and moans with painful stimuli. Which of the following is the most appropriate next step?

A. CT scan
B. 2000 mL IV fluid bolus
C. Contact the neurosurgeon
D. Endotracheal intubation

ANSWERS

12.1 **A.** This patient has a GCS of 7 (E1, V2, M4). Low GCS can be contributed by alcohol intoxication; however given the reported oxygen saturation of 91%, the degree of mild hypoxia is unlikely to be a factor responsible for his low GCS. Chronic neurosyphilis infection usually causes balance issues or sometimes the Argyll Robertson papillary reflex. A history of a seizure disorder will not typically affect level of consciousness, except in the immediate post-ictal state.

12.2 **B.** The patient now has a GCS of 6T (E1, V1T, M4). His hypotension and hypoxia has been improved with his initial management. At this time he is found to have frontal contusions, cerebral swelling, and subarachnoid hemorrhage. Although the brain CT findings are causes for alarm, these finding are not amendable to operative treatment; midline shift and focal hemorrhage would be possible indications for surgical decompression. Optimizing the patient's condition providing best supportive care to prevent secondary brain injury is the most effective treatment at this time for his brain injury.

12.3 **B.** Moderate closed head injury with GCS of 11 (E3, V3, M5). Given this level of brain injury, intubation and mechanical ventilation is not mandatory. However, all precautions should be taken to avoid hypotension, hypoxia, and hypercapnea.

12.4 **D.** This patient has an initial GCS of 6 (E1, V2, M3), which places him in the category of severe brain injury. Early intubation to optimize oxygenation and ventilation is critical in the prevention of secondary brain injury. While CT scans and neurosurgical consultations are important aspects of this patient's care, airway management takes precedence over these other measures

Clinical Pearls

- Prevention of secondary brain injury begins with optimizing the patient's oxygenation, ventilation, and brain perfusion, particularly correcting hypoxemia, hypoventilation, and hypotension.
- The initial GCS determined at the emergency department and the patient's age are the most important indicators of outcome in head-injured patients.
- Pupillary reflex and the GCS (eye opening, motor response, and verbal response) are the cornerstones of initial neurologic assessment.
- The side with the dilated pupil is usually the side on which the intracranial mass is located.

REFERENCES

Burgess JE. Critical care of patients with traumatic brain injury. In: Irwin RS, Rippe JM, eds. *Intensive Care Medicine*. 5th ed. Philadelphia, PA: Lippincott Williams & Wilkins; 2003:1789-1799.

Weingart JD. Head injuries. In: Cameron JL, ed. *Current Surgical Therapy*. 9th ed. Philadelphia, PA: Mosby Elsevier; 2008: 949-953.

Case 13

A 63-year-old man is rescued from a house fire and brought to the emergency department. According to paramedics responding to a three-alarm fire, the victim was found unconscious in an upstairs bedroom of a house. The patient's past medical problems are unknown. His pulse is 112 beats/min, blood pressure 150/85 mm Hg, and respiratory rate 30 breaths/min. A pulse oximeter registers 92% O_2 saturation with a face mask. His face and the exposed portions of his body are covered with a carbonaceous deposit. The patient has blistering and open burn wounds involving the circumference of his left arm and left leg and more than 80% of his back and buttocks. He does not respond verbally to questions and reacts to painful stimulation with occasional moans.

- What is the most appropriate next step?
- What are the immediate and late complications associated with thermal injuries?

ANSWERS TO CASE 13: Thermal Injury

Summary: A 63-year-old man presents with an approximately 40% total body surface area (TBSA) burn injury and inhalation injuries.

- **Next step:** Definitive airway management by intubation is appropriate in this patient with possible inhalation injuries and carbon monoxide (CO) poisoning.
- **Immediate and late complications:** Airway compromise and tissue hypoperfusion are common early complications, and sepsis and functional loss are possible late complications.

ANALYSIS

Objectives

1. Be familiar with the initial assessment and treatment of patients with thermal injuries.
2. Be familiar with the assessment and management of burn wounds.
3. Be familiar with the prognosis associated with thermal injuries.

Considerations

Given the circumstances surrounding the injury (a house fire), the size of the burn, and the age of patient, all of which indicate a high likelihood of pulmonary complications, immediate intubation is clearly indicated. Persons at risk for upper airway thermal damage include this particular patient because he was found unconscious in a closed-space fire. Fluid resuscitation with lactated Ringer solution should be initiated based on 2 to 4 mL/kg/% burn. Unless the patient is already at a facility that specializes in burn care, immediate arrangements should be made for a transfer after initial stabilization.

APPROACH TO Thermal Injury

The skin is the largest organ of the body. It allows the body to maintain fluid balance, temperature regulation, and protein regulation and provides a barrier against bacteria and fungi. It is a necessary organ for living. Knowledge of the initial resuscitation and treatment, along with the late complications, can help minimize the morbidity and mortality of these injuries.

CLINICAL APPROACH

Initial Assessment

The initial assessment of a burn patient is the same as for a trauma patient (attention to the airway, breathing, and circulation—the ABCs), with additional considerations. Along with their burns, patients can acquire thoracic and abdominal trauma, fractures, or head injuries from associated falls or crashes. This case focuses on the particulars of burn injuries, but one must be mindful that associated injuries must be managed concurrently.

Airway

As for other traumas, airway assessment is the initial consideration. Although patients do not receive "pulmonary burns" (unless they inhale live steam or explosive gases), the upper airway can be burned as it cools the hot gases from a fire. Additional signs of potential airway involvement include facial and upper torso burns and carbonaceous sputum. If **the oropharynx is dry, red, or blistered, the patient will probably require intubation.** When indicated, endotracheal intubation should be performed early, before a surgical airway is required secondary to pharyngeal and laryngeal edema. Smoke inhalation can also cause tracheobronchitis and edema from exposure to the incomplete combustion of carbon particles and other toxic fumes.

CO poisoning can cause hypoxia because CO has a 240-fold greater affinity for hemoglobin than O_2, thus shifting the oxyhemoglobin curve to the left. **All patients injured in closed-space fires should have their carboxyhemoglobin (COHgb) level determined. A COHgb level of greater than 30% may indicate significant central nervous system dysfunction** that may also be permanent. **A COHgb level of greater than 60% may portend coma and death.** Note that one can develop a 30% COHgb level within 3 minutes in a moderately smoky fire. When associated with cutaneous burns, smoke inhalation doubles the risk of mortality. Patients with a COHgb greater than 10% with carbonaceous sputum from a closed-space fire have a greater than 90% chance of needing ventilator support if they have associated burns of more than 20% TBSA. The half-life of CO in the blood on room air is 250 minutes. If the patient is receiving 100% O_2, the half-life is approximately 40 to 60 minutes. Therefore, calculation of the patient's initial COHgb level is estimated by knowing the transport time and the time prior to the arterial blood draw, as well as the oxygen concentration the patient is receiving. A request for the COHgb level can be sent to the laboratory along with the request for a baseline arterial blood gas analysis. In the scenario described here, where the patient is found unconscious in a building with 40% TBSA burns, carbonaceous sputum, signs of hypoxia (abnormal oxygen saturation), and neurologic deficits (responding only to painful stimuli), intubation is needed.

Resuscitation

Cutaneous burns result in accelerated fluid loss. Mediators such as prostaglandins, thromboxane A2, and reactive oxygen radicals are released from injured tissue, which cause local edema, increased capillary permeability, decreased perfusion, and end-organ dysfunction. Burn sizes exceeding 20% TBSA can result in a systemic response, with significant interstitial edema in distant soft tissues. With these large burns, an initial decrease in cardiac output is seen, followed by a hypermetabolic state. These intravascular fluid losses make resuscitation an important part of burn management. Organs, including skin, can progress from a hypoperfused state to more permanent end-organ damage if resuscitation is not accomplished.

Calculating Resuscitation Fluid Requirements

Most patients with burns involving **less than 15% TBSA can be resuscitated with oral fluids.** For larger burns, isotonic intravenous fluids such as lactated Ringer solution should be used (large volumes of normal saline can cause hyperchloremic metabolic acidosis). Fluid needs are estimated by the Parkland or Baxter formula. Based on the **Parkland formula, for adults and children weighing more than 10 kg, the total 24-hour volume is calculated using 4 mL/kg/% burn. Half of this amount is given in the first 8 hours, and the remainder in the next 16 hours.** Intravenous fluid hydration given by the paramedics en route should be considered part of this volume. Children weighing less than 10 kg should be given 2 to 3 mL/kg/% burn divided similarly over the next 24 hours. In addition, they should receive a maintenance fluid that includes 5% dextrose. Because of the increased capillary permeability, colloids such as albumin are generally avoided for the first 12 to 18 hours but can be used subsequently if resuscitation is not being achieved with the crystalloid regimen. **Inhalational injuries, extensive and/or deep burns, and delayed resuscitation usually result in larger fluid requirements than initially calculated.**

Assessing the Adequacy of Resuscitation

Measuring urine output (UOP) is a helpful way of assessing the adequacy of the resuscitation. Adults should achieve 0.5 mL/kg/h of UOP, children should produce 0.5 to 1 mL/kg/h, and infants should produce 1 to 2 mL/kg/h because they have a higher volume-to-surface area ratio. Generally, UOP is averaged over 2 to 3 hours before changes are made. Excess UOP should also be avoided unless one is treating myoglobinuria.

Calculating the Burn Area

The "rule of nines" is a useful guide in assessing the extent of a person's burns (Table 13–1). The body can be fairly accurately divided into anatomic regions that represent 9% or multiples of 9% of the total body surface. In estimating

Table 13–1 RULE OF NINES

LOCATION	ADULT(%)	INFANT(%)
Front of head with neck	4.5	9
Back of head with neck	4.5	9
Front of torso	18	18
Back of torso	18	18
Front of one arm	4.5	4.5
Back of one arm	4.5	4.5
Front of one leg (full length)	9	7
Back of one leg (full length)	9	7

irregular outlines or distributions, note that the palm of a patient's hand (not including the fingers) represents approximately 1% of the patient's total body surface.

Burn Depth

When calculating the total percentage of burn involvement in a patient with more serious burns, first-degree burns are not included. Different burn depths (see Table 13–2) should be noted on a burn diagram form. As burns marginate, the assessment of depth may change from the value calculated initially, particularly in the case of scald burns, where the initial depth may not appear as severe.

Fourth-degree burns are those that extend through skin and subcutaneous fat, even involving deep structures.

Temporary Wound Coverings

Because the skin serves in temperature regulation and as a barrier against bacterial and fungal organisms, attention must be given to the prevention of hypothermia and monitoring for infection. Because **a burn site can become infected and allow microbes systemic access, steroids should not be used for any burn greater than 10% TBSA.** Prophylactic intravenous antibiotics are usually not recommended because they select for resistant organisms. The different creams commonly used topically have local broad antimicrobial activity that can resist colonization. **Silver sulfadiazine** (SS) does not penetrate the eschar and so is not helpful in an infected burn. It can rarely cause leukopenia, requiring cessation of use. Patients who are allergic to sulfa are

Table 13–2 BURN DEPTH

	LOCATION AFFECTED	CHARACTERISTICS	COURSE	TREATMENT
First-degree	Epidermis	Erythema and pain	Heals in 3-4 d without scarring. The dead epidermal cells desquamate (peel). Sunburns that blister are actually superficial dermal burns.	Lotions (like aloe) and nonsteroidal anti-inflammatory drugs
Second-degree or partial thickness	Through epidermis and into dermis	Pink/red,weepy, swelling and blisters, very painful	Superficial dermal heal within 3 wk without scarring or functional impairment. Deep dermal heal in 3-8 wk but with severe scarring and loss of function.	Excise and graft deep dermal burns
Third-degree or full thickness	All the way through dermis	White or dark, leathery, waxy, painless	Burns can heal only by epithelial migration from periphery and contraction. Unless they are tiny (cigarette burn size), they will need grafting.	Excise and graft

usually not affected by SS because the silver molecule is attached to the antigenic portion of the sulfadiazine molecule; however, if this cream is chosen, it is prudent to try a test patch for patients with a sulfa allergy. A rash or pain (rather than the usual soothing) will ensue if they are truly allergic to SS. **Sulfamylon (mafenide)** is less commonly used because it is painful on application. Furthermore, it can cause severe systemic metabolic acidosis through carbonic anhydrase inhibition. It penetrates the eschar and is therefore useful for full-thickness infected burns (there is less pain on application) and for unexcised burns with colonization. **Silver nitrate** does not penetrate the eschar and turns the burn area black. Usage can result in severe leaching of sodium and chloride, which can lead to profound hyponatremia and hypochloremia, particularly when used on large areas on children. **Pigskin** can be used on flat, clean wounds. Its growth factors can encourage epithelialization in partial-thickness burns.

BURN COMPLICATIONS

NEUROLOGIC: Transient delirium commonly occurs, but an altered mental status requires evaluation to identify other etiologies such as anoxia and metabolic abnormalities.

PULMONARY: Pneumonias and respiratory failure requiring mechanical ventilation are frequently seen.

CARDIOVASCULAR: Venous thrombosis can occur. Suppurative thrombophlebitis can lead to bacteremia, which may cause endocarditis along with the local venous abscess.

GASTROINTESTINAL: Stomach and duodenal ulcers can develop secondary to decreased mucosal defenses resulting from the decrease in splanchnic blood flow. Early gastric tube feedings before atony occurs may help improve nutrition or prevent stress ulcers. Early feeding may prevent the development of nosocomial pneumonias by inhibiting bacterial overgrowth. As the result of regional hypoperfusion, critically ill burn patients are at risk for the development of acalculous cholecystitis, pancreatitis, and hepatic dysfunction.

RENAL: Acute tubular necrosis can develop because of inadequate resuscitation or myoglobinuria.

INFECTION: Can arise from the burns themselves or from treatments used in critical care: urinary tract infections from Foley catheters and sinusitis or otitis from feeding or nasogastric tubes.

OPHTHALMIC: Corneal abrasions or ulcerations may be seen, resulting either from the initial injury or from exposure. Patients with potential eye injuries, particularly those caused by explosions, should be examined early in the emergency department using fluorescein for corneal abrasions, which should be treated with antibiotic lubrication. Early examination is important before edema makes the examination difficult. Eyelid problems also may require treatment.

MUSCULOSKELETAL AND SOFT TISSUE: Scarring can cause functional or cosmetic defects. Physical and occupational therapy, scar releases, regrafting, and silicone prostheses can help.

PSYCHOLOGICAL: Burns can be very traumatic as well as defacing. Adequate support should be provided.

Because of the specialized care required and the multidisciplinary aspects of burn treatment, the American Burn Association recommends that certain patients receive their care at burn centers (Table 13–3).

Table 13–3 AMERICAN BURN ASSOCIATION RECOMMENDATIONS FOR TRANSFER TO BURN CENTERS
< 10 y or > 50 y with full-thickness burn > 10% TBSA
Any age with TBSA burn? 20%
Partial- or full-thickness burn involving face, eyes, ears, hands, genitalia, perineum, and over joints
Burn injury complicated by chemical, electrical, or other forms of significant trauma
Any patient requiring special social, emotional, and long-term rehabilitative support

Abbreviation: TBSA, total body surface area.

Comprehension Questions

13.1 Which of the following is the most appropriate definitive wound management option for a 30-year-old man with second-degree burns over the anterior chest and abdomen measuring approximately 20% TBSA?

A. Excision of entire burn wound with autologous split-thickness skin graft application

B. Burn wound excision and split-thickness skin graft coverage to be performed in 3 separate stages

C. Excision of burn wound with application of cadaveric skin for temporary coverage, followed by definitive coverage with autologous skin graft in 8 days

D. Application of silver sulfadiazine to wound until epithelialization of wound is complete

13.2 Which of the following burn victims is best managed in a specialized burn center?

A. A 40-year-old man with a 10% TBSA burn to the anterior abdomen, who is also a member of the Jehovah's Witness Church

B. A 6-year-old boy with second-degree burn to the front of the left arm

C. A 55-year-old man with second- and third-degree burn to the anterior chest and abdomen sustained when his clothes caught on fire at a barbecue.

D. A 3-year-old boy with a scalding burn to the left forearm after he accidentally pulled a pan of hot grease of the stove and whose mother is extremely tearful and guilt-ridden.

13.3 Which of the following is the most appropriate resuscitation strategy for a 30-year-old man weighing 70 kg with a 40% total body surface area burn wound? Use the Parkland formula for this determination.

A. $D_5$0.45 NS at an initial rate of 700 mL/hr for the initial 8 hours followed by a rate of 350 mL/hr for the next 16 hours

B. Lactated Ringer solution at 350 mL/hour for the initial 8 hours followed by an infusion rate of 700 mL/hour for the next 16 hours

C. Lactated Ringer solution at an initial rate of 700 mL/hour for the first 8 hours followed by an infusion rate of 350 mL/hour for the next 16 hours

D. Lactated Ringer solution at 500 mL/hour for the first 8 hours and then titrate the IV infusion rate to an hourly urine output of 0.5 mL/kg

13.4 Which of the following is the most appropriate next step, if the patient described in 13.3 has an average hourly urine output of <15 mL/hours during the first 4 hours of his burn resuscitation?

A. Initiate volume resuscitation with 5% salt-free albumin.

B. Adjust IV fluid rate to achieve an average urine output of 3 mL/kg/hour for the next few hours.

C. Adjust IV fluid rate to achieve average urine output of 0.5-1.0 mL/kg/hour.

D. Initiate dopamine drip at 0.3 microgram/kg/min to improve renal perfusion.

13.5 Which of the following is a complication associated with sulfamylon application to a 30% TBSA burn wound?

A. Bacterial colonization of the wound

B. Arterial blood gas findings: pH 7.32, PaO_2 92, $PaCO_2$ 48, HCO_3 30

C. Seizures

D. Arterial blood gas finding: pH 7.32, PaO_2 88, $PaCO_2$ 38, HCO_3 21

ANSWERS

13.1 **A.** Early excision of the burn wound followed by autologous skin graft application is the most appropriate definitive wound management approach for this patient, because this approach reduces septic complications associated with wound sepsis, and early skin grafting also provides patients with the best functional recovery. Cadaveric skin and porcine skin are useful for temporary coverage of burn wounds when there is insufficient autologous skin (eg 80% TBSA burn). Staged burn wound excision and skin graft coverage is another strategy applied for patients who do not have sufficient autologous skin for initial coverage. Definitive treatment of burn wounds with dressing changes and healing by secondary intention (wound contraction) is not acceptable for most burn patients because of increased wound infection risks associated with uncovered burn wounds, and because the poor cosmetic and functional results associated with this type of healing.

13.2 **C.** The estimated size of the burn wound in this 55-year-old man is 18%, and given the patient's age and burn size, the American Burn Association has recommended that patients such as this one would be best treated at a specialized burn center.

13.3 **C.** The Parkland formula recommends an initial fluid resuscitation over the first 24 after a major burn to consist of Lactated Ringers solution with a 24 hour volume = 4 mL/kg/% burn. Half of this calculated volume is recommended for the first 8 hours, followed by infusion of the remaining 50% of the volume over the next 16 hours. For this 70 kg man with 40% TBSA burn, the total volume = 4 mL × 70 kg × 40% = 11200 mL. Half over the first 8 hours would be 5600 mL/8 = 700 mL/hour. For the subsequent 16 hours, infusion volume = 5600 mL/16 = 350 mL/hour.

13.4 **C.** A patient who does not respond to initial fluid resuscitation with the calculated fluid amount should be reassessed for possible complicating factors including coronary artery disease, intrinsic renal disease, and possible miscalculation of burn wound size. Given this patient's young age, the patient's low urine output is possibly related to inadequate fluid administration; therefore, adjustment of IV fluid infusion rate may be appropriate. If the patient continues to respond inadequately, CVP monitoring may become needed to guide therapy. The infusion of colloids such as albumin may potentiate capillary leak and tissue swelling during the initial 8 hours of resuscitation. Dopamine therapy should not be initiated until intravascular volume has been adequately restored.

13.5 **D.** Sulfamylon application may cause metabolic acidosis, as demonstrated by the arterial blood gas. Another unattractive quality associated sulfamylon is that it causes pain when applied.

Clinical Pearls

- When the oropharynx is dry, red, or blistered, the patient will probably require intubation.
- All patients injured in closed-space fires should have their COHgb values determined in the emergency department to assess for CO poisoning.
- The rule of nines is a useful guide to determine the extent of a person's burns in that the body can be divided into anatomic regions that represent 9% or multiples of 9% of the total body surface.

REFERENCES

Gamelli RL, Siver GM. Burn wound management. In: Cameron JL, ed. *Current Surgical Therapy*. 9th ed. Philadelphia, PA: Mosby Elsevier, 2008:1066-1071.

Heimbach D, Gibran N. *Burn pearls*. 18th ed. Seattle,WA: University of Washington Burn Center at Harborview. 2000:12-57.

Milner SM, Singh VA, Eldred J. Fluid management and nutritional support of the burn patient. In: Cameron JL, ed. *Current Surgical Therapy*. 9th ed. Philadelphia, PA: Mosby Elsevier; 2008:1072-1074.

Case 14

A 62-year-old man with chronic hypertension presents with pain and fatigue in his legs that occur whenever he walks. The patient says his symptoms have been present for the past 12 months and have progressively worsened. The patient currently has pain and tightness in both calves that develop after walking less than one block but routinely resolve after a short period of rest. His past medical history is significant for hypertension. He smokes approximately one pack of cigarettes per day. On examination, his feet are warm and without lesions. The femoral pulses are normal bilaterally. The popliteal, dorsalis pedis, and posterior tibial pulses are absent bilaterally. Doppler examination of the lower extremities reveals the presence of Doppler signals in both his feet with ankle-brachial indexes (ABIs) showing moderately severe disease: ABI 0.5 on the left, and 0.54 on the right.

- What is the most likely diagnosis?
- What is the most appropriate next step?
- What is the best initial treatment for this patient?

ANSWERS TO CASE 14: Claudication Syndrome

Summary: A 62-year-old nondiabetic man presents with bilateral leg claudication. Based on the physical examination, the patient most likely has bilateral superficial femoral artery (SFA) occlusion.

- **Most likely diagnosis:** Atherosclerosis with bilateral superficial artery occlusions.
- **Next step:** Assessment of disability and adequate counseling on the risks and benefits of therapy.
- **Best initial treatment:** Lifestyle modification with smoking cessation, exercise training, and risk factor control.

ANALYSIS

Objectives

1. Know the differential diagnosis for claudication caused by arterial insufficiency.
2. Be able to recognize the indications for lower extremity revascularization and the benefits and limitations of open surgical and endovascular techniques.
3. Learn the noninvasive modalities available for the evaluation and follow-up of patients with claudication.

Considerations

This patient's presentation is similar to that of typical vascular disease patients with lower extremity peripheral arterial disease: a history of slowly increasing exertional pain in conjunction with multiple risk factors for atherosclerosis. Lower extremity peripheral vascular occlusive disease (LEPVOD) represents a continuum of regional signs and symptoms of the systemic disease state of atherosclerosis. Patients with claudication are at risk for the developing complications related to the lower extremities, as well as coronary and cerebral vascular complications. Most patients with intermittent claudication can be managed with lifestyle modifications and pharmacologic therapy directed at reducing the patients' overall atherosclerotic risk factors. Aspirin has not been shown to improve claudication but has been shown to reduce the risk of myocardial infarctions, strokes, and the progression of claudication symptoms. The antiplatelet agent, clopidogrel is more effective than aspirin in the prevention of cardiovascular ischemic events; however, this medication is associated with increased cost and increased bleeding complications. Lipid-lowering medications (statins) have been found highly effective in reducing the risk of major cardiovascular events in patients with peripheral vascular disease.

For patients with more advanced stages of ischemia, interventional treatments for limb salvage becomes the desired goal. The recommended standard of LEPVOD classification can help stratify patients according to their presentation and treatment (Table 14–1). More advanced disease generally implies more anatomic levels with occlusive or stenotic pathology. The patient's ABIs of 0.5 and 0.54 are consistent with exertional pain.

Table 14–1 FONTAINE CLASSIFICATION OF LOWER EXTREMITY PERIPHERAL VASCULAR OCCLUSIVE DISEASE

STAGE	SYMPTOMS	SIGNS	NONINVASIVES	TREATMENT
I	None	None	0.8 < ABI < 1.0	Lifestyle and risk factors
II	Claudication, exertional pain	Decreased or absent distal pulses	0.41 < ABI < 0.8	Stage I plus potential intervention
III	Rest pain	Stage II plus elevation pallor	0.2 < ABI < 0.4	Stage II plus probable bypass
IV	Ulceration	Stage III plus distal skin breakdown	ABI < 0.2	Stage III plus wound care
V	Minor gangrene	Stage III plus digital gangrene	ABI < 0.2	Stage IV plus possible minor amputation
VI	Major gangrene	Stage III plus gangrene proximal to forefoot	ABI < 0.2 to not obtainable	Stage IV plus possible major or minor amputation

Abbreviation: ABI, ankle-brachial index.

APPROACH TO
Lower Extremity Vascular Disease

DEFINITIONS

LOWER EXTREMITY PERIPHERAL VASCULAR OCCLUSIVE DISEASE: Ischemia in the lower extremities caused by arterial stenosis. Acute ischemia is typically characterized by a sudden onset of **pain, pallor, and pulselessness.** Chronic arterial ischemia manifests as lower extremity pain with exercise and resolves with rest.

ARTERIAL BYPASS: Surgical procedure in which one artery is connected to another artery with a conduit (such as a saphenous vein or prosthetic material).

ABI: Ratio of Doppler signals of the ankle systolic blood pressure to those of the brachial artery, normally > 0.95; intermittent disease correlates with 0.5 to 0.95, and severe disease with < 0.5.

CLINICAL APPROACH

An understanding of the arterial circulation helps one to localize the pathology in LEPVOD. Increasing levels of arterial involvement usually suggest a greater need for interventional therapy. One must also keep in mind that patients with LEPVOD have systemic atherosclerosis; thus, there is a higher probability of concomitant coronary artery and carotid artery disease. The other manifestations of atherosclerosis impact long-term survival in patients with LEPVOD. Diabetes is important in LEPVOD, both because of its presence as an independent risk factor and because it can alter the clinical presentation. Neuropathy can confound an impression of ischemic rest pain. Additionally, the susceptibility of a diabetic patient to infection can enhance the risk of tissue loss.

Lifestyle therapy is essential for all patients. Because **any intervention can cause possible limb- or life-threatening complications, the clinician needs to weigh the risks and benefits of intervention for a patient with claudication differently than for a patient with digital gangrene.** The patient with claudication should be severely disabled and not merely inconvenienced before being considered for either endovascular treatment or an arterial bypass. Conversely, the patient with digital gangrene is in a limb-threatening situation, requiring definitive revascularization if the limb is to be salvaged. Tissue loss is a limb-threatening presentation that requires revascularization. True ischemic rest pain with multilevel LEPVOD also requires revascularization for definitive treatment. A patient with claudication with severe lifestyle limitations (such as the loss of a job) may be a candidate for revascularization if the risk profile is not too unfavorable.

All interventional therapy carries a spectrum of risks and benefits. Angioplasty techniques work best for proximal vessels with short, focal, concentric, noncalcified atherosclerotic stenosis. In selective cases, when there is residual gradient or dissection following angioplasty, stent placement may help improve short-term patency. The more unfavorable the lesion is with respect to length, number, location, and morphology, the less successful percutaneous therapy will be. As a general rule, outright arterial occlusions require bypass to achieve revascularization. More proximal-level bypasses at the aortoiliac level can achieve 90% 5-year patency, whereas distal femoral-tibial bypasses can achieve less than 65% 5-year patency.

Comprehension Questions

14.1 A 57-year-old man who works as a deliveryman is able to walk only 40 yards before stopping because of right calf and thigh cramping. He is worried that he will lose his job. He is a diabetic and takes an oral hypoglycemic agent, a long-acting β-blocker, and a statin-class lipid-lowering agent. He smokes one pack of cigarettes a day. He has normal right leg pulses but no pulses in the left groin and leg. Which of the following is the most likely site of arterial occlusion?

A. His left aortoiliac system
B. His left SFA
C. His right SFA
D. His left internal carotid artery

14.2 A patient has the symptoms described earlier, as well as nonhealing ulcers between his left third and fourth toes. Which of the following arteries is most likely to be involved?

A. An occlusion in his left internal iliac artery
B. An occlusion in his left SFA
C. An occlusion in his right SFA
D. An occlusion in his right aortoiliac artery

14.3 A patient has the symptoms and ulcers described above, as well as documented left iliac artery occlusion for the entire left external iliac artery and full-length occlusion of his left SFA with reconstitution of his popliteal artery just below the adductor hiatus. Which of the following is the most appropriate treatment?

A. Lifestyle counseling and risk factor control
B. A femoral–femoral bypass from the left leg to the right leg
C. A femoral popliteal bypass with a reversed saphenous vein if available
D. All of the above

14.4 An 82-year-old woman with history of severe dementia and left CVA is noted to have a gangrenous toes and erythematous left foot. She is severely debilitated by her dementia and CVA and is bed-bound. Her physical examination reveals normal temperature, normal femoral pulses, diminished left popliteal pulse and non-palpable left pedal pulses. Her right lower extremity vascular examination reveals normal femoral pulse, diminished popliteal and pedal pulses. Her left great toe and second toe have dark eschars at the tip with surrounding erythema extending to the mid-foot. Which of the following is the most appropriate treatment option?

A. Obtain an angiogram of the aorta and left lower extremity to identify the areas of occlusion and treat the blockage with angioplasty and stent placement. After blood flow is restored to the foot, proceed with toe amputation and wound care.
B. Obtain an angiogram of the aorta and left lower extremity, followed by an arterial bypass operation to restore flow to the lower extremity. After blood flow is restored to the foot, proceed with toe amputation and wound care.
C. Initiate systemic heparin therapy.
D. Perform left below-the-knee amputation.

14.5 A 57-year-old man presents with acute onset of right foot pain. He states that he had been in his usual state of health until 6 hours ago, when he developed sudden onset of right foot and leg pain, associated with the pain the patient has noted the onset of numbness in his right toes. His past medical history is significant for hypertension. Physical examination reveals irregular pulse rate of 120 beats/min, blood pressure of 130/82 mm Hg, respiratory rate of 24 breaths/min. His rhythm on the cardiac monitor shows irregularly, irregular rate without the presence of p-waves. His right lower extremity has a bluish discoloration and is cool to the touch below the mid-thigh. His aortic pulse is normal, his right femoral pulse is normal, and the right popliteal and pedal pulses are absent. The femoral, popliteal, and pedal pulses are normal on the left. Which of the following is the most appropriate management option for this patient?

A. Systemic heparinization, right femoral artery thrombectomy
B. Systemic heparinization, angiography, and placement of right SFA stent
C. Systemic heparinization
D. Systemic thrombolytic therapy

ANSWERS

14.1 **A.** His symptoms imply occlusive disease above the common femoral level, confirmed by the absence of a femoral pulse.

14.2 **B.** When tissue loss is noted, multilevel disease is usually present. There is likely to be disease in both the aortoiliac and superficial femoral arteries.

14.3 **D.** All patients require lifestyle modification, but the patient in question needs a complete multilevel revascularization.

14.4 **D.** Left below-the-knee amputation may be the most appropriate treatment for this elderly, nonambulatory patient with artery occlusion at the femoral artery level. Given the ischemic changes in the left 1st and 2nd toes, it is highly probable that the patient also has occlusive disease in the tibial arteries as well. Revascularization of the lower extremities is generally not indicated in nonambulatory patients, and given the evidence of soft tissue infection of the foot, an amputation may be the best option for this patient at this time.

14.5 **D.** This patient's acute onset of symptoms and the presence of normal vascular examination in the left lower extremity are highly suggestive of a recent embolic event leading to occlusion of the right SFA. It is important to initiate heparin therapy to prevent the propagation of thrombus in the right lower extremity, at the same time, because the process has bee in place for several hours and the patient has clear signs of ischemia, additional vascular imaging may actually delay treatment. An additional procedure to consider in this individual following re-establishment of blood flow is right lower leg fasciotomy to prevent the development of compartment syndrome. The patient may be best served by early operative thrombectomy. In some patients with acute embolic events and no significant ischemia, arteriography with intra-arterial delivery of thrombolytics may be indicated.

Clinical Pearls

- Pulses are diminished distal to an arterial stenosis and are absent distal to an occluded artery.
- Claudication is extremely reproducible, with the same exertional load producing the same symptom complex.
- Rest pain is better called "metatarsalgia" to understand where the pain should be, making it different from pain in a foot with diabetic neuropathy.

REFERENCES

Belkin M, Owens CD, Whittemore AD, et al. Peripheral arterial occlusive disease. In: Townsend CM, Beauchamp RD, Evers BM, et al, eds. *Sabiston Textbook of Surgery*. 18th ed. Philadelphia, PA: Saunders Elsevier; 2008:1941-1979.

Kirk HA, O'Mara CS. Nonoperative treatment of claudication. In: Cameron JL, ed. *Current Surgical Therapy*. 9th ed. Philadelphia, PA: Mosby Elsevier, 2008:806-809.

Case 15

A 22-year-old man presents to the hospital 1 hour after sustaining two stab wounds during an altercation. On examination, the patient appears intoxicated and grimaces during manipulation of the wounds. His temperature is 36.8°C (98.2°F), pulse rate 86 beats/min, blood pressure 128/80 mm Hg, and respiratory rate 22 breaths/min. A thorough physical examination reveals two stab wounds. One wound is located at the anterior axillary line, 1 cm above the left costal margin; the second wound is located 4 cm left of the umbilicus. There is no active bleeding from either wound site. The breath sounds are present and equal bilaterally. The abdomen is tender only in the vicinity of the injuries. The patient claims that the knife used in the attack was approximately 5 in (12.7 cm) in length.

- ➤ What is your next step?
- ➤ What are the potential injuries?

ANSWERS TO CASE 15: Penetrating Abdominal Trauma

Summary: A 22-year-old hemodynamically stable, intoxicated man presents with stab wounds to the left thoracoabdominal region and abdomen.

- **Next step:** Perform primary and secondary assessments focusing on the abdominal examination and obtain an upright chest radiograph (to assess for pneumothorax, hemothorax, and free intra-abdominal air).
- **Potential injuries:** Heart, lung, diaphragm, intra-abdominal injury.

ANALYSIS

Objectives

1. Learn the various possible approaches in the selective treatment of patients with a penetrating abdominal injury.
2. Learn the benefits and potential limitations associated with the various diagnostic strategies for detecting intra-abdominal injuries.

Considerations

This patient has sustained penetrating thoracoabdominal and abdominal injuries. Initial attention should be directed to the primary survey, which includes assessment of the airway, breathing, and circulation (ABCs). These appear to be stable based on the scenario. For this patient, the concerns include possible injury to the thoracic structures, diaphragm, and intra-abdominal structures. There are a number of different acceptable management options, but a reasonable approach for this patient may include an initial upright chest radiograph to rule out pneumothorax, hemothorax, and free air, with a study repeated in 6 hours if no abnormalities are seen initially. **Subsequently, a focused abdominal sonography for trauma (FAST) examination can be performed to exclude pericardial effusion, which would indicate a cardiac injury.** The patient could then undergo diagnostic laparoscopy to determine if there is peritoneal penetration of the stab wound and if there is a diaphragm injury. **Any suspicion of a hollow viscus injury during laparoscopy should result in a celiotomy.**

APPROACH TO Penetrating Abdominal Trauma

CLINICAL APPROACH

Primary Survey

Patient treatment always begins with an evaluation and management of the airway, breathing, and circulation (the ABCs, a primary survey). Listening to the patient allows the examiner to determine the adequacy of the airway and brain perfusion and to make certain there are no obvious neurologic deficits. **Breathing is evaluated by listening to the patient's breath sounds.** The finding of obvious decreased breath sounds on the left side is an indication for the placement of a chest tube. In addition to measuring vital signs, the examiner can evaluate the circulation by palpating the skin and observing the capillary refill. **Cool skin or a capillary refill for more than 2 seconds is an indication of shock.** The circulation evaluation includes an examination **for distended neck veins or muffled heart tones,** which are indications of **cardiac tamponade and require immediate treatment.**

A determination of the extent of disability is the equivalent of a rapid neurologic examination, and it includes assessing the pupillary response as well as the patient's response to verbal stimuli. The patient's clothes should be removed to look for evidence of other injuries. During the primary survey, an **upright chest radiograph** should be obtained. This chest radiograph is useful in the evaluation of **pneumothorax or hemothorax, the cardiac silhouette for evidence of cardiac injury, and intra-abdominal free air** consistent with a hollow viscus injury. If the chest radiograph shows no abnormalities, it should be repeated at 4 to 6 hours to rule out a delayed pneumothorax. **FAST** should also be performed to rule out blood in the pericardium. The **sensitivity of FAST in detecting pericardial** blood is **as high as 100%,** but **its sensitivity in detecting abdominal injury approximates only 50%.**

Secondary Survey

Following the primary survey, a careful secondary survey should be performed to ascertain the extent of the patient's injuries. The most important part of the secondary survey in this patient is the abdominal examination. The presence of prominent physical findings such as **rigidity, guarding, or significant tenderness distant from the stab wounds is an indication for celiotomy.** It is important to note that the physical examination may not be reliable in patients with penetrating abdominal trauma, especially in those who are intoxicated.

Treatment Options

Patients with penetrating abdominal trauma have historically undergone mandatory surgical exploration, resulting in a high nontherapeutic celiotomy rate and a high complication rate. The practice of selective celiotomy currently has become widely accepted. This change in practice has resulted in alternative methods of evaluation, including admission to the hospital for serial abdominal examinations, local exploration of the wound followed by diagnostic peritoneal lavage (DPL), and abdominal computed tomography (CT) or exploratory laparoscopy.

Observation of asymptomatic patients with abdominal stab wounds for the development of positive physical findings results in a low nontherapeutic celiotomy rate. Patients who are observed require frequent evaluations for peritoneal findings or hemodynamic instability. Patients should be observed for a minimum of 24 to 48 hours. A policy of observing patients with stab wounds is associated with the reduction in nontherapeutic laparotomy; however, this approach could lead to the delay in treatment of injuries.

Local wound exploration of stab wounds permits a determination of fascial penetration. A sterile field is prepared around the stab wound, and the area is infiltrated with a local anesthetic. The stab wound is enlarged to permit adequate exploration, and the tract of the wound is followed. If the **anterior abdominal fascia has been penetrated, further evaluation is indicated.**

Diagnostic peritoneal lavage was designed to sample the intra-abdominal contents for blood, inflammation (white blood cell [WBC] count), or fecal matter. A catheter is placed in the abdomen using the Seldinger (catheter over a guidewire) technique. The catheter is aspirated after placement to look for evidence of gross blood or fecal contents. If the aspiration results are negative, 1 L of warmed normal saline is instilled into the abdomen and then removed by gravity. The criteria for a **positive DPL results in patients with blunt trauma** are well established and include **gross aspiration of 10 mL of blood, aspiration of fecal contents, or the presence of > 100,000/mm^3 red blood cells (RBCs) or 500/mm^3 WBCs in the lavage fluid.**

Diagnostic Peritoneal Lavage Criteria

Although the criteria for grossly positive DPL results and the WBC count criteria (500 cells/mm^3) for penetrating are the same as for blunt trauma, the RBC count criteria have not been standardized. The published thresholds range from 1000/mm^3 to 100,000/mm^3. The use of low RBC count criteria results in sensitivities approaching 100% but in nontherapeutic celiotomy rates as high as 30%. The use of higher erythrocyte thresholds is associated with a reduced sensitivity and a reduced nontherapeutic celiotomy rate. DPL is not a sensitive test for injuries to the diaphragm or retroperitoneal structures.

The use of **CT** has been described for the evaluation of penetrating torso injuries in hemodynamically normal patients. Oral, intravenous, and rectal contrasts are often used to help detect intraperitoneal fluid and enteric content leakage. Results from a CT scan are considered positive if there is evidence of peritoneal penetration, free intraperitoneal fluid or air, intraperitoneal extravasation of contrast material, or injury to an intraperitoneal hollow organ. Abdominal CT imaging can be used to follow a stab wound tract or bullet path accurately, allowing determination of the structures that are at risk for injury. Some solid organ injuries can be managed nonoperatively if a hollow viscus injury can be ruled out and the patient remains stable. CT scanning is noninvasive and specific for injury, but it is not sensitive in detecting diaphragm injuries.

Diagnostic laparoscopy is also an option in assessing patients with penetrating abdominal trauma. It is extremely useful in evaluating peritoneal penetration, solid organ injury, and diaphragm injury. Laparoscopy is not sensitive in detecting hollow viscus injury. **If there is any possibility of a hollow viscus injury based on the presence of peritoneal penetration and the trajectory of the stab wound tract, celiotomy should be performed.** Laparoscopy is unique in that it is accurate in the detection of diaphragm injuries and injuries that can be repaired using laparoscopic techniques. Laparoscopy obviates the need for a full celiotomy in approximately 50% of stable patients with abdominal stab wounds. The disadvantages of laparoscopy are its lack of sensitivity in detecting hollow viscus injuries and the requirement for an operative procedure.

Comprehension Questions

15.1 A 25-year-old man sustains a stab wound to the abdomen 8 cm superior to the umbilicus. His skin is cool, and he is diaphoretic. His blood pressure is 74/40 mm Hg, and his pulse is 130 beats/min. His abdomen is distended and diffusely tender. Which of the following management possibilities is most appropriate?

A. Abdominal CT scan
B. Laparoscopy
C. Celiotomy
D. Local wound exploration

15.2 A 47-year-old man sustains a stab wound to the left upper quadrant of his abdomen. He complains of minimal pain. He is alert and hemodynamically normal, and the results from his abdominal examination show no abnormalities. Which of the following statements is true?

A. Abdominal CT is sensitive in the detection of diaphragm injuries.
B. The FAST examination reliably rules out intra-abdominal injury.
C. Local wound exploration revealing fascial penetration is an absolute indication for celiotomy.
D. The patient should be admitted for a 24- to 48-hour observation period.

15.3 A 37-year-old woman sustains a stab wound located at the anterior axillary line, 3 cm superior to the costal margin. She is alert and has normal mentation. Her blood pressure is 104/60 mm/Hg, and pulse is 110 beats/min. Which of the following is the most appropriate next step?

A. Listen to the patient's breath sounds.
B. Obtain a chest radiograph.
C. Perform a FAST examination.
D. Examine her abdomen.

15.4 A 56-year-old man was stabbed in the right lower quadrant of his abdomen. He complains of pain at the wound site. His vital signs are normal, and the findings from his abdominal examination are normal. Local wound exploration reveals penetration of the anterior fascia, and DPL reveals 7000 RBCs/mm^3 and 750 WBCs/mm^3. Which of the following is the most appropriate next step?

A. Repeat the DPL in 4 hours.
B. Obtain an abdominal CT scan.
C. Perform a laparoscopy.
D. Perform a celiotomy.

ANSWERS

15.1 **C.** The patient tachycardia and hypotension suggest that he has a life-threatening intra-abdominal hemorrhage, and after the ABCs and volume resuscitation, he needs immediate celiotomy. Based on the location of the patient's stab wound, it is also conceivable that his clinical picture could be due to a cardiac injury and cardiac tamponade, therefore preparations should also be made to address that possibility.

15.2 **D.** Asymptomatic stab wounds can be observed for the development of abdominal symptoms or hemodynamic instability. The sensitivity of the FAST examination is only 50%.

15.3 **A.** The primary survey (ABCs) should be performed first. Rather than focusing on radiological studies or abdominal exam, the first priority should be assessing airway and breathing (air exchange).

15.4 **D.** The DPL results are positive by WBC criteria, and hollow viscus injury is suspected. Celiotomy is the best method of excluding this type of injury.

Clinical Pearls

- The sensitivity of the FAST examination in detecting pericardial blood is as high as 100%, but its sensitivity in detecting abdominal injury approximates 50%.
- An abdominal examination revealing prominent findings such as rigidity, guarding, or significant tenderness distant from the stab wounds is an indication for celiotomy.
- Selected patients who have sustained penetrating abdominal injury may be observed for a minimum of 24 to 48 hours.
- If the anterior abdominal fascia is penetrated by a wound, further evaluation is needed.
- Positive DPL results in blunt trauma patients include gross aspiration of 10 mL of blood, aspiration of fecal contents, or the presence of > 100,000 RBCs/mm^3 or 500 WBCs/mm^3 in the lavage fluid.

REFERENCES

American College of Surgeons. Abdominal trauma. In: *Advanced Trauma Life Support for Doctors*. 7th ed. Chicago, IL: American College of Surgeons Committee on Trauma Staff; 2004:131-145.

Britt LD, Rushing GD. Penetrating abdominal trauma. In: Cameron JL, ed. *Current Surgical Therapy*. 9th ed. Philadelphia, PA: Mosby Elsevier; 2008:964-970.

Case 16

A 37-year-old man is brought to the emergency department after being involved in a high-speed motor vehicle collision. The patient's vehicle crashed into a tree when he fell asleep at the wheel. The patient was restrained, his vehicle sustained severe front-end damage, and the air bags deployed in the vehicle. In the emergency center, his vital signs were blood pressure 110/80 mm Hg, pulse 110 beats/min, respiration rate 28 breaths/min, Glasgow Coma Score (GCS) 14. The primary survey revealed a patent airway, diminished breath sounds on the left with exquisite chest wall tenderness, and subcutaneous emphysema. The heart sounds are normal and there is no jugular venous distension. The secondary survey revealed no abdominal tenderness, a stable pelvis, and no extremity abnormalities. A chest radiograph revealed several rib fractures on the left, a large pulmonary contusion, a left pneumothorax, and widening of the mediastinal structures.

➤ What are the most likely diagnoses?

➤ How would you confirm the diagnosis?

ANSWERS TO CASE 16:
Chest Trauma (Blunt)

Summary: A 37-year-old man presents with multiple blunt chest injuries following a high-speed motor vehicle collision. In addition to injuries that have already been demonstrated by chest radiography, a major concern at this point is the possibility of thoracic aortic disruption.

➤ **Most likely diagnoses:** Blunt chest trauma with pulmonary contusion, pneumothorax, rib fractures, and possible thoracic aortic disruption.

➤ **Confirmation of diagnosis:** All of the diagnoses except for the aortic injury have been confirmed by chest radiography. The aortic injury can be diagnosed by angiography, CT angiography, or transesophageal echocardiography.

ANALYSIS

Objectives

1. Know the priorities in the treatment of patients with multiple blunt trauma.
2. Learn the diagnosis and treatment of pneumothorax, pulmonary contusion, and thoracic aortic injury following blunt trauma.

Considerations

The initial assessment of the patient should begin with the airway, breathing, and circulation (ABCs), followed by the secondary survey. Simultaneously, intravenous lines should be placed, blood collected, and vital signs monitored. With the presence of diminished breath sounds, chest wall tenderness, and left-sided soft tissue crepitation, it would have been appropriate to place a left chest tube even without radiographic confirmation of left pneumothorax. Reassessment of the patient's respiratory status should be made and repeated chest radiographs obtained immediately following chest tube placement. If the patient's respiratory status worsens or fails to improve dramatically, intubation should be considered to help improve cardiopulmonary stability while efforts are made to identify other potential life-threatening injuries. Once all the injuries have been identified (Table 16–1), they can be addressed according to their urgency.

Table 16–1 CAUSES OF INSTABILITY AFTER BLUNT CHEST TRAUMA

INJURY	TREATMENT
Tension pneumothorax	Tube thoracostomy Needle decompression
Hemothorax	Tube thoracostomy resuscitation Possible exploration, repair
Cardiac tamponade	Decompression (open, needle) Exploration repair
Blunt cardiac injury	Supportive care (inotropes); operative repair for cardiac rupture
Air emboli	Exploration, repair
Injury to great vessels	Exploration, repair

APPROACH TO Blunt Chest Trauma

CLINICAL APPROACH

In the evaluation and treatment of patients with blunt chest trauma, it is critical to assess the magnitude of energy transfer that the accident has delivered to the injured victim. For instance, patients involved in a frontal impact collision with the deployment of air bags should be presumed to have absorbed a tremendous amount of kinetic energy to the chest wall and underlying structures. After the ABCs have been assessed, a secondary survey accomplished, and intravenous lines and blood studies performed, the patient should be examined for any change in clinical status (ie, mental status, vital signs, respiratory status). Often subtle changes forebode a looming catastrophe and require prompt reevaluation. As the assessment continues and injuries are identified, prioritizing attention depends on the severity and type of injury. A simple question to ask is "What will kill the patient **first?**" and address these issues first (Table 16–2).

The identification of **rib fractures,** especially fractures of the upper ribs (first and second), may indicate the presence of more severe associated injuries such as vascular injuries. The treatment of rib fractures is focused on management of the associated pain and the chest wall splinting that may lead to hypoventilation, atelectasis, and pneumonia. Therefore, adequate pain control may require the use of epidural anesthetic.

Table 16–2 ASSESSMENT OF CASE NO. 16's INJURIES, DIAGNOSIS, AND TREATMENT

INJURY	DIAGNOSIS	TREATMENT	COMMENT
Rib fractures	PE, chest radiograph rib series	Conservative, pain management	Possible harbinger for other injuries, goal → pain control (epidural anesthesia) to prevent hypoventilation and associated pulmonary complications
Pneumothorax	PE, chest radiograph	Tube thoracostomy	Should achieve full reexpansion Failure to reexpand or persistent air leak → consider major tracheobronchial injury
Pulmonary contusion	Chest radiograph, CT scan	Supportive care with or without intubation	Ventilatory support on clinical grounds
Traumatic aortic rupture	Aortogram CT angiography TEE	Urgent repair	See Figure 16–2

Abbreviations: PE, physical examination; CT, computed tomography; TEE, transesophageal echo cardiography.

Pneumothorax as identified by the chest radiograph results from disruption of the pleural surface. In general, simple traumatic pneumothorax may have been caused by a fractured rib penetrating the pleura or by direct injury to the pulmonary parenchyma. Proper insertion of a chest tube (tube thoracostomy) into the pleural space generally results in reexpansion of the lung parenchyma. **If the lung fails to reexpand after chest tube placement and significant air leakage is noted, one should consider the possibility of a major tracheobronchial injury.**

Blunt cardiac injury may range from myocardial contusion to cardiac rupture. When this occurs, 40% present with arrhythmia, 45% with cardiogenic shock, and 15% with anatomic defects; most patients with cardiac defects die before reaching the hospital.

Pulmonary contusion results from hemorrhage into the alveolar and interstitial spaces. The clinical condition is determined by the severity of the injury and the extent of lung parenchyma involved. Severe pulmonary contusions may result in significant shunting and hypoxia. In general, supportive measures should be undertaken and the decision for ventilatory support made on clinical

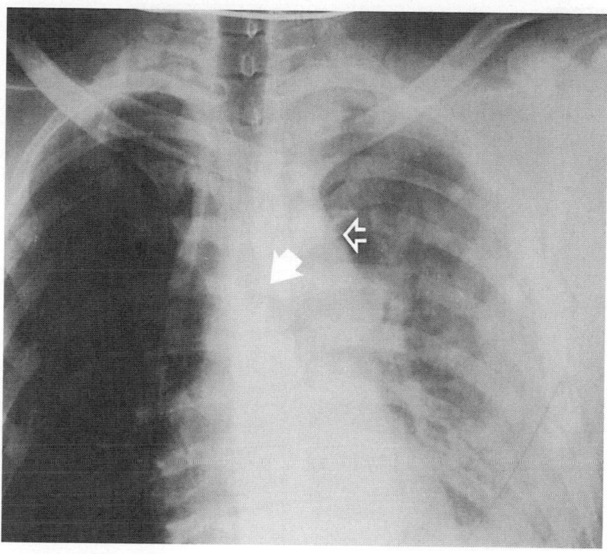

Figure 16–1. Traumatic rupture of the aorta. A widened mediastinum (*open arrow*) on the chest radiograph of a patient who had blunt trauma to the descending aorta. The left mainstem bronchus is depressed (*solid arrow*). *Reproduced, with permission, from Mattox KL, Feliciano DV, Moore E.* Trauma. *4th ed. New York, NY: McGraw-Hill; 2000:562.*

grounds. Because of capillary leakage, fluid restriction is usually advised but does not take precedence over adequate fluid resuscitation and oxygen delivery. This injury occurs most commonly from direct compression of the heart between the thoracic wall and the spine.

In the case of blunt chest trauma, *a widened mediastinum as revealed by a screening chest radiograph should raise a suspicion for traumatic rupture of the aorta (TRA)* (Figure 16–1). Although TRA is classically considered in the case of frontal impact (acceleration-deceleration) injuries, 25% of TRAs occur as a result of side impact collisions. The outcome with TRA is determined by whether the rupture is contained by the mediastinal pleura. Most patients with a free rupture into the pleural space die at the scene of the accident and never arrive at a hospital to receive medical attention. Thus, those who arrive for medical attention may need immediate diagnosis and treatment to prevent impending rupture. Debate exists as to the best tool for diagnosis. Although **the gold standard for the diagnosis of TRA remains an aortogram,** limitations in access (ie, a separate team is usually required to perform the test) and the invasiveness of the procedure have led to **CT angiography becoming more widely accepted for confirming the diagnosis of TRA.** Transesophageal echocardiography, not mentioned in the algorithm (see Figure 16–2), can be used for diagnosis but remains operator dependent and is relatively invasive.

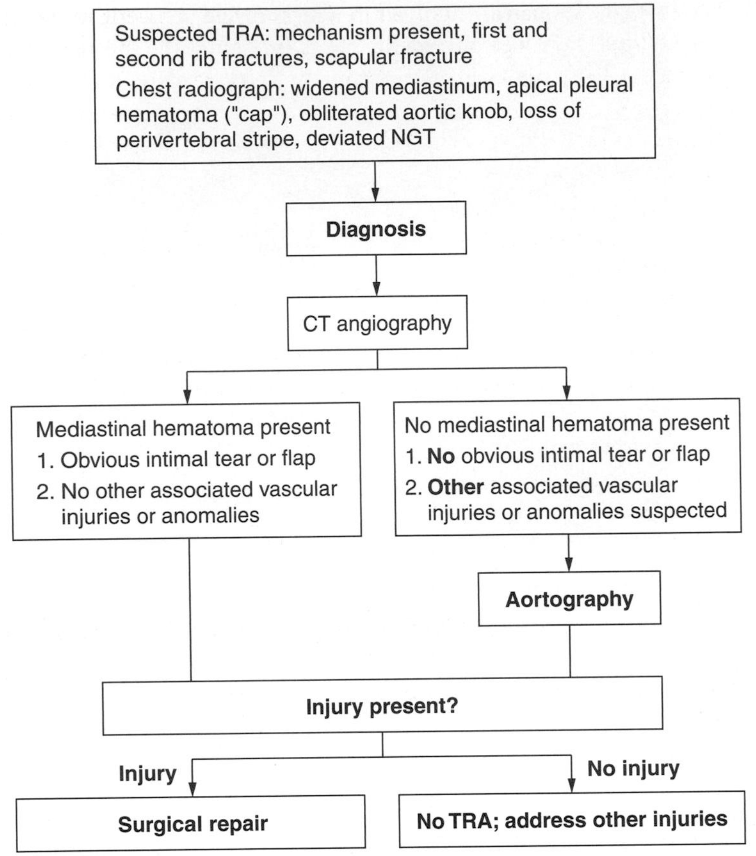

Figure 16–2. Algorithm for the management of traumatic rupture of the aorta (TRA). NGT, nasogastric tube; CT, computed tomography.

Comprehension Questions

16.1 A 16-year-old adolescent male is brought into the intensive care unit (ICU) for multiple blunt trauma approximately 12 hours previously. His injuries included a femur fracture. He is noted to have a PO_2 of 60 mm Hg, despite the use of 100% oxygen by rebreather mask, and has become confused. The chest radiograph reveals clear lung fields and a normal cardiac size. Which of the following is the most likely diagnosis?

A. Pulmonary contusion
B. Fat embolism
C. Atelectasis
D. ICU psychosis

16.2 A 43-year-old man is involved in a motorcycle accident in which his bike slipped on wet pavement. He is brought into the hospital and noted to have multiple rib fractures, a tibial fracture, and significant contusions. The cardiac monitor reveals multiple premature atrial contractions. Which of the following is the most likely etiology for the cardiac arrhythmias?

A. Anxiety
B. Lower extremity fractures
C. Rib fractures
D. Blunt cardiac injury

16.3 A radiologist evaluates a chest radiograph of a 19-year-old woman who was upended while riding her bicycle by a pickup truck. Which of the following findings is most likely to suggest a diagnosis of ruptured thoracic aorta?

A. A loss of aortic knob contour
B. Pneumomediastinum
C. Fracture of the sternum
D. Markedly enlarged cardiac silhouette

16.4 Which of the following remains the gold standard in diagnosing TRA?

A. CT angiography
B. Magnetic resonance imaging
C. Chest radiograph
D. Aortogram

ANSWERS

16.1 **B.** Fat embolism syndrome is an exceedingly uncommon problem that may occur with major long bone fracture, and it can cause hypoxemia and central nervous system effects such as confusion or coma. Other findings include petechiae and retinal lesions. Pulmonary contusion is a possibility in patients with blunt chest injuries, however patients with pulmonary contusions generally have chest x-ray findings of non-anatomic opacification. Pulmonary atelectasis generally has chest x-ray finding as well.

16.2 **D.** Blunt cardiac injuries may result in tachyarrhythmias or cardiac (pump) failure. Rib fractures are associated with pain, atelectasis, and pneumonia but rarely with atrial arrhythmias.

16.3 **A.** Chest radiographic findings consistent with thoracic aortic rupture include apical cap, deviated nasogastric tube, obliteration of the aortic knob, and hemomediastinum (not pneumomediastinum).

16.4 **D.** Aortography is considered the gold standard for diagnosis of TRA, although at many centers CT angiography is used.

Clinical Pearls

- Understanding the amount of energy absorbed by the injured victim is important in treating blunt trauma victims.
- The approach to chest trauma is to prioritize by identifying the injury that will kill the patient **first** (after the ABCs are assessed): tension pneumothorax, pericardial tamponade, hypovolemia from exsanguination.
- Identification of **rib fractures,** especially fractures of the upper ribs (first and second) may indicate the presence of more severe associated injuries (ie, vascular injuries).
- A widened mediastinum on a chest radiograph in a patient who has undergone blunt chest trauma, including injury in a deceleration accident, strongly suggests TRA.
- CT angiography and aortography are both effective tests to confirm TRA.

REFERENCES

Estrera AL, Mattox KL, Wall MJ Jr. Thoracic aortic injury. *Semin Vasc Surg*. 2000;13:345-352.

Haut ER. Blunt cardiac injury. In: Cameron JL, ed. *Current Surgical Therapy*. 9th ed. Philadelphia, PA: Mosby Elsevier, 2008:1063-1066.

Hirschberg A, Mattox KL. Vascular trauma. In: Townsend CM, Beauchamp RD, Evers BM, et al, eds. *Sabiston Textbook of Surgery*. 18th ed. Philadelphia, PA: Saunders Elsevier, 2008:1980-2001.

Case 17

A 20-year-old woman with abdominal pain is evaluated in the emergency department. She describes the gradual onset of pain 24 hours previously, which has been persistent in its location in the lower abdomen. Shortly after the onset of pain, the patient developed nausea. She denies any diarrhea, dysuria, or previous abdominal symptoms. She had her last normal menstrual period 7 days ago, and she denies any abnormal patterns in her menses. The patient is sexually active with one partner. Her past medical and surgical history is unremarkable. She takes oral contraceptives and consumes alcohol socially. On physical examination, her temperature is 100.8°F (38.2°C) and her blood pressure, pulse, and respiration rate are normal. The cardiopulmonary examination is unremarkable. Her abdomen is soft, with tenderness to palpation in the right lower quadrant and suprapubic region. No peritoneal irritation or masses are detected. Her bowel sounds are hypoactive. The rectal examination reveals tenderness on the right side. Pelvic examination reveals no purulent discharge; however, there is tenderness in the right adnexal region. Laboratory studies reveal a white blood cell (WBC) count of 14,600/mm^3, normal hemoglobin and hematocrit values, and normal electrolyte and amylase levels. Urinalysis reveals concentrated urine with 3 to 5 red blood cells (RBCs per hpf), 5 to 10 WBCs per hpf, and negative results for leukocyte esterase. The result from a serum pregnancy test is negative.

➤ What should be your next step?

ANSWER TO CASE 17:
Abdominal Pain (Right Lower Quadrant)

Summary: A 20-year-old woman has a 24-hour history of abdominal pain that is **atypical** for acute appendicitis. She has a low-grade fever and lower abdominal tenderness, with maximal tenderness in the right lower quadrant. Her laboratory tests are significant for leukocytosis, microscopic hematuria, and pyuria.

➤ **Next step:** Obtain a CT scan of the abdomen and pelvis.

ANALYSIS

Objectives

1. Learn the pathophysiology of acute appendicitis.
2. Learn the diagnostic approaches for patients with suspected acute appendicitis.

Considerations

The diagnosis of acute appendicitis is frequently made on the basis of clinical history, physical findings, and laboratory data. However, **when a patient presents with an atypical history, atypical physical and/or laboratory findings, it is important to determine whether the atypical presentation is related to another disease process or to atypical positioning of the diseased appendix.** Further diagnostic options (see Table 17–1) for an "atypical" patient include imaging studies (a CT scan, ultrasonography), clinical observation with serial laboratory evaluations, and diagnostic laparoscopy. The CT scan is selected in this case because it is sensitive for identifying inflammatory changes and thickening of the appendix. In a patient with fever, lower abdominal tenderness, and leukocytosis, these radiographic changes should be present if the findings are indeed caused by appendicitis. A factor that favors the use of a CT scan over ultrasonography in this case is that the patient's history and examination results are not suggestive of pelvic pathology, which is more effectively evaluated by ultrasonography. For this patient, clinical observation with serial laboratory evaluation is not a good option because she already has localized abdominal pain, fever, and leukocytosis, and therefore continued observation for regression of these symptoms would lead to a delay in diagnosis. Diagnostic laparoscopy is an operative procedure with associated morbidity and is mainly indicated for patients with nonspecific clinical or radiographic evidence of inflammation or pathology that cannot be further delineated by additional imaging studies.

Table 17–1 DIAGNOSTIC OPTIONS FOR ACUTE APPENDICITIS

	ADVANTAGES	DISADVANTAGES	RECOMMENDED USE
CT imaging	Identifies appendicitis changes or other pathology (~95% accuracy)	Limited sensitivity for early appendicitis and pelvic pathology	Inflammatory process not related to pelvic pathology
Ultrasonography	Greater sensitivity and specificity for gynecologic pathology than CT	Limited by body habitus; appendicitis signs less well defined	Suspected gynecologic pathology; young children
Clinical observation with serial laboratory studies	Allows the natural history of disease evolution	Limited application if localized pain, fever, and leukocytosis are already present	Possible early appendicitis and without localized signs
Diagnostic laparoscopy	Allows accurate assessment of pathology	Invasive; some morbidities	Inflammatory or pathology of uncertain source

Abbreviation: CT, computed tomography.

APPROACH TO Suspected Acute Appendicitis

DEFINITIONS

CHRONIC OR RECURRENT APPENDICITIS: Occurs in 5% of patients with appendicitis and may result from antibiotic administration in patients with early acute appendicitis.

INTERVAL APPENDECTOMY: This procedure generally is for the treatment of appendicitis complicated by abscess or phlegmon. The patient is treated initially with broad-spectrum antibiotic therapy and CT-guided drainage of the abscess to resolve the infectious process, followed by appendectomy after several weeks. Since some patients with appropriate nonoperative treatment do not develop appendicitis recurrences, the role of interval appendectomy remains unclear.

MESENTERIC ADENITIS: An inflammatory condition occurring with a viral illness, resulting in painful lymphadenopathy in the small bowel mesentery. This process can be associated with right lower quadrant pain and tenderness and is especially common in children.

CLINICAL APPROACH

Pathogenesis and Clinical Presentation of Appendicitis

The appendix arises from the cecal diverticulum during embryonic development. During this process, it rotates from its posterior location toward the iliac fossa. Incomplete rotation occurs frequently, leading to variable appendiceal positioning and variations in clinical presentation. The development of appendicitis generally begins with luminal obstruction by a fecalith, lymphoid hyperplasia, or food matter. With this obstruction there is an increase in mucous secretion, venous and lymphatic congestion, and bacterial overgrowth (see Table 17–2). When unabated, this process leads to ischemic necrosis and perforation. **The classic history of acute appendicitis begins with vague pain in the periumbilical region, nausea, vomiting, and the urge to defecate;** these symptoms **are followed by localization of the pain in the right lower quadrant** associated **with localized peritonitis.** Approximately 20% of patients with acute appendicitis experience perforation within 24 hours of the onset of symptoms. Recognition of appendicitis can be delayed because of atypical presentations caused by retrocolic or pelvic locations. Similarly, antibiotic administration during the early course of appendicitis may alter the clinical course. **Only approximately 50% of patients with acute appendicitis show a classic presentation.**

Table 17–2 CLINICAL-PATHOLOGIC CORRELATION

PATHOLOGIC CONDITION	CLINICAL SIGNS AND SYMPTOMS
Luminal obstruction	Poorly localized periumbilical pain, nausea, vomiting, and urge to defecate
Inflammation	Location of pain depending on the position of the appendix; peritonitis is present only if the inflamed appendix or inflammatory changes involve the peritoneum
Perforation	Transient improvement in pain but an increase in systemic toxicity

Diagnosis

Patients with the classic presentation generally require only a thorough history and physical examination, a CBC with a differential count, urinalysis, and a pregnancy test (women only) for diagnosis. When patients with an atypical history, physical examination, or laboratory findings are encountered, selective application of diagnostic imaging is indicated to avoid delays in therapy and minimize the occurrence of nontherapeutic operations.

Comprehension Questions

17.1 A 19-year-old woman presents with a 2-day history of right lower quadrant pain and no fever. She has a tender right adnexal mass, a normal WBC count, negative findings from a pregnancy test, and normal urinalysis results. Which of the following is the most appropriate management?

A. CT of the abdomen and pelvis
B. Abdominal and pelvic ultrasonography
C. Diagnostic laparoscopy
D. Observation with serial laboratory studies

17.2 A 24-year-old man complains of colicky intermittent umbilical and right lower quadrant abdominal pain of 24 hours' duration. He complains of anorexia and nausea. His temperature is 36.7°C (98°F). Which of the following is the most likely diagnosis?

A. Acute appendicitis
B. Chronic appendicitis
C. Gastroenteritis
D. Acute pancreatitis

17.3 An 18-year-old woman has a 1-day history of worsening lower abdominal pain, nausea and vomiting, and a low-grade fever. Her temperature is 37.2° (99°F), and she has mild lower abdominal tenderness and no rebound. She has possible right adnexal tenderness. Which of the following tests would most definitively differentiate pelvic inflammatory disease from acute appendicitis?

A. CT scan of the abdomen and pelvis
B. Magnetic resonance imaging of the abdomen and pelvis
C. Ultrasound examination of the pelvis
D. Laparoscopy

17.4 A 43-year-old woman presents with 1-day history of right flank and right lower quadrant pain. She has a history of nephrolithiasis and indicates that the pain she experiences now is not similar to those experienced before. Her temperature is 38.5°C, and her abdomen and right flank are tender to deep palpation. Her urinalysis shows 10-20 WBC/HPF and 10-20 RBC/HPF. Which of the following is the best management strategy?

A. Hospitalization, IV hydration, analgesics, and antibiotic therapy for UTI
B. Perform pelvic ultrasound to rule out ovarian torsion
C. Perform CT scan of the abdomen
D. Diagnostic laparoscopy

17.5 A 14-year-old boy present with right lower quadrant abdominal pain of two days duration. He indicates that he has been ill for the past 10 days with cough, runny nose, and fever, and over the past two days his lower abdomen has become painful. Over the past 12 hours the pain has been improving slowly. His temperature is 37.8°C. His abdomen is tender in the right lower quadrant, without masses or signs of peritonitis. His WBC is 11,000/mm^3 and urinalysis is normal. CT of the abdomen reveals no inflammatory changes in the area around the cecum. There are several prominent lymph nodes measuring approximately 2 cm in size in the mesentery of the small bowel. The bowel wall is not thickened. What is your diagnosis and treatment?

A. Mesenteric andenitis. Discharge from ED with follow-up.
B. Probable mesenteric adenitis. Perform diagnostic laparoscopy to ruleout appendicitis
C. Crohn' disease. Consult a gastroenterology colleague for definitive long-term management.
D. Mesenteric adenitis. Admit the patient for IV antibiotic therapy.

ANSWERS

17.1 **B.** For this patient with findings suggestive of pelvic pathology (an adnexal mass), ultrasonography is an accurate modality in defining the pathology.

17.2 **C.** Intermittent pain is not typical for appendicitis. Acute pancreatitis typically presents as constant boring pain radiating to the back.

17.3 **D.** Laparoscopy is the most accurate test to assess for acute pelvic inflammatory disease (an erythematous tube with purulent drainage from the fimbria) and to visualize the appendix.

17.4 **C.** Perform a CT scan of the abdomen. This patient has right flank and right lower quadrant pain and history of kidney stones; however the patients states that her pain now is dissimilar to her prior pain with kidney stones. A CT scan without contrast may be useful to help identify kidney stones, and if this does not visualize kidney stones, a CT with contrast may also be performed to help rule-out appendicitis and pylonephritis.

17.5 **A.** This patient's history, physical findings, and CT findings are compatible with mesenteric adenitis, which is nonspecific, and self-limiting inflammation of the mesenteric lymph nodes. No antibiotics treatment is necessary for the condition. Since CT of the abdomen has good negative predictive value in ruling-out acute appendicitis, a diagnostic laparoscopy is unnecessary in this patient.

Clinical Pearls

- The options in assessing atypical presentations for appendicitis include imaging tests, clinical observation with a serial laboratory evaluation, and diagnostic laparoscopy.
- The classic history of acute appendicitis begins with vague pain in the periumbilical region, nausea, vomiting, and the urge to defecate; these symptoms are followed by localization of the pain in the right lower quadrant associated with localized peritonitis.
- Only approximately 50% of patients with acute appendicitis have the classic presentation.
- Ultrasonography is generally the best modality to assess pelvic pathology, whereas a CT scan is the best way to assess nongynecologic abdominal processes.

REFERENCES

Jaffe BM, Berger DH. The appendix. In: Brunacardi FC, Adersen DK, Billiar TR, et al, eds. *Schwartz's Principles of Surgery*. 8th ed. New York, NY: McGraw-Hill, 2005:1119-1137.

Maa J, Kirkwood KS. The Appendix. In: Townsend CM, Beauchamp RD, Evers BM, et al, eds. *Textbook of Surgery: The Biological Basis of Modern Surgical Practice*. 18th ed. Philadelphia, PA: Saunders Elsevier; 2008:1333-1347.

Case 18

A 58-year-old woman complains of the sudden onset of right chest pain and shortness of breath 6 days following an uncomplicated left hemicolectomy for adenocarcinoma of the descending colon. The patient has had an uncomplicated postoperative course until this time. During your evaluation, she appears anxious and is unable to remain comfortable. Her temperature is 37.9°C (100.2°F), pulse rate 105 beats/min, blood pressure 138/80 mm Hg, and respiratory rate 32 breaths/min. She is receiving O_2 by nasal canula with an O_2 saturation of 96% by pulse oximetry. Despite this oxygen saturation, the patient continues to complain of difficulty breathing. There is no jugular venous distension. Her lungs are clear, with diminished breath sounds in both bases. Her cardiac examination reveals sinus tachycardia. Her abdomen is slightly tender and without distension, and the surgical incision is normal in appearance. Her legs reveal mild edema bilaterally and tenderness in the left calf. Laboratory evaluations reveal a white blood cell (WBC) count of 11,000/mm^3 with a normal differential, normal hemoglobin and hematocrit values, and a normal platelet count. The electrolyte levels are likewise normal. An arterial blood gas study reveals pH 7.45, PO_2 73 mm Hg, PCO_2 34 mm Hg, and HCO_3 24 mEq/L. A 12-lead electrocardiogram (ECG) reveals sinus tachycardia. The creatine kinase and troponin levels are within normal limits. A portable chest radiograph (CXR) demonstrates no infiltrates or effusions and minimal atelectasis in both lower lung fields.

- What is the most likely diagnosis?
- What should be your next step?

ANSWERS TO CASE 18: Venous Thromboembolic Disease

Summary: A 58-year-old woman has acute chest pain and dyspnea postoperatively. The results from cardiopulmonary and abdominal examinations are nonspecific. She has a minimally elevated leukocyte count and normal cardiac enzyme levels. Arterial blood gas studies indicate respiratory alkalosis and hypoxemia. The CXR and ECG show no obvious pathology.

- **Most likely diagnosis:** Pulmonary embolism (PE) is very likely with the sudden onset of chest pain and shortness of breath in a patient without pulmonary or cardiac pathology.
- **Next step:** Empirical systemic anticoagulation with confirmatory imaging pending.

ANALYSIS

Objectives

1. Know the risk factors and causes of venous thromboembolic disease.
2. Know the applications and effectiveness of prophylactic measures for deep vein thrombosis (DVT).
3. Learn the diagnostic and therapeutic approaches for patients with suspected venous thromboembolism.

Considerations

The differential diagnosis for a 58-year-old woman with the sudden onset of chest pain and shortness of breath during the postoperative period includes cardiac ischemia, respiratory tract infection, acute lung injury, and PE. In this case, PE should be strongly considered based on the history of acute dyspnea and chest pain with a normal WBC count, normal ECG and CXR results, and normal cardiac enzyme levels. As for most patients, making a definitive diagnosis of PE based on clinical criteria is difficult. However, this evaluation is vital in determining the level of clinical suspicion (pretest probability), which influences the diagnostic precision of subsequent imaging studies. In this case, the clinical picture indicates a high clinical probability of PE. The decision to **initiate systemic anticoagulation without a confirmed diagnosis of PE is justifiable based on a high clinical suspicion and the absence of contraindications to anticoagulation.** As one decides whether to initiate empirical treatment, it is important to bear in mind that **patients treated with early aggressive anticoagulation therapy are less likely to experience treatment failure or develop recurrences.**

APPROACH TO
Deep Venous Thrombosis and Pulmonary Embolism

DEFINITIONS

VENOUS DUPLEX IMAGING: An accurate, noninvasive imaging modality combining ultrasonography and Doppler technology to assess the patency of veins and the presence of blood clot in veins; it is especially useful for the lower extremities.

VENTILATION-PERFUSION (V/Q) SCAN: A radioisotope scan used to identify V/Q mismatches, which can indicate PE and other pulmonary conditions. Results must be interpreted based on coexisting pulmonary pathology and the clinical picture.

COMPUTED TOMOGRAPHY: A vascular contrast study involving CT imaging with a sensitivity for PE detection ranging widely from 64% to 93%; it is highly sensitive for PE involving the central pulmonary arteries but insensitive for subsegmental clots. Some advocate that it not be used as the initial imaging study and that it is perhaps best used with venous duplex or pelvic CT venography for better accuracy.

PULMONARY ANGIOGRAPHY: Considered the gold standard for the diagnosis of PE. It is accurate (approximately 96%), carries a false-negative rate of 0.6%, and especially has greater sensitivity than CT for subsegmental and chronic PE. The significant drawbacks are a major procedural complication rate of 1.3%, mortality rate of 0.5%, and the time delay associated with the procedure.

THROMBOLYTIC THERAPY: Thrombolysis for PE has survival advantages in patients with massive PE, especially when it is associated with right heart dysfunction. Tissue plasminogen activator (TPA) is the most commonly used agent and may be given systemically or by catheter-directed infusion into the clot. Recent major surgery (such as within a 10-day period) and recent severe closed head injury are contraindications to systemic thrombolytic therapy.

PULMONARY EMBOLECTOMY: Surgical retrieval of clots in the pulmonary artery through a median sternotomy, requiring cardiopulmonary bypass. Major indication: massive PE with hemodynamic instability and hypoxia, where thrombolytic therapy is contraindicated. It is associated with 30% to 60% mortality.

CLINICAL APPROACH

Prophylaxis

The development of acute thromboembolic complications is presumed to be related to stasis, hypercoagulability, and vein wall injury that occur as the

Table 18–1 APPROXIMATE DEEP VENOUS THROMBOSIS PREVALENCE WITH AND WITHOUT PROPHYLAXIS

TREATMENT	GENERAL SURGERY (%)	TOTAL HIP REPLACEMENT (%)	TRAUMA (%)
No therapy	25	51	50-58
Low-dose heparin	8	31	44
Low-molecular-weight heparin	7	15	30; proximal deep vein thrombosis reduced to 6
Elastic stockings	9 (data include only low-risk patients)	22	No evidence available
Intermittent pneumatic compression device	10 (only low- to moderate-risk patients)	38	No evidence available

result of local and systemic effects of trauma and operative injuries, aging, and preexisting medical conditions. The incidence of DVT in general surgery patients is estimated at approximately 25%, with most being asymptomatic.

Major orthopedic surgery and major trauma are associated with a significantly greater risk of this complication. Most patients with DVT have involvement of the tibial-level veins and may remain asymptomatic; however, involvement of the femoral and/or iliac veins dramatically increases the risk of PE and symptoms, such that approximately 30% to 50% of these patients may develop PE. All patients with identifiable risk factors should undergo prophylaxis against DVT/PE, which is effective in reducing the complication rate. In high-risk patients, prophylaxis is effective in reducing the occurrence of DVT/PE (Table 18–1).

Diagnosis

A suggested diagnostic approach is shown in Figure 18–1.

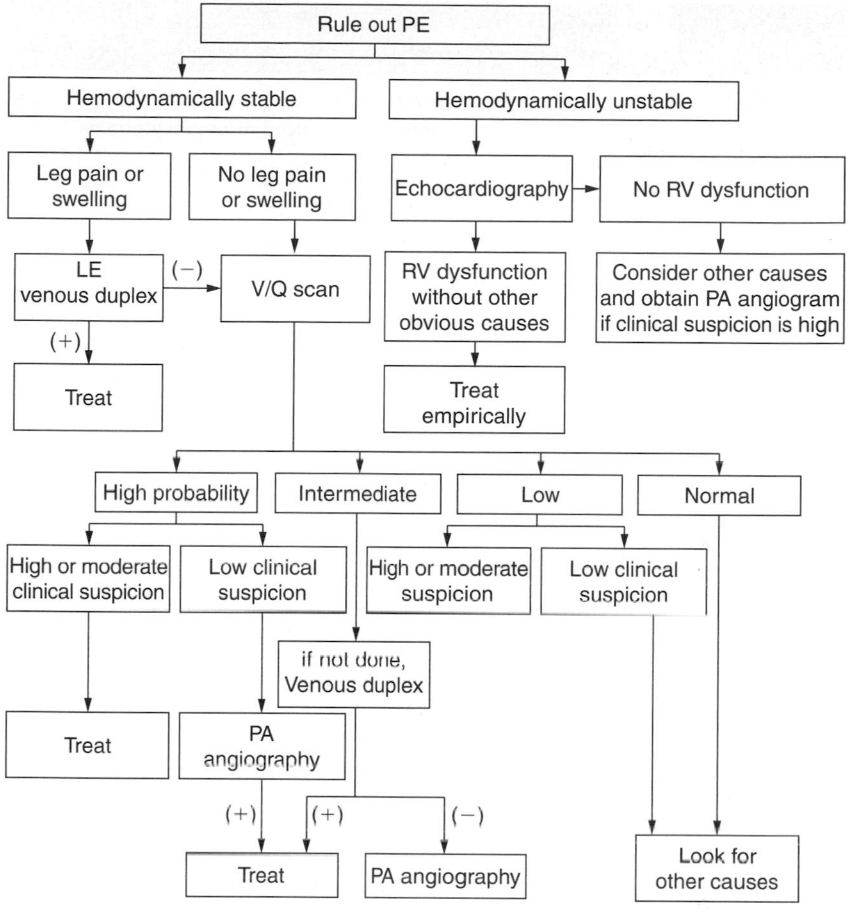

Figure 18–1. Diagnostic flowchart for treatment of a patient with suspected pulmonary embolism. *Adapted, with permission, from Shepard AD, Shin LH. Pulmonary thromboembolism. In: Cameron JL, ed.* Current Surgical Therapy. *7th ed. St Louis, MO: Mosby-Year Book; 2001;1016.*

Treatment

In general, all patients with documented DVT and PE should undergo treatment with systemic anticoagulation therapy with heparin infusion, oral warfarin, or subcutaneous low-molecular-weight heparin. The duration of therapy for uncomplicated DVT is generally 3 months. Patients with PE and no identifiable hypercoagulability state should be treated for 6 months, and patients with documented hypercoagulability should be considered for lifelong therapy (Table 18–2). Recurrent PE despite adequate anticoagulation, complications from anticoagulation, and contraindication to anticoagulation are the three major indications for vena cava filter placement.

Table 18–2 DEEP VEIN THROMBOSIS TREATMENT AND EFFICACY

Unfractionated heparin	6% recurrence; 3% major bleeding; 1%-3% risk of heparin-induced thrombocytopenia
Low-molecular-weight heparin	3% recurrence; 1% major bleeding; associated with a lower risk of heparin-induced thrombocytopenia
Thrombolysis therapy	Indicated for iliofemoral deep vein thrombosis; contraindicated in recently postoperative patients or after recent head trauma

Comprehension Questions

18.1 A 45-year-old man with diabetes complains of pain and swelling in the right calf and thigh of 2 days' duration. Which of the following is the next appropriate step in the treatment of this patient?

A. Begin systemic thrombolytic therapy.
B. Perform a lower extremity venous duplex scan.
C. Perform CT pulmonary angiography.
D. Determine the D-dimer level. Perform pulmonary angiography if this level is elevated.

18.2 In which of the following patients with confirmed femoral venous thromboses is fractionated heparin therapy contraindicated?

A. A hemodynamically stable 80-year-old man with a documented PE
B. A 20-year-old man who sustained a closed head injury 14 days ago
C. A 23-year-old woman in her third trimester of pregnancy
D. A 44-year-old woman with heparin-induced thrombocytopenia

18.3 A 35-year-old man complains of dyspnea and left leg pain. He undergoes a V/Q scan, interpreted as being of low probability for PE. Which of the following is the most accurate statement?

A. The probability of PE is less than 1%.
B. The probability of PE is as high as 40%.
C. The next test should be a determination of the serum D-dimer level.
D. Pulmonary angiography should be performed to rule out PE definitively.

18.4 Which of these is the most appropriate DVT prophylactic measure for a 36-year-old man who just underwent an exploratory laparotomy, distal pancreatectomy, splenectomy, and gastric repair for a gunshot wound to the abdomen? The patient had approximately 3000 mL of blood loss prior to surgical control of his bleeding and repairs of his injuries. Following his operation, he has been stable in the ICU with a hematocrit of 28% and INR of 1.7.

A. Low molecular weight heparin
B. 5000 units of fractionate heparin TID
C. 5000 units of fractionate heparin BID
D. Pneumatic compression devices

ANSWERS

18.1 **B.** Obtain a venous duplex scan of the legs. Systemic thrombolytic therapy is indicated only if patients have proven proximal DVT. D-dimer levels are elevated in 99.5% of all patients with DVT/PE, but this is also seen following trauma and surgery, and so the test is highly sensitive but nonspecific.

18.2 **D.** Heparin-induced thrombocytopenia, which is usually an immunoglobin G–mediated reaction, is a contraindication to heparin therapy. Heparin does not cross the placenta and is not contraindicated during pregnancy. Generally, at 14 days following a closed head injury, there is no contraindication to anticoagulation.

18.3 **B.** The probability of PE can be as high as 40% in a patient with a low-probability V/Q scan. The probability of PE in a patient with a low-probability V/Q scan and low clinical suspicion is approximately 4%. If the patient's V/Q scan indicates a low probability and the clinical suspicion is intermediate or uncertain, the risk for PE is approximately 16%. A venous duplex scan is indicated for further evaluation of intermediate- and high-risk patients.

18.4. **A.** Low molecular heparin is more effective than fractionated heparin in the prevention of DVT in high-risk individuals. Trauma patients with history of significant blood loss are considered extremely high-risk patients. Pneumatic compression devices have no proven efficacy in the prevention of DVT in the high-risk trauma population.

Clinical Pearls

- Up to 95% of patients with venous thromboembolic complications have recognizable risk factors and therefore would benefit from prophylactic measures.
- The benefits of prophylactic measures against DVT/PE are additive and should be applied together to reduce risk maximally in very-high-risk patients.
- A serial surveillance duplex scan should be obtained in very-high-risk patients despite prophylactic measures.
- Heparin-induced thrombocytopenia is a contraindication to heparin therapy.
- The main indication for pulmonary embolectomy is massive PE with hemodynamic instability or refractory hypoxemia.
- Upper extremity DVT (such as subclavian vein thrombosis) carries a much higher PE risk than lower extremity DVT.

REFERENCES

Lam EY, Giswold ME, Moneta GL. Venous and lymphatic disease. In: Brunacardi FC, Adersen DK, Billiar TR, et al, eds. *Schwartz's Principles of Surgery*. 8th ed. New York: McGraw-Hill; 2005:809-833.

Smith ST, Clagett P. Pulmonary thromboembolism. In: Cameron JL, ed. *Current Surgical Therapy*. 9th ed. Philadelphia, PA: Mosby Elsevier; 2008:903-907.

Case 19

A 65-year-old man presents with dyspnea on exertion and angina. The patient's current symptoms have been present for approximately 3 to 4 weeks. He denies any cough, weight loss, and gastrointestinal (GI) tract symptoms. His past medical history is significant for hypertension, stable angina, and colonic polyps that were removed 7 to 8 years ago by colonoscopy. The physical examination reveals a well-nourished man who is in no acute distress. The findings from head and neck, cardiopulmonary, and neurologic examinations are unremarkable. Examination of the abdomen reveals an obese abdomen without tenderness or palpable masses. The rectal examination reveals no masses, a smooth and enlarged prostate, and strongly Hemoccult-positive stool in the vault. The complete blood count reveals a normal white blood cell (WBC) count, hemoglobin 8.7 g/dL, hematocrit 29%, and mean cell volume 72 fL (normal, 76-100 fL). The electrolyte levels and liver function studies are within normal limits. A 12-lead electrocardiogram reveals normal sinus rhythm and mild left ventricular hypertrophy. A chest radiograph reveals a normal cardiac silhouette, no pulmonary infiltrate, no pleural effusion, and no pulmonary mass.

- What is the most likely mechanism causing this process?
- How would you confirm the diagnosis?

ANSWERS TO CASE 19:
Colorectal Cancer and Polyps

Summary: A 65-year-old man presenting with dyspnea on exertion and worsening angina pectoris related to anemia produced by occult GI tract bleeding.

- **Most likely mechanism:** Anemia caused by occult GI tract bleeding.
- **Confirmation of diagnosis:** Esophagogastroduodenoscopy (EGD) to evaluate the upper GI tract and colonoscopy to evaluate for a possible colorectal source of bleeding.

ANALYSIS

Objectives

1. Learn the clinical presentation and management of colorectal cancer.
2. Know the risk factors for and surveillance of high-risk patients.

Considerations

This patient presents with angina, dyspnea on exertion, microcytic anemia, and guaiac-positive stool. His presentation is strongly indicative of occult GI tract blood loss. The lower GI tract is the most likely source of bleeding in patients who are not consuming aspirin or other nonsteroidal anti-inflammatory drugs. In this case, the initial treatment should consist of transfusion to improve the patient's anemia, followed by endoscopic evaluation of the upper and lower GI tract with EGD and colonoscopy. If the source of the blood loss is not identified after these diagnostic procedures, evaluation of the small bowel for a blood loss source by contrast radiography should be performed. Given his previous history of colonic polyps requiring endoscopic removal, this man is at risk for the development of polyps as well as colorectal cancer. Thus, he should have been placed on a regular surveillance schedule 8 years ago, with repeated colonoscopy after 3 years. If negative results were obtained, he should subsequently have been placed on surveillance colonoscopy at 5-year intervals.

APPROACH TO
Colorectal Cancer and Polyps

DEFINITIONS

ABDOMINOPERINEAL RESECTION: Resection of the rectum and anal canal including anal sphincter complex for a low-lying rectal carcinoma. The procedure leaves the patient with a permanent colostomy.

LOW ANTERIOR RESECTION: Resection of the rectum to the level of the levator ani muscles leaving the anal canal and anal sphincter muscles intact so that a stapled or hand-sewn anastomosis can be performed.

BOWEL PREPARATION FOR ELECTIVE COLON SURGERY: A mechanical preparation consisting of a large volume of polyethylene glycol solution or a smaller volume of phosphosoda and a broad-spectrum intravenous and/or oral nonabsorbable antibiotic. The goal is to decrease the bacterial count in the event of spillage of colonic contents.

CLINICAL APPROACH

Epidemiology

Colorectal cancer is the fourth most common internal malignancy and the second most common cause of cancer death in the United States. (Lung cancer is the most common.) The average American has an approximately 5.5% to 6% lifetime risk of developing colorectal cancer. This cancer is predominantly a disease of the middle-age and elderly population, with only 5% of cancers occurring in patients younger than 40 years. Roughly 70% of colorectal cancers initially develop as adenomatous polyps. Through a series of mutations in protooncogenes and tumor suppressor genes, a malignant transformation occurs leading to the development of carcinoma. Based on the polyp-carcinoma sequence of cancer development, it is possible to prevent cancer by identifying and removing polyps prior to the development of invasive cancer. The rectum and sigmoid colon have long been the most common site of malignancy; however, this is changing as right-sided colon cancers are steadily increasing in number.

Screening

Disease screening can most effectively be accomplished by complete colonoscopy.

For average risk individuals, the American College of Gastroenterology screening recommendation is colonoscopy every 10 years beginning at 50 years of age. If an adenomatous polyp bigger than 1 cm is identified and removed, repeat colonoscopy should be done in 3 years. When the colon is clear of polyps, colonoscopy can be done every 5 years.

Clinical Presentation

Symptoms of colorectal cancer vary depending on the location of the tumor. The most common presenting symptom is rectal bleeding (occult or gross). After bleeding, symptoms include chronic changes in bowel habits in 77% to 92% of patients, obstruction in 6% to 16%, and perforation with peritonitis in 2% to 7%. Characteristic changes in bowel habits are a decrease in the caliber of stools and diarrhea. These are more commonly seen with left-sided tumors and rectosigmoid tumors. Tumors of the right side are less likely to cause obstructive symptoms until late in the course of the disease. Anemia is a more common presentation in these patients.

Cancer Staging

The tumor-node-metastasis (TNM) system and the Astler-Coller modification of the Duke classification are the most common staging systems used for colorectal carcinoma (Tables 19–1 and 19–2).

Treatment

Patients with colonic polyps can be treated with endoscopic resection. Endoscopic therapy is considered definitive when the resection of the polyp is complete.

Table 19–1 TNM STAGING SYSTEM

STAGE	DEPTH	NODAL STATUS	DISTANT METASTASIS
Stage 1	T1, T2	N0	M0
Stage 2	T3, T4	N0	M0
Stage 3	Any T	N1, N2, N3	M0
Stage 4	Any T	Any N	M1

TX: Primary tumor cannot be assessed
T0: No evidence of primary tumor
Tis: Carcinoma in situ
T1: Tumor invasion into submucosa
T2: Tumor invasion into muscularis propria
T3: Tumor invasion through muscularis propria
T4a: Tumor perforation of visceral peritoneum
T4b: Tumor invasion of adjacent structure
NX: Regional lymph nodes cannot be assessed
N1: 1-3 regional lymph nodes
N2: ≥ 4 regional lymph nodes involved
N3: Regional lymph nodes involved along a major vascular structure
M0: No distant metastatsis
M1: Any distant metastatsis

Table 19–2 ASTLER-COLLER MODIFICATION OF THE DUKE CLASSIFICATION

	TUMOR	NODES	DISTANT METASTASIS
A	Tis, T1, T2, T3	N0	M0
B	T4	N0	M0
C1	T1, T2, T3	N1, N2, N3	M0
C2	T4	N1, N2, N3	M0
D	Any T	Any N	M1

Cancer risks increase with larger polyps, with the risk of carcinoma approximately 1.3% for adenomatous polyps smaller than 1 cm, 9.5% for polyps 1 to 2 cm, and 46% for polyps bigger than 2 cm. Polypectomy alone is considered curative if the tumor has not penetrated the submucosa, whereas submucosal penetration increases the likelihood of regional lymph node metastasis.

Invasive adenocarcinoma of the colon requires segmental resection of the involved colon. A patient with a reasonable life expectancy should undergo a preoperative metastatic workup including chest radiography and abdomen and pelvic computed tomography (CT) scans. The amount of colon resected is based on blood supply and regional lymphatic drainage (Figure 19–1). Primary anastomosis can be performed with stapling devices or via a hand-sewn technique. Both methods have equal risks of anastomotic dehiscence and stricture. Following recovery from colon resection, patients with lymph node involvement (stage III disease) have improved survival and a reduced possibility of recurrence when they are given adjuvant chemotherapy. Current standard therapy is the FOLFOX4 regimen: 5-FU (fluorouracil), leucovorin, and oxaliplatin. The approximate 5-year survival of patients by stage is as follows: stage I, 80% to 90%; stage II, 60% to 70%; stage III, 40% to 60%; and stage IV, 4% to 9%.

Invasive adenocarcinoma of the rectum accounts for approximately 30% of all colorectal carcinoma. The rectum is classically described as the lowest 15 cm of the GI tract. Because of the close proximity of the rectum to the surrounding structures, patients with rectal cancer are not only at risk for distant metastasis but also for local tumor recurrence. Preoperative evaluation of patients with rectal carcinoma should include chest radiography and a CT scan of the abdomen and pelvis. In addition, endoscopic ultrasonography should be performed to determine the depth of tumor invasion and the status of the perirectal lymph nodes. Several surgical treatment options for rectal cancer are available depending on the location in the rectum and the depth of invasion. For most patients with superficial invasion (T1), the risk of lymph node metastasis is low. If the tumor is low in the rectum, a transanal

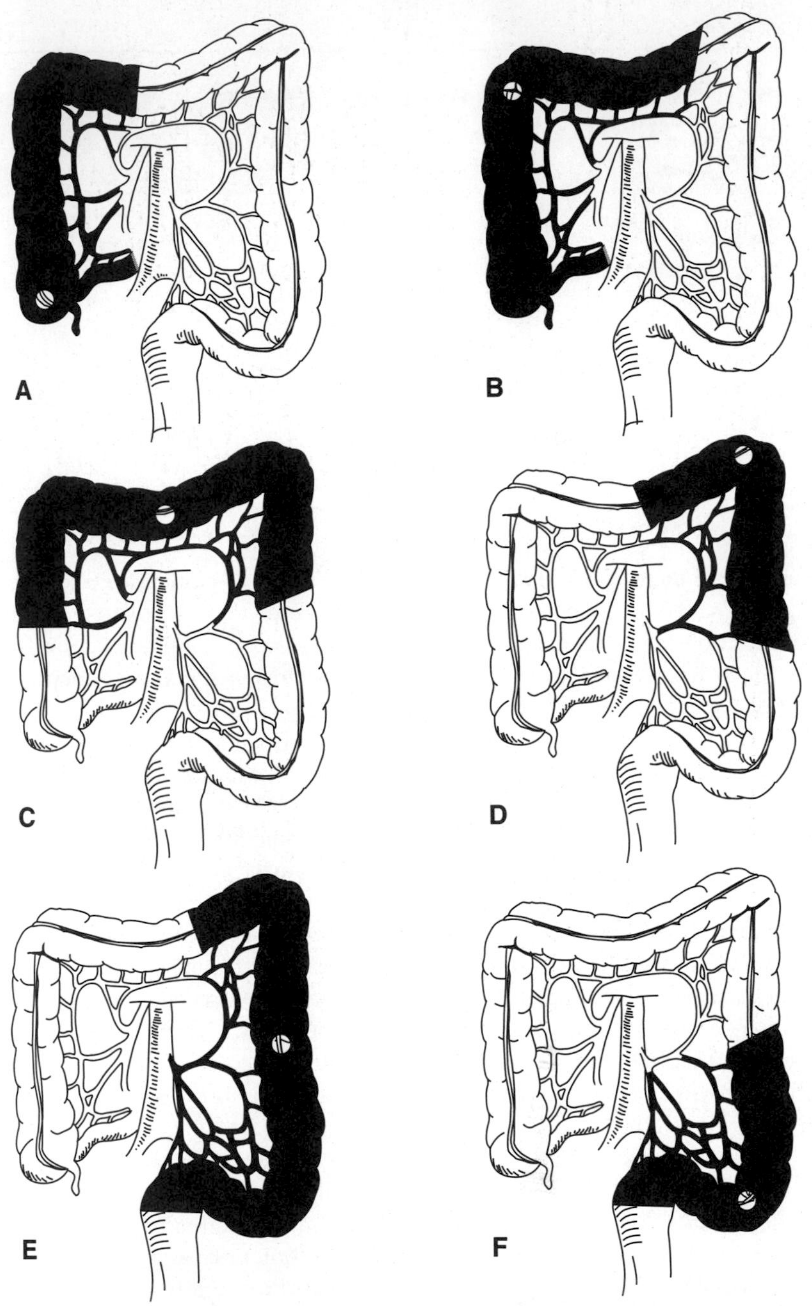

Figure 19–1. Resection of colon cancer. Right colectomy (**A**), right hemicolectomy with division of middle colic pedicle (**B**), transverse colectomy (**C**), resection of splenic flexure sparing left colic artery (**D**), left hemicolectomy (**E**), sigmoid colectomy sparing left colic artery (**F**) *Reproduced, with permission, from Niederhuber JE, ed.* Fundamentals of Surgery. *Stamford, CT: Appleton & Lange; 1998:322 as modified from Schwartz SI, Ellis H.* Maingot's Abdominal Operations. *10th ed. Norwalk, CT: Appleton & Lange; 1989:1053.*

resection of the tumor with tumor-free margins is the standard therapy. For maximal benefit from this approach, patients generally should have a tumor involving less than a third of the rectal circumference, less than transmural involvement, a well to moderately differentiated histologic grade, and unaffected rectal lymph nodes. For patients with deeper invasion (T2 and T3) and higher risk of lymph node metastases, surgical resection of the involved rectum and surrounding lymph nodes is necessary. A low anterior resection (LAR) is performed for rectal cancers above the anal sphincter complex. For those tumors near the sphincter complex, an abdominoperineal resection (APR) with permanent colostomy is usually necessary.

Patients with locally invasive rectal carcinoma (stage III) experience a reduction in pelvic tumor recurrence when they complete a course of chemoradiation therapy prior to surgical resection (neoadjuvant therapy). Neoadjuvant therapy appears to have additional benefits over postoperative chemoradiation therapy in rectal carcinoma in preventing local recurrence. Patients with stage III rectal carcinoma who have not received neoadjuvant therapy may derive benefits from postoperative chemoradiation therapy.

Postoperative Follow-Up

The incidence of metachronous (subsequent) colorectal cancer is 1.1% to 4.7%. It is not clear how often and by what means patients should be evaluated following the successful treatment of colorectal cancers. One such surveillance colonoscopy program advocates initial colonoscopy at 6-month intervals up to 1 year, followed by yearly colonoscopy for 2 years, and subsequent surveillance colonoscopy every 3 years. In addition, patients should undergo a regular evaluation involving history and physical examinations and serial carcinoembryonic antigen (CEA) measurements.

High-Risk Patient Groups

Patients at high risk for colorectal cancer include those with familial adenomatous polyposis (FAP) syndrome, familial cancer (first-degree relatives), hereditary nonpolyposis colorectal cancer (HNPCC) syndrome, and a history of inflammatory bowel disease, particularly ulcerative colitis. Screening recommendations differ depending on the disease. Children of persons with FAP should have a flexible sigmoidoscopy every 1 to 2 years beginning at 10 to 12 years of age. Individuals with a strong family history of colorectal cancer should have an initial colonoscopy at 40 years of age or when they are 10 years younger than the age at which the relative was diagnosed, whichever comes first. For patients with HNPCC syndrome, the initial colonoscopy is recommended at 25 years of age, followed by yearly fecal occult blood testing and colonoscopy every 3 years (see Table 19–3). Patients with a history of ulcerative colitis of more than 7 to 8 years' duration should have a colonoscopy with biopsies every 1 to 2 years.

Table 19–3 RECOMMENDED SCREENING AND SURVEILLANCE GUIDELINES

Sporadic adenomatous polyposis
- Complete colonoscopy and clearance of all polyps along with index polyp
- Repeat colonoscopy in 3 y (selectively—patients with tubular adenoma < 1 cm may not require long-term follow-up)
- If initial examination and clearance are suboptimal, initial follow-up colonoscopy should be at 1 y

Familial adenomatous polyposis
- Flexible upper endoscopy for all first-degree relatives of FAP, Gardner syndrome, and Turcot syndrome patients
- Screening colonoscopy should begin for known FAP patients at age 10-12 y and performed every 1-2 y until age 40, and then every 3 y thereafter
- Initial upper endoscopy at age 20 or at age of prophylactic colectomy
  a. For mild duodenal disease, upper endoscopy every 2-3 y.
  b. For severe duodenal disease, upper endoscopy every 6 mo to 1 y
- Surveillance of all first-degree relatives of FAP patient with abdominal CT for desmoid tumors
- Surveillance of first-degree relatives of Turcot syndrome patients with CT scan of the brain

Abbreviations: FAP, familial adenomatous polyposis; CT, computed tomography.

Metastatic Disease

The presence of metastatic disease to the liver or lungs generally indicates the presence of disseminated disease. There are small subsets of patients who may develop isolated metastasis to these sites who can be treated appropriately by surgical resection.

Comprehension Questions

19.1 Which of the following patients has the highest risk of developing colorectal cancer?

A. A 45-year-old man whose younger brother has a history of colon cancer
B. A 30-year-old woman with a BRCA1 mutation
C. A 55-year-old man with a 15-year history of ulcerative colitis
D. A 50-year-old man with a history of resected adenomatous colonic polyps
E. A 44-year-old man with FAP syndrome (polyposis coli)

19.2 Which of the following is the most appropriate treatment for a 40-year-old man with a T3 N1 carcinoma of the cecum?

A. Preoperative chemoradiation therapy followed by right hemicolectomy
B. Right hemicolectomy and postoperative chemotherapy with 5-FU, leucovorin, and oxaliplatin
C. Endoscopic removal of the tumor followed by chemoradiation therapy
D. Right hemicolectomy and postoperative tamoxifen therapy

19.3 Which of the following is the most appropriate follow-up for a 60-year-old man who underwent a colonoscopy and complete endoscopic removal of a 2-cm adenomatous polyp from the sigmoid colon?

A. Annual colonoscopy
B. Repeated colonoscopy at 3 years and, if the results are negative, repeated every 5 years
C. CT scan and repeated colonoscopy at 3 years and, if the results are negative, repeated every 5 years
D. Repeated colonoscopy every 2 years

ANSWERS

19.1 **E.** BRCA1 does not confer an increased risk of colon cancer, whereas BRCA2 does. The other conditions are associated with increased risks of developing colorectal cancer, but a patient with FAP syndrome (the colon is filled with thousands of polyps) has nearly a 100% risk of developing colon cancer.

19.2 **B.** Right hemicolectomy with postoperative adjuvant chemotherapy using FOLFOX4 (5-FU, leucovorin, and oxaliplatin) is indicated for this patient with stage III colon cancer. Radiation therapy is generally indicated for patients with rectal carcinoma. Tamoxifen therapy is not useful for colorectal carcinoma.

19.3 **B.** The current recommendations for colonic polyp follow-up are as follows: Once the colon is cleared of polyps, repeated colonoscopy at 3 years and, if the results are negative, repeated colonoscopy every 5 years. A CT scan is not recommended for the follow-up of patients with polyps.

Clinical Pearls

- Many of the symptoms associated with colorectal cancer are nonspecific, including postprandial bloating, distension, and constipation.
- Patients with FAP syndrome are at high risk for adenomas and adenocarcinomas of the duodenum in addition to colorectal cancers, and these patients require surveillance EGD.
- Approximately 70% of colon cancers are thought to arise from adenomatous polyps. The larger the adenomatous polyp, the greater the risk of colon cancer.
- For rectal cancer, neoadjuvant chemotherapy seems to be helpful in reducing local recurrence.

REFERENCES

Andre T, Boni C, Mounedji-Boudiaf L, et al. Oxaliplatin, fluorouracil, and leucovorin as adjuvant treatment for colon cancer. *N Engl J Med*. 2004;350:2343-2351.

Fry RD, Mahmoud N, Maron DJ, Ross HM, Rombeau J. Colon and rectum. In: Townsend CM Jr, Beauchamp RD, Evers BM, et al. *Sabiston Textbook of Surgery*. 18th ed. Philadelphia, PA: Saunders Elsevier; 2008:1348-1432.

Levin B, Lieberman DA, McFarland B, et al. Screening and surveillance for early detection of colorectal cancer and adenomatous polyps, 2008: A joint guideline from the American Cancer Society, the US Multi-society Task Force on Colorectal Cancer and the American College of Radiology. *Gastroenterol*. 2008;134:1570-1595.

Case 20

A 33-year-old man presents for evaluation of swelling in his right thigh. He first noticed the swelling 8 to 10 weeks ago and attributed it to injuries incurred during long-distance running. The patient has no known medical problems. He is physically fit and runs approximately 3 to 5 miles daily. On examination, he is found to have a 6 × 5 cm, firm, nontender mass in the anterior portion of the right thigh. There are no skin or motor/sensory changes in the right leg and no lymphadenopathy in the right groin. A radiograph of the thigh reveals no bony abnormalities.

➤ What is the most likely diagnosis?

➤ How would you confirm the diagnosis?

➤ What is the best therapy?

ANSWERS TO CASE 20: Sarcoma (Soft Tissue)

Summary: A 33-year-old man presents with a large, nontender, soft tissue tumor that is highly suggestive of an extremity sarcoma.

- **Most likely diagnosis:** Soft tissue sarcoma (STS) should be highly suspected.
- **Confirmation of diagnosis:** A core needle biopsy of the mass should be obtained for tissue diagnosis.
- **Best therapy:** Surgical excision is the mainstay of therapy. Multimodality therapy, including radiation and chemotherapy delivered either preoperatively or postoperatively, may be indicated for selected high-grade, large STSs.

ANALYSIS

Objectives

1. Know the presentation of extremity, truncal, and retroperitoneal sarcomas and the importance of obtaining tissue for early diagnosis and treatment.
2. Learn the treatment options and outcome for patients with sarcomas.
3. Learn the genetic conditions and risk factors associated with sarcoma development.

Considerations

The initial approach in this patient should include biopsy of the mass for pathologic diagnosis. The biopsy can be performed using a core needle biopsy or by open incision if a needle biopsy fails to obtain adequate tissue. **Excisional biopsy should never be attempted with lesions suspected to be STSs because of the difficulty in achieving adequate resection margins, which would compromise the definitive care of the patient.** Young, healthy, active individuals under age 30 with extremity STSs are frequently misdiagnosed as having a hematoma or a bruised muscle because sarcomas are infrequently encountered by physicians in most medical practices. Therefore, it is imperative to **consider STS whenever an unexplained soft tissue mass or swelling is identified** in an individual of any age. Certain clinical features in this case should further raise a **suspicion of STS,** including the **size of the lesion (6 × 5 cm), the absence of a specific event to account for a hematoma of this size, the firmness of the mass, and the absence of surrounding skin changes to suggest an inflammatory or infectious process.** As a rule, most patients with STS present without any regional lymphadenopathy or systemic symptoms such as weight loss, night sweats, or cachexia. STS may manifest occasionally as local pain, erythema, or tenderness over the mass and can be easily misdiagnosed as a soft tissue abscess; these symptoms are caused by rapid tumor growth leading to partial necrosis of the STS.

APPROACH TO Sarcomas

DEFINITIONS

SARCOMA: One of a group of tumors usually arising from connective tissue, and are characterized as extremity, truncal, or retroperitoneal.

LI-FRAUMENI SYNDROME (LFS): A cancer predisposition syndrome associated with soft-tissue sarcoma, breast cancer, leukemia, osteosarcoma, melanoma, and cancer of the colon, pancreas, adrenal cortex, and brain. Individuals with LFS are at increased risk for developing multiple primary cancers. LFS is diagnosed in individuals meeting established clinical criteria. More than 50% of individuals diagnosed clinically have an identifiable TP53 gene.

CLINICAL APPROACH

Sarcomas can be categorized as extremity, superficial truncal, and visceral/retroperitoneal. Diagnostic delays associated with extremity STSs are not uncommon, in part because of the failure of the patient to seek treatment and because of misdiagnoses by physicians. The typical presentation is that of a new area of swelling in the arm or leg frequently thought to be a hematoma or bruised muscle and often noticed after trivial trauma to the area. It is important to note that trauma is not the cause of STS but rather the event that brings attention to the mass itself. The differential diagnosis for a soft tissue mass include benign lipoma, which is much more common; however, STS should be suspected in any patient with a new fixed mass, a mass that is increasing in size, or a mass bigger than 5 cm in diameter.

Approximately 50% of STS are found in the extremities, but the distribution can involve any site. Sarcomas arise from mesodermal tissue and can exist as one of many pathologic subtypes (eg, liposarcoma, fibrosarcoma, leiomyosarcoma, and malignant fibrohistiocytoma). The diagnosis of STS begins with development of a high index of suspicion based on the history and physical examination, followed by either a core needle biopsy or a fine-needle biopsy for diagnosis. **Patients with tumors of large size or high grade (highly mitotic) based on histologic study are at increased risk for pulmonary metastasis. These individuals should undergo CT imaging of the lung.** Staging of an extremity STS is based on size, grade, and superficial versus deep location. Table 20–1 outlines favorable and unfavorable characteristics of extremity and superficial trunk STSs. The staging for STS is still evolving.

Table 20–1 CHARACTERISTICS OF EXTREMITY SOFT TISSUE SARCOMAS

CHARACTERISTIC	FAVORABLE	UNFAVORABLE
Size	≤ 5 cm	> 5 cm
Grade	Low	High
Depth	Superficial	Deep

In general, sarcomas with three favorable signs are stage 0, those with two favorable signs are stage 1, those with one favorable and two unfavorable signs are stage 2, and those with three unfavorable signs are stage 3. All sarcomas with either lymph node or distant metastasis are considered stage 4. **Lymph node metastasis is rare in STS; however, when it occurs, patient survival is similar to that for individuals with distant metastasis. Distant metastasis occurs most commonly in the lungs.** Disease-specific survival (DSS) for patients with extremity STS varies depending on the site, histology, grade, and size. Basically, patients with low-grade tumors smaller than 5 cm have greater than 90% 5-year DSS, whereas those with high-grade tumors bigger than 5 cm have approximately a 50% 5-year DSS. Patients with stage 4 STSs have a 10% to 15% 5-year DSS. Nevertheless, when pulmonary metastases are amenable to complete resection, the 5-year DSS may be as high as 35%.

The **treatment of extremity STSs** has evolved substantially over the past several decades. Previously, amputation was the standard of care. A landmark prospective randomized study by the National Cancer Institute comparing limb-sparing surgery with radiation to amputation, however, found no survival benefits in performing amputations. **The current standard treatment is wide local excision, with all efforts made to obtain negative microscopic margins.** Complete resection of a muscle compartment results in greater functional loss and is generally unnecessary. Complete resection with a **2-cm gross margin** is reasonable to ensure negative microscopic margins. Patients with stage 0 disease rarely experience a recurrence or die of the disease, but the risk of local recurrence increases with the stage. Radiation therapy should be considered for stage 2 and 3 disease to reduce local recurrence. Generally, brachytherapy (radioactive catheters placed directly in the tumor resection bed) is given for high-grade tumors, and external beam therapy is given for larger, low-grade, and more deeply located tumors. Because brachytherapy catheters are placed intraoperatively, a tissue diagnosis should be obtained by core biopsy preoperatively whenever such therapy is considered.

Local recurrence of STS takes place despite resection with grossly clear margins. For this reason, every attempt should be made to obtain negative microscopic margins during the initial resection. With large tumors in deep locations, magnetic resonance imaging or computed tomography (CT) imaging performed preoperatively can help more clearly define the tumor's relationship to major structures. Patients with tumors encasing bone, major vessels, or nerves may be more appropriately treated with preoperative (neoadjuvant) chemoradiation to shrink the tumor to allow for limb-sparing surgery.

The role of adjuvant chemotherapy in patients following the complete resection of extremity sarcoma is not clear. While the individual clinical trials have not demonstrated any survival advantage with treatment, a meta-analysis has demonstrated a survival advantage for patients receiving chemotherapy.

Postoperative Follow-Up

Recommendations for follow-up after surgical resection currently are not standardized. A reasonable practice is to follow patients with a low risk for recurrence biyearly with a physical examination and yearly with a chest radiograph. Patients at high risk for recurrence are usually examined every 3 months, with chest radiographs obtained every 3 to 6 months indefinitely.

Retroperitoneal Sarcoma

Sarcomas arising from retroperitoneal structures tend to remain asymptomatic until they reach a large size. Most patients have late presentations, commonly with tumor involvement of contiguous structures. **Patients with high-grade and/or incompletely resected primary tumors have a substantial recurrence risk.** Unlike high-risk extremity STS, more likely to result in death because of recurrence at a distant site, **retroperitoneal sarcomas are much more likely to recur locally** and cause death as a result of local involvement. Lewis and colleagues evaluated 231 patients following the resection of retroperitoneal sarcomas and found 2- and 5-year survivals of 80% and 60%, respectively. **Complete resection is best achieved during the initial surgery,** and the probability of complete resection is reduced with each subsequent operative attempt. Distant metastasis from retroperitoneal sarcoma, which infrequently occurs, often involves the liver and lungs. Postoperative follow-up for retroperitoneal sarcoma is not clearly defined. CT scans performed at 6-month intervals may be considered reasonable.

Genetic and Environmental Predisposition to Sarcomas

Both physical and genetic factors can predispose to the development of sarcomas. Physical factors include prior radiation, lymphedema, and chemical exposure (including prior chemotherapy). Table 20–2 lists the genetic predisposing factors. Patients with neurofibromatosis are prone to develop sarcomas arising from nerve structures, as well as paragangliomas and pheochromocytomas. The development of retinoblastoma in patients with the Li-Fraumeni syndrome

Table 20–2 GENETIC PREDISPOSITION ASSOCIATED WITH SARCOMAS
Neurofibromatosis
Li-Fraumeni syndrome
Retinoblastoma
Familial polyposis coli (Gardner syndrome)

(an autosomal dominant disorder with predisposition to the early onset of many types of cancers) has been genetically linked to mutations in *Rb-1* and *p53* genes, respectively. Whereas patients with the Li-Fraumeni syndrome have an increased risk for several cancers, those with retinoblastoma are prone to develop osteosarcomas. Patients with familial polyposis coli have an increased risk of developing desmoid tumors, which are generally considered benign tumors with a predilection for local recurrence following excision.

Comprehension Questions

20.1 A 35-year-old man notices a firm, nontender, 10-cm mass in his thigh after falling off a ladder. Which of the following is the most appropriate first step following a history and a physical examination?

A. Observation to see if it changes over the next month
B. Core needle biopsy followed by a CT scan of the extremity
C. Immediate resection with wide margins
D. Ultrasonography of the mass

20.2 A 41-year-old woman underwent excision of what was thought to be a superficial lipoma of the upper extremity. Findings from pathology studies subsequently revealed a 3-cm low-grade sarcoma with positive histologic margins. Which of the following treatments is most appropriate?

A. Follow-up physical examination in 6 months
B. External beam radiation
C. Chemotherapy
D. Re-excision to obtain negative margins

20.3 A 28-year-old man is noted to have a leiomyosarcoma of the right leg. Upon investigation, he is noted to have metastatic involvement. Which of the following is the most likely site of metastasis?

A. Lymph nodes
B. Liver
C. Lung
D. Bone

20.4 A 54-year-old woman is seen in a follow-up after resection of a large retroperitoneal sarcoma. Which of the following locations is the most likely site of recurrence?
A. Peritoneal or retroperitoneal space.
B. Liver.
C. Lung.
D. Recurrence is unlikely following complete resection.

ANSWERS

20.1 **B.** This patient noted a large nontender mass of the thigh. The finding of a **nontender** mass is inconsistent with a soft tissue injury despite the history of a fall; therefore, a core biopsy is indicated.

20.2 **D.** Surgical resection to achieve negative margins is the best treatment in this case. In general, surgical therapy is the best treatment of sarcomas.

20.3 **C.** The lungs are the most common site of metastasis for extremity STS.

20.4 **A.** Local and regional recurrence is the most likely cause of treatment failure for retroperitoneal sarcomas.

Clinical Pearls

- Features of an extremity mass that are suggestive of sarcoma include the size of the lesion (0.5 cm), the absence of a specific event to account for a hematoma, firmness of the mass, and the absence of surrounding skin changes suggesting an inflammatory or infectious process.
- The diagnosis of STS begins with a high suspicion based on the history and physical examination, followed by performance of a diagnostic core biopsy or fine-needle biopsy.
- The current standard therapy for sarcomas is wide local excision with all efforts made to obtain negative microscopic margins, followed by radiation therapy in high-risk patients.
- Prior radiation or chemotherapy and genetic factors such as neurofibromatosis are risk factors for STS.

REFERENCES

Lewis JJ, Leung D, Woodruff JM, et al. Retroperitoneal soft tissue sarcoma: analysis of 500 patients treated and followed at a single institution. *Ann Surg*. 1998;228:355.

Singer S, Canter RJ. Soft tissue sarcoma. In: Cameron JL, ed. *Current Surgical Therapy*. 9th ed. Philadelphia, PA: Mosby Elsevier; 2008:1101-1107.

Case 21

A 23-year-old female medical student presents for the evaluation of an asymptomatic neck mass that was found during a practice head and neck examination performed by a fellow medical student. The student is otherwise healthy and denies any previous medical problems. Evaluation of her neck reveals a 4-cm discrete, nontender, firm mass in the inferior pole of the right lobe of her thyroid gland. The remainder of the thyroid is normal. No other abnormalities are noted during the rest of her physical examination. The patient denies any family history of thyroid disease or other endocrinopathies. She denies any unusual exposure to ionizing radiation. Thyroid function studies are obtained and reveal normal serum thyrotropin (thyrotropin-stimulating hormone [TSH]) and thyroxine (T_4) levels.

➤ What is your next step?

ANSWER TO CASE 21: Thyroid Mass

Summary: A 23-year-old medical student presents for the evaluation of an asymptomatic 4-cm, discrete, nontender, firm mass in the inferior pole of the right lobe of the thyroid gland. She denies any previous medical problems, a prior history of head or neck irradiation, or a family history of thyroid cancer or other endocrinopathies. Her serum TSH level is normal.

➤ **Next step:** Fine-needle aspiration for a cytologic assessment for malignancy.

ANALYSIS

Objectives

1. Learn the approach to evaluate thyroid nodules, especially concerning cancer risks.
2. Review the diagnostic evaluation of a patient with a thyroid nodule.
3. Identify the indications for surgical treatment of a thyroid nodule.

APPROACH TO Thyroid Nodules

DEFINITIONS

MULTIPLE ENDOCRINE NEOPLASIA (MEN) 2 SYNDROME: An autosomal dominant syndrome with medullary thyroid carcinoma, pheochromocytoma, and parathyroid hyperplasia or adenomas.

FOLLICULAR ADENOMA: Benign thyroid nodules noted to be fairly common in adults; they usually take up radioactive iodine.

PAPILLARY THYROID CARCINOMA: The most common type of thyroid carcinoma, usually well differentiated.

MEDULLARY CARCINOMA: A type of thyroid cancer occurring sporadically or in familial clusters (MEN); it usually does not take up radioactive iodine.

CLINICAL APPROACH

In the United States, the prevalence of thyroid nodules detected by physical examination is 4% to 7%, and prevalence of nodules detected by ultrasonography or autopsy is 19% to 67%. Thyroid nodules that are bigger than 1 cm

Table 21–1 MULTIPLE ENDOCRINE NEOPLASIA

Multiple endocrine neoplasia 2A
- Medullary thyroid cancer
- Pheochromocytoma
- Hyperparathyroidism
- Lichen planus amyloidosis
- Hirschsprung disease

Multiple endocrine neoplasia 2B
- Medullary thyroid cancer
- Pheochromocytoma
- Marfanoid habitus
- Mucosal neuromas
- Ganglioneuromatosis of the gastrointestinal tract

are considered clinically significant and require further evaluation. A patient with a thyroid nodule should be questioned about symptoms of hyper- or hypothyroidism, compressive symptoms such as dyspnea, coughing or choking spells, dysphagia or hoarseness, and a prior history of head or neck irradiation. Patients should also be asked about a family history of thyroid cancer, hyperparathyroidism, or pheochromocytoma. Symptoms of hyper- or hypothyroidism may be present in patients with thyroiditis. Symptoms of hyperthyroidism are also seen in patients with benign functioning follicular adenomas. The presence of **compressive symptoms,** which occur from thyroid enlargement and impingement on **adjacent structures, most notably the trachea, esophagus, and recurrent laryngeal nerve, are indications for surgery.** A patient with a **solitary thyroid nodule and a prior history of low-dose head or neck irradiation** has a **40% risk of carcinoma.** A **family history of thyroid cancer** should increase the physician's suspicion of carcinoma in a patient with a thyroid nodule. An estimated 20% to 30% of medullary thyroid cancers occur as part of a familial syndrome; the most notable are MEN 2A and MEN 2B (Table 21–1). Five percent of papillary cancers are familial.

On physical examination, the size and character of the thyroid nodule should be noted. The thyroid gland should be examined for other nodules, and the neck for associated cervical lymphadenopathy and the position of the trachea. The **presence of associated adenopathy should increase suspicion of malignancy.**

The primary challenge in the management of a thyroid nodule is selecting for surgery those patients with a high risk for cancer and avoiding operations in patients with benign disease. **Currently, fine-needle aspiration biopsy (FNAB) is the initial and most important step in the diagnostic evaluation of a dominant thyroid nodule.** Management of nodular thyroid disease depends on the results from the FNAB (Figure 21–1). Patients with a malignant FNAB are treated with thyroidectomy. A cytologic diagnosis of malignancy is very

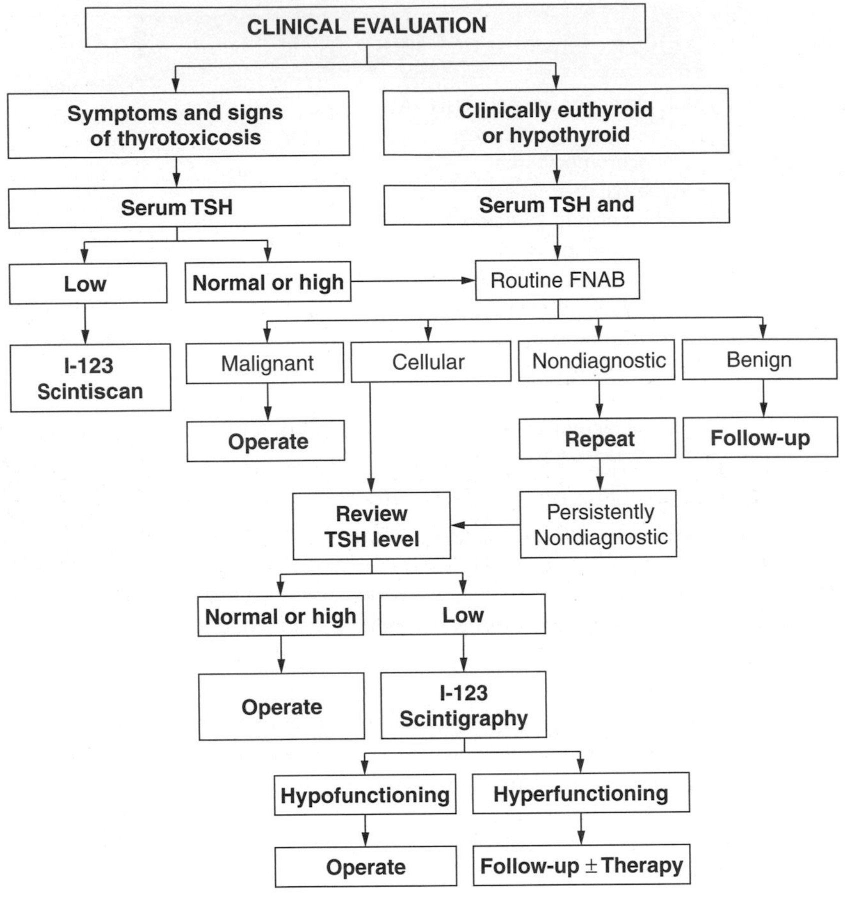

Figure 21–1. Algorithm for the evaluation of patients with a dominant thyroid nodule. *Reproduced, from McHenry CR, Sgusarczyk SJ, Askari AT, et al. Refined use of scintigraphy in the evaluation of nodular thyroid disease.* Surgery. *1998;124:660, with permission from Elsevier.*

reliable with only a 1% to 2% incidence of false-positive results. Patients with benign FNAB results are followed with a yearly physical examination of the neck and a serum TSH-level test. Thyroidectomy is reserved for progressive nodule enlargement or compressive symptoms. The incidence of false-negative FNAB results is approximately 2% to 5%.

A cellular FNAB result refers to a specimen with cytologic features consistent with either a follicular or a Hürthle cell neoplasm. A follicular or Hürthle cell carcinoma cannot be distinguished from a follicular or Hürthle cell adenoma using cytologic criteria alone. A diagnosis of follicular or Hürthle cell carcinoma is based on the presence of capsular or vascular invasion as observed in a tissue sample. For patients with a cellular FNAB, the results of a serum TSH level test are reviewed. A solitary nodule in a patient with a normal or an increased serum TSH level is almost always hypofunctioning, whereas in approximately 90% of patients with a hyperfunctioning nodule, the serum TSH level is low. **Clinically significant carcinoma occurs in less than 1% of patients with hyperfunctioning nodules compared to 10% to 20% of patients with hypofunctioning nodules.** As a result, iodine-123 thyroid scintigraphy is recommended for patients with a cellular FNAB when the serum TSH level is low. **Thyroidectomy** is recommended for patients with a **cellular FNAB when the serum TSH level is normal or high or when a hypofunctioning nodule** is demonstrated on thyroid scintigraphy. Patients with a solitary hypofunctioning nodule and a cellular FNAB have a 20% to 30% incidence of carcinoma.

In patients with nondiagnostic FNAB results, the biopsy should be repeated because an adequate specimen is obtained with a repeated biopsy in more than 50% of patients. For patients with **persistently nondiagnostic FNAB results, an operation is recommended when the serum TSH level is normal or high,** and iodine-123 scintigraphy is performed in patients with a low serum TSH level. **Surgery is recommended for patients with persistently nondiagnostic FNAB results and a hypofunctioning nodule.** A 9% incidence of carcinoma has been reported in this subset of patients.

Comprehension Questions

21.1 A 38-year-old woman is noted to have a 1.2 cm thyroid nodule. In which of the following situations would the results of thyroid scintigraphy most likely impact treatment?

A. Fine needle aspiration biopsy (FNAB) results consistent with a malignant neoplasm
B. FNAB results consistent with a benign neoplasm
C. FNAB results consistent with a follicular neoplasm
D. Prior history of head or neck irradiation

21.2 A 40-year-old woman presents with a single thyroid nodule. Which of the following situations would be associated with the highest risk of malignancy?

A. A prior history of head or neck irradiation
B. Hyperfunction of the nodule seen on thyroid scintigraphy
C. Hypofunctioning of the nodule seen on scintigraphy (cold nodule)
D. History of Graves disease

21.3 A 55-year-old man is noted to have a 1.4-cm nodule in the right thyroid lobe. In which of the following situations is thyroidectomy the best choice for treatment of this thyroid nodule?

A. Initial nondiagnostic FNAB results
B. Hypothyroidism
C. A mother who had papillary carcinoma
D. FNAB results consistent with a benign neoplasm when compressive symptoms are present

21.4 Which of the following procedures should be performed routinely in a patient with a thyroid nodule who is clinically euthyroid?

A. FNAB and determination of a screening serum TSH level
B. Measurement of radioiodine uptake and thyroid scintiscanning
C. Measure of serum T_4, triiodothyronine (T_3), and TSH levels
D. Ultrasound examination of the thyroid gland to distinguish a solid from a cystic nodule

21.5 A 60-year-old man is noted to have a 2-cm nodule in the right lobe of the thyroid. He is asymptomatic, and FNA biopsy has been attempted on 2 separate occasions demonstrating nondiagnostic findings. Ultrasound has shown a solid thyroid nodule without other abnormalities, and iodine-123 scintigraphy has revealed a nonfunctioning nodule. Which of the following management approaches is most appropriate?

A. Place patient on suppressive dose of levothyroxine and repeat FNA in 3 months.
B. Right thyroidectomy.
C. Place patient on suppressive dose of levothyroxine and repeat ultrasound in 3 months.
D. Total thyroidectomy with bilateral functional neck dissection.

21.6 A 52-year-old woman with history of asymptomatic carotid stenosis undergoes follow-up ultrasound of the neck that revealed stable stenosis of the carotid and an incidental finding of several solid and fluid-filled nodules seen in both lobes of the thyroid gland. The largest of these nodules measure 0.3 cm in diameter. Her serum TSH is within normal range of values. Which of the following is the most appropriate management for this patient?

A. Total thyroidectomy
B. I131-radioablation of the thyroid
C. Observation
D. Placement on suppressive dose of levothyroxine

ANSWERS

21.1 **C.** Radionuclide scanning can determine the function of the nodule. With a fine-needle aspirate showing a follicular pattern, a "cold" hypofunctioning pattern is associated with a significant risk of cancer, whereas a "warm or hot" functioning pattern is associated with a low (1%) risk of cancer.

21.2 **A.** A history of head and neck irradiation greatly increases the risk of a thyroid nodule being malignant. A cold nonfunctioning nodule does increase the risk of cancer, but not as significantly as the history of irradiation.

21.3 **D.** Compressive symptoms are life threatening, and urgent surgical intervention is considered the best therapy.

21.4 **A.** FNAB and a TSH level test for the assessment of thyroid function and determination of the histology of the lesion are the two most important initial tests for evaluating a thyroid nodule.

21.5 **B.** Right thyroidectomy is appropriate option for this patient, because an overall cancer rate of 9% has been reported for this population. Thyroxine suppression would not change the fact that this is a nonfunctioning nodule. Total thyroidectomy is not indicated, since a diagnosis is not yet ascertained.

21.6 **C.** Thyroid nodules less than 1 cm in diameter are common findings in women, and most of these are of no clinical consequences, do not progress, and have low probability of being malignant. The probability of cancer in this patient is further reduced because there are multiple nodules seen. Observation with repeat ultrasound is generally appropriate for these patients.

Clinical Pearls

- Currently, FNAB is the initial and most important step in the diagnostic evaluation of a dominant thyroid nodule.
- Thyroid enlargement and impingement on adjacent structures, most notably the trachea, esophagus, and recurrent laryngeal nerve, are indications for surgery.
- A patient with a prior history of neck irradiation or a family history consistent with MEN syndromes has a high risk of thyroid cancer.
- A nonfunctioning "cold" thyroid nodule has significantly more risk for cancer than a "hot" functioning nodule.

REFERENCES

McHenry CR. Goiter and nontoxic benign thyroid conditions. In: Bland KI, ed. *The Practice of General Surgery*. Philadelphia, PA: Saunders; 2002:1041-1048.

Mittendorf EA, McHenry CR. Management of thyroid nodules. In: Cameron JL, ed. *Current Surgical Therapy*. 9th ed. Philadelphia, PA: Mosby Elsevier; 2008: 602-608.

Case 22

A 33-year-old man presents with a sudden onset of left chest pain and shortness of breath that occurred while he was working in his yard. The patient denies any trauma to his chest and any cough or other respiratory symptoms prior to the onset of pain. His past medical history is unremarkable. He takes no medications. He consumes one pack of cigarettes a day and two to three beers a day. On physical examination he appears anxious. His temperature is normal, his pulse rate 110 beats/min, his blood pressure 124/80 mm Hg, and his respiratory rate 28 breaths/min. The pulmonary examination reveals diminished breath sounds on the left and normal breath sounds on the right. A cardiac examination demonstrates no murmurs or gallops. Results from the abdominal and extremity examinations are unremarkable. The laboratory examination reveals a normal complete blood count and normal serum electrolyte levels. The chest radiograph shows a 50% left pneumothorax, without effusion or pulmonary lesions.

- What is your next step?
- What are the risk factors for this condition?

ANSWERS TO CASE 22: Pneumothorax (Spontaneous)

Summary: An otherwise healthy 33-year-old man presents with a large primary spontaneous pneumothorax.

- **Next step:** Perform either tube thoracostomy or needle aspiration to allow reexpansion of the left lung.
- **Risk factors for this condition:** Primary spontaneous pneumothorax is caused by the rupture of subpleural blebs. Secondary spontaneous pneumothorax may be caused by bullous emphysematous disease, cystic fibrosis, primary and secondary cancers, and necrotizing infections with organisms such as *Pneumocystis carinii*.

ANALYSIS

Objectives

1. Learn to distinguish between primary and secondary spontaneous pneumothorax.
2. Learn the treatment and diagnostic strategies for patients presenting with spontaneous pneumothorax.

Considerations

The patient is a young man, the type of individual most likely to develop spontaneous pneumothorax. The most common cause is the rupture of a subpleural bleb. This patient does not have any risk factors for secondary causes of spontaneous pneumothorax such as malignancy, tuberculosis, or chronic obstructive pulmonary disease. The best management would be insertion of a chest tube or needle aspiration to allow for reexpansion of the lung.

APPROACH TO Spontaneous Pneumothorax

DEFINITIONS

PNEUMOTHORAX: Condition whereby air enters the pleural space, thus preventing expansion of the lung parenchyma.

TENSION PNEUMOTHORAX: Caused by a flap-valve effect such that air enters the pleural space but cannot exit until the pleural pressure is so great that it prevents blood from entering the chest.

OPEN PNEUMOTHORAX: Injury to the full thickness of the chest wall such that the negative intrapleural pressure results in air being sucked directly though the chest wall defect, preventing air from being taken in through the trachea; it requires a mechanical covering over the chest wound.

FLAIL CHEST: Injury to multiple ribs leading to a paradoxical inward movement of the affected chest region on inspiratory effort, resulting in little air movement. Concerns in patients with this condition are lung dysfunction associated with injuries to the lungs under the flail segment and the development of atalectasis secondary to pain from the rib fractures.

TUBE THORACOSTOMY: Placement of a catheter (chest tube) into the pleural space to evacuate air, blood, or fluid to permit better ventilation.

CLINICAL APPROACH

The initial management of pneumothorax requires reexpansion of the lung. This often requires tube thoracostomy, but thoracentesis or pleural catheter drainage can be attempted for smaller pneumothoraces (<30% of the width of the hemithorax). Small asymptomatic pneumothoraces (<15% of the width of the hemithorax) can be initially observed with serial chest radiographs. If the pneumothorax does not improve or the patient develops symptoms (chest pain, dyspnea), tube thoracostomy will be required.

Spontaneous pneumothorax can be classified as either primary or secondary. **Primary pneumothorax is usually caused by the rupture of subpleural pulmonary blebs.** This condition is more commonly observed in young men (15 to 35 years of age) without other risk factors for spontaneous pneumothorax. **Secondary spontaneous pneumothorax** results from an **acquired process** and is most commonly seen in **older (>50 years) patients with chronic obstructive pulmonary disease.** These patients may present with severe respiratory difficulty because of the already present diffuse lung disease. Other reasons for secondary spontaneous pneumothorax include malignancy, infection (tuberculosis, *P carinii*), catamenial (pulmonary endometriosis, occurring usually with menstruation), asthma, and cystic fibrosis. For management of these problems see Figure 22-1.

Chest tube management is sufficient treatment for most cases of spontaneous pneumothorax, with 15% to 20% requiring surgical intervention. Surgery is indicated for first-time spontaneous pneumothorax when there is persistent air leakage (3 to 5 days), when the lung fails to reexpand, in patients who are at high risk for recurrence (bilateral pneumothoraces, a previous history of contralateral pneumothorax, significant bullous disease on radiographs), in patients who have limited access to medical care (those living

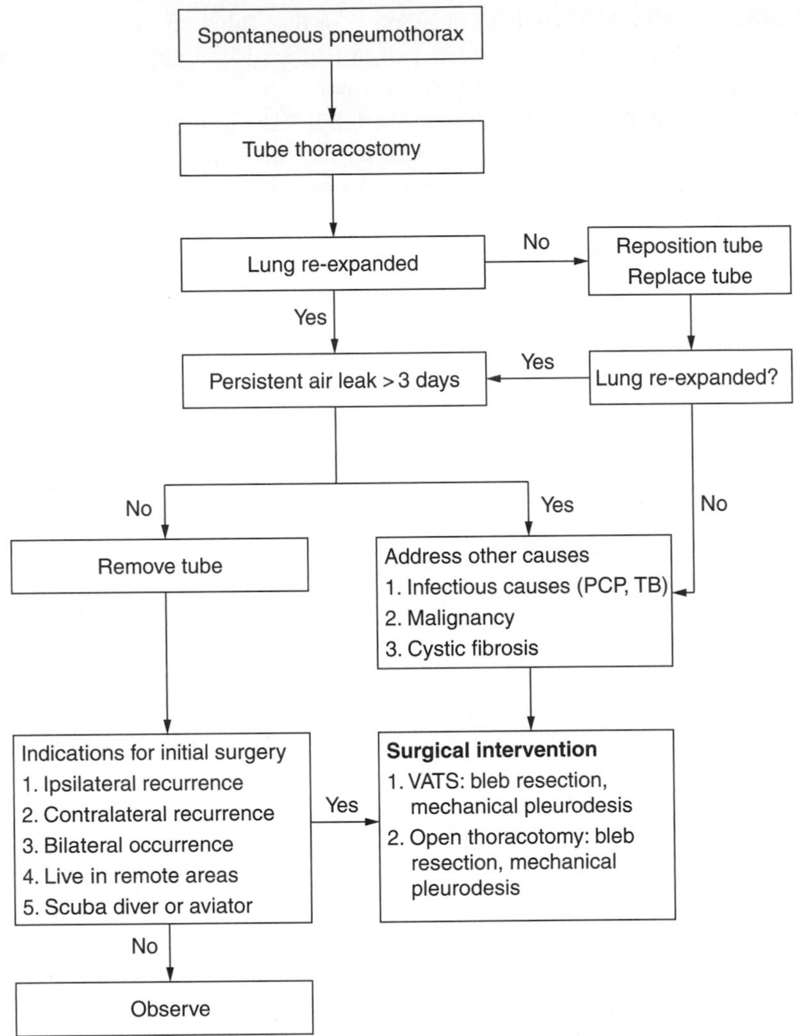

Figure 22–1. Algorithm for the management of spontaneous pneumothorax. PCP, *Pneumocystis jiroveci* pneumonia; TB, tuberculosis, VATS, video-assisted thoracoscopy.

in remote areas), and in patients whose occupation produces an increased risk (scuba divers, pilots).

The recurrence rate for spontaneous pneumothorax is 30% after the first occurrence, 50% after the second, and 80% after the third. Therefore, **immediate surgical intervention is indicated after the second recurrence.** Surgical treatment in these patients consists of pleurodesis and resection of the blebs by either thoracoscopic approach or thoracotomy.

Comprehension Questions

22.1 A patient is seen by the pulmonologist for recurrent spontaneous pneumothorax. Which of the following is the most likely risk factor for this condition?
A. Female gender
B. Age 55 to 70 years
C. Tall, thin physique
D. History of tuberculosis

22.2 The patient in 22.1 asks about recurrence risk. Which of the following factors is most predictive of the recurrence of pneumothorax?
A. Patient's occupation
B. Location of blebs
C. Presence of chronic obstructive pulmonary disease
D. Number of previous episodes of pneumothorax

22.3 A 33-year-old woman who underwent multiple enterotomies for penetrating abdominal trauma has a subclavian central line placed and subsequently develops "air hunger." Which of the following is the most likely etiology?
A. Acute psychosis
B. Panic disorder
C. Hemothorax
D. Pneumothorax
E. Pulmonary embolism

22.4 Which of the following presentations is most consistent with tension pneumothorax?
A. Hypotension, distended neck veins, midline trachea, and muffled heart sounds
B. Hypotension, open wound measuring 10x10 cm in the left lateral chest
C. Hypotension, diminished breath sounds on left, tracheal deviation to the right, and chest x-ray demonstration of opacification of the left hemi-thorax
D. Diminished left breath sounds, tracheal deviation to the right

22.5 An emergency center physician is assessing a 38-year-old man who has respiratory complaints. The physician's differential diagnosis is pleural effusion versus pneumothorax. Which one of the following findings is more likely to be found in pleural effusion and not pneumothorax?
A. Respiratory rate of 33/minute
B. Agitation
C. Somnolence
D. Dullness to percussion over the chest wall on the affected side

ANSWERS

22.1 **C.** Spontaneous pneumothorax occurs more commonly in young men who are thin and tall and in smokers. These are processes that are primary events, not due to disease processes.

22.2 **D.** The number of prior episodes of pneumothorax is more predictive of a recurrence, with an 80% recurrence rate after three previous episodes.

22.3 **D.** A fairly common complication of the placement of central venous catheters is pneumothorax.

22.4 **D.** Diminished breath sound on the left and tracheal deviation to the right. Findings described in "A" are compatible with cardiac tamponade. Findings in "B" are compatible with an open pneumothorax. Findings in "C" are compatible with left tension hemothroax or hydrothorax leading to mediastinal structures shifting to the right.

22.5 **D.** Dullness to percussion of chest wall on the affected side is not a finding consistent with pneumothorax. Tachypnea can be associated with the increased work of breathing associated with pneumothorax. Agitation is a finding that could be produced by the hypoxmia associated pneumothorax. Somnolence can develop in the setting of profound hypoxia just prior to the onset of respiratory arrest.

Clinical Pearls

- Although most cases of pneumothorax can be managed with a tube thoracostomy, aggressive surgical intervention is indicated for cases where there is a high risk of recurrence.
- The general therapeutic goal is to address the underlying problem (blebs, infection, etc) and to achieve pleural apposition (reexpansion of the lung).
- Failure to achieve pleural apposition or persistent air leakage requires surgical intervention.

REFERENCES

Sugarbaker DJ, Lukanich JM. Chest wall and pleura. In: Townsend CM, Beauchamp RD, Evers BM, et al, eds. *Sabiston Textbook of Surgery*. 18th ed. Philadelphia, PA: Saunders Elsevier; 2008: 1655-1676.

Todd SR, Vercruysse GA, Moore FA. Pneumothorax. In: Cameron JL, ed. *Current Surgical Therapy*. 9th ed. Philadelphia, PA: Mosby Elsevier; 2008:702-705.

Case 23

A 38-year-old man fell 15 ft from a ladder while trying to rescue a cat. During the evaluation at the hospital, he was found to have a closed fracture of the right femur, a fracture of the right radius and ulna, and soft tissue contusions and abrasions. The patient underwent open reduction and internal fixation of his femur and external fixation of his forearm without apparent complications. On postinjury day 2, he began to complain of difficulty in breathing. On physical examination, his temperature is found to be 38.4°C (101°F), pulse rate 120 beats/min, blood pressure 148/86 mm Hg, respiratory rate 34 breaths/min, and Glasgow Coma Score 15. The patient appears anxious and complains of difficulty breathing but is without chest pain. Auscultation of the chest reveals diminished breath sounds bilaterally with scattered rhonchi. The results of a cardiac examination are unremarkable. The abdomen is nondistended and nontender. Examination of the extremities reveals postinjury soft tissue swelling. Laboratory studies reveal the following: white blood cell (WBC) count 16,000/mm^3, hemoglobin 10.8 g/dL, platelet count 185,000/mm^3. Arterial blood gas studies reveal pH 7.4, Pao_2 55 mm Hg, $Paco_2$ 40 mm Hg, and HCO_3 24 mEq/L. A chest radiograph (CXR) reveals bilateral nonsegmental infiltrates and no effusion or pneumothorax.

➤ What are your next steps?

➤ What is the most likely diagnosis?

ANSWERS TO CASE 23:
Postoperative Acute Respiratory Insufficiency

Summary: A previously healthy young man develops acute respiratory insufficiency after being injured in a fall and undergoing operative repair of traumatic orthopedic injuries.

- **Next steps:** Administration of supplemental oxygen and transfer to the intensive care unit for closer observation and possible mechanical ventilation if the patient's condition does not improve or deteriorates.
- **Diagnosis:** Acute respiratory insufficiency caused by acute lung injury (ALI).

ANALYSIS

Objectives

Learn the presentations and differential diagnosis of acute respiratory insufficiency surgical patients.

1. Learn the pathophysiology of ALI.
2. Know the types of invasive and noninvasive modes of pulmonary support.

Considerations

The timing of the development of respiratory insufficiency is relatively early for pulmonary embolism (PE) but within the expected time frame for ALI. The patient's pulmonary examination reveals diminished breath sounds and scattered rhonchi, nonspecific findings compatible with ALI. The CXR reveals bilateral nonsegmental infiltrates, and an arterial blood gas study shows moderate hypoxemia. PE typically presents with a relatively normal CXR. By strict definition, ALI requires the respiratory insufficiency to be acute in onset, associated with a PaO_2:FIO_2 value < 300, bilateral infiltrates, and a pulmonary capillary wedge pressure of less than 18 mm Hg. Although many features of this case suggest a diagnosis of ALI, other potential diagnoses must be considered and excluded, including aspiration pneumonitis, atypical pneumonia, atelectasis, and PE. During the initial evaluation of any patient with acute respiratory insufficiency, it is important to consider the diagnosis, but the primary consideration should be to determine the most appropriate level of respiratory support. For this patient, even though he does not appear to require immediate mechanical ventilatory support, his oxygenation and pulmonary compliance defects may progress and cause further respiratory embarrassment.

APPROACH TO Acute Respiratory Insufficiency

DEFINITIONS

ASPIRATION: Spillage of gastric contents into the bronchial tree causing direct injury to the airways, which can progress to a chemical burn or pneumonitis (especially when pH < 3) and predispose to bacterial pneumonia. When the aspirated gastric contents contain particulate matter, bronchoscopy may be helpful in clearing the airway. Half of affected patients develop subsequent pneumonia not prevented by empirical antibiotics.

PNEUMONIA: Pulmonary infection caused by impairment of the lung's defense mechanisms. Incisional pain frequently affects the patient's ability to clear airway mucus, leading to small airway obstruction and ineffective bacteria clearance. Most commonly, nosocomial organisms are those that colonize patients during hospitalization.

PULMONARY EMBOLISM: A major source of morbidity and mortality in surgical patients. The prophylaxis, diagnosis, and treatment of PE are continuous concerns for the surgeon. Bed rest, cancer, and trauma increase the risk of deep vein thrombosis (DVT) and PE occurrence. PE may be clinically silent or symptomatic. In high-risk surgical patients, the risk of developing a clinically significant PE is 2% to 3%, and the risk of developing a fatal PE approaches 1%. The clinical hallmarks include acute-onset hypoxia associated with anxiety leading to tachypnea and hypocarbia without significant CXR abnormalities.

LUNG CONTUSION: Blunt trauma to the chest is a common cause of pulmonary dysfunction resulting from direct parenchymal injury and impaired chest wall function. An injured chest wall leads to impaired breathing mechanics that can range from splinting secondary to a rib fracture to the severe impairment of a flail chest. The morbidity from lung contusion is attributed to direct parenchymal injury and bronchoalveolar hemorrhage, causing ventilation-perfusion (V/Q) mismatch leading to hypoxia. This condition is worsened by chest wall injury pain, leading to atelectasis in the uninvolved lung.

ACUTE RESPIRATORY DISTRESS SYNDROME (ARDS): The most severe form of ALI (PaO_2:FIO_2 < 200), this condition encompasses a spectrum of lung injuries characterized by increasing hypoxia and decreased lung compliance. Initially, an injury to the pulmonary endothelial cells leads to an intense inflammatory response. Inhomogeneous involvement of the lung occurs, with interstitial and alveolar edema, loss of type II pneumocytes, surfactant depletion, intra-alveolar hemorrhage, hyaline membrane deposition, and eventual fibrosis. These changes manifest clinically as severe hypoxia, decreased lung compliance, and increased dead space ventilation.

ATELECTASIS: The collapse of alveolar units in patients who undergo general anesthesia, which causes a reduction in functional residual capacity that is further reduced because of incisional pain. The subsegmental atelectasis may progress to obstruction and inflammation, leading to larger airway obstruction and segmental collapse. Most patients have only a low-grade fever and mild respiratory insufficiency.

CARDIOGENIC PULMONARY EDEMA: Myocardial dysfunction most frequently resulting from ischemia can produce left ventricular dysfunction, fluid overload, and pulmonary interstitial edema. The increase in the amount of interstitial water compresses the fragile bronchovascular structures, thereby increasing the V/Q mismatch and resulting in hypoxia.

CLINICAL APPROACH

Patient Assessment

In treating patients with acute respiratory insufficiency, the first priority is to assess and stabilize the airway, breathing, and circulation (ABCs). Patients with lethargy and diminished mentation may benefit from immediate endotracheal intubation to protect against aspiration. The assessment of each patient should be directed toward the immediate status as well as toward the anticipated future status of the patient's ventilation and oxygenation. The adequacy of oxygenation is evaluated by pulse oximetry or PaO_2 measurement by arterial blood gas (ABG) studies. The inability to maintain **a PaO_2 of 60 mm Hg or an oxygen saturation of more than 91% with a supplemental nonrebreathing O_2 mask is indicative of a significant alveolar-arterial (A-a) gradient, and intubation and mechanical ventilation may be needed.** Hypoxemia frequently causes agitation and confusion, and an uncooperative patient can contribute to delays in diagnosis. The adequacy of ventilation is generally assessed by observing the patient's respiratory efforts and subjective symptoms, and quantified by the measurement of $PaCO_2$ by ABG analysis. It is important to bear in mind that ventilation assessment requires the use of all these data and should not be made on the basis of a blood gas value alone.

Pathophysiology of Acute Lung Injury

Acute lung injury encompasses a spectrum of lung disease from mild forms to severe lung injury or ARDS. The inciting event can be a direct or indirect pulmonary insult (Figure 23-1). The resultant cascade of events includes both cellular and humoral components that produce an inhomogeneous injury. The inflammatory response involves activated polymorphonucleocytes that generate oxygen radicals, cytokines, lipid mediators, and nitric oxide. The complement, kinin, coagulation, and fibrinolytic systems are also involved.

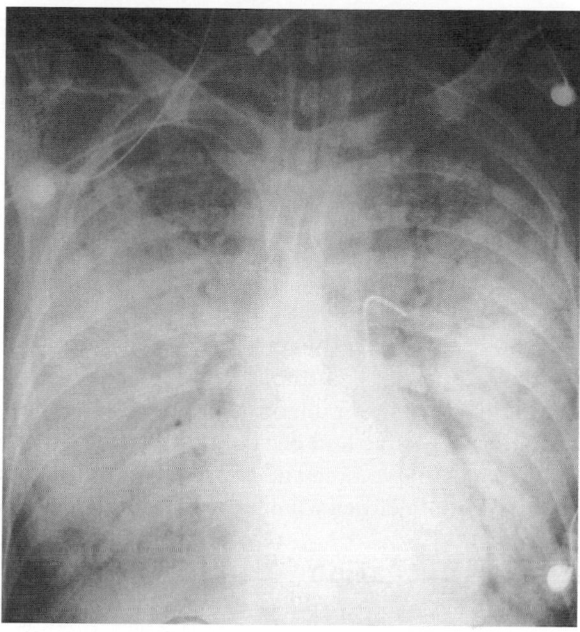

Figure 23–1. Chest radiography revealing the bilateral dense pulmonary infiltrates typical of acute respiratory disease syndrome. *Reproduced, with permission, from Mattox KL, Feliciano DV, Moore EE, eds.* Trauma. *4th ed. New York, NY: McGraw-Hill; 2000:526.*

Endothelial damage ensues with an increase in microvascular permeability leading to the accumulation of extravascular lung water. This soon results in diminished lung volume and decreased lung compliance. Lung compliance is further hampered because of the sloughing of type I pneumocytes and a decrease in surfactant production by type II pneumocytes. The process continues, further aggravating interstitial edema, alveolar collapse, and lung consolidation. In the pathogenesis, inflammatory cells and fluid are sequestered within the lungs, leading to a decrease in pulmonary compliance and an increase in the work of breathing. During the prodromal phase of ALI, patients may simply complain of difficulty in catching their breath, leading to tachypnea. **Ventilation is reflected by the $Paco_2$, but the patient's appearance, respiratory rate, and respiratory efforts are equally important endpoints.** Hypercapnia is not associated with anxiety or agitation; therefore, patients with an altered level of consciousness should have $Paco_2$ (by ABG) or end-tidal CO_2 (by capnography) monitoring to assess ventilation.

Noninvasive Pulmonary Support

Patients with acute postoperative respiratory insufficiency can be provided with supplemental oxygen and noninvasive respiratory support, including a continuous positive airway pressure mask (useful for atelectasis) and chest physiotherapy, including bronchodilators and mucolytic agents (useful for atelectasis, pneumonia, and reactive airway disease). Patients with a significant A-a gradient may benefit from mechanical ventilator support for oxygenation.

MECHANICAL VENTILATION MODES

Conventional Ventilation

Conventional ventilation or positive pressure ventilation fills the lungs via supra-atmospheric pressure applied through an endotracheal tube to the airways. This creates a positive transpulmonary pressure that ensures inflation of the lungs. Exhalation is passive and occurs after release of the positive pressure. The major settings are volume and pressure controlled, where the tidal volume delivery is based on either volume- or pressure-limiting settings.

High-Frequency Ventilation

High-frequency ventilation also uses an endotracheal tube to facilitate gas exchange; however, high-frequency ventilation delivers very small tidal volumes, on the order of 1 mL/kg body weight at a very high rate, approximately 100 to 400 breaths per minute. Although this mode has an important role in the treatment of respiratory insufficiency in neonates, it has not had the same success in adults.

Liquid Ventilation

The theoretical advantage of liquid ventilation lies in its ability to reduce the amount of energy necessary to overcome surface tension at the gas-liquid interface of alveoli. Because diseased lungs have less surfactant, liquid ventilation can improve lung compliance. Studies are needed to document the clinical benefits of this ventilation mode.

Extracorporeal Life Support

Cardiopulmonary bypass or extracorporeal life support uses a heart-lung machine to take over pulmonary and/or cardiac function. If cardiac function is adequate, a venovenous circuit can be used to remove CO_2 and oxygenate the blood. As in the case of high-frequency ventilation, the early success achieved in neonates has not been duplicated in adult populations.

Comprehension Questions

23.1 A 57-year-old woman develops an acute onset of respiratory distress 7 days following colectomy for adenocarcinoma of the colon. She had been doing well up until this time. The physical examination reveals diminished breath sounds at the lung bases. The CXR reveals atelectasis of the left lower lobe segment. Which of the following is the most appropriate treatment at this time?

A. Provide supplemental oxygen and begin chest physiotherapy.
B. Provide supplemental oxygen and initiate chest physiotherapy and antibiotic therapy.
C. Begin antibiotic therapy and immediate bronchoscopy to open up the lungs.
D. Provide supplemental oxygen, obtain venous duplex scans of the lower extremities and a lung V/Q scan, and consider starting heparin therapy.

23.2 Diagnostic bronchoscopy is most appropriate in which of the following patients?

A. A 33-year-old man with right lower lobe hospital-acquired pneumonia
B. A 40-year-old man with AIDS who develops fever, acute respiratory distress, and bilateral pulmonary infiltrates
C. A 66-year-old man with dementia who develops a right upper lobe infiltrate following an episode of aspiration
D. A 30-year-old man who develops ARDS associated with fever and a loculated right pleural effusion

23.3 A 34-year-old woman is hospitalized for septic shock caused by toxic shock syndrome. She is treated with intravenous nafcillin and noted to have hypoxemia. A CXR reveals diffuse infiltrates in bilateral lung fields. Which of the following would most likely differentiate ARDS from cardiogenic pulmonary edema?

A. Pulmonary artery catheter readings
B. Serum colloid osmotic pressure
C. Urinary electrolytes and partial excretion of sodium
D. V/Q scan

23.4 A 46-year-old man sustained multiple left rib fractures after having fallen off a horse. He is otherwise healthy and has a one pack/day smoking history for the past 24 years. Approximately one hour after arrival to the emergency room, the patient's breathing appears to be more labored, and despite having received several doses of morphine sulfate for pain, he continues to complain of severe chest pain. At this time, his respiratory rate is 36 breaths/min, and shallow, blood pressure is 160/100 mm Hg, pulse rate is 115 beats/min, and the pulse oximeter monitor indicates 92% saturation on 40% oxygen facemask. His breath sounds are diminished bilaterally but significantly less audible on the left. Which of these options is most appropriate for this patient at this time?

A. Obtain a chest x-ray.
B. Endotracheal intubation and initiate mechanical ventilation.
C. Replace his oxygen mask with a continuous positive airway pressure mask.
D. Obtain an arterial blood gas, and intubate patient if the PaO_2 is less than 50 mm Hg and/or if the $PaCO_2$ is greater than 50 mm Hg.

23.5 A 34-year-old man slipped and fell in the bathroom at home and struck his anterior neck on the edge of some shelves. When he arrived in the emergency center, he had significant anterior neck pain, soft tissue crepitance, and stridor. He was successfully intubated after several difficult attempts. His chest x-ray immediately following intubation demonstrated satisfactory endotracheal tube placement, diffuse bilateral nonsegmental infiltrates, and no evidence of pneumothorax or pleural effusions. Which of the following is the most appropriate treatment option at this time?

A. Bronchoscopy to identify injury to the tracheal-bronchial tree
B. Supportive care including mechanical ventilation, fluid management
C. Initiate antimicrobial therapy for aspiration pneumonia
D. Consult a thoracic surgeon

ANSWERS

23.1 **D.** Provide supplemental O_2, perform a workup for PE, and consider empirical treatment. This patient develops a sudden onset of respiratory distress 7 days postoperatively. The clinical presentation is highly suggestive of PE. The diagnosis of atelectasis as the primary cause of this patient's clinical picture should not be readily accepted until PE can be ruled out.

23.2 **B.** Diagnostic bronchoscopy and bronchoalveolar lavage are indicated in an immunocompromised individual with new-onset fever and bilateral pulmonary infiltrates.

23.3 **A.** The pulmonary capillary wedge pressure (PCWP) approximates the left ventricular end-diastolic pressure. A low-normal pulmonary artery wedge pressure (<18 mm Hg) supports leaky capillaries (ARDS) as the etiology, whereas a high PCWP suggests a hydrostatic mechanism, cardiogenic pulmonary edema.

23.4 **A.** This patient's current clinical picture is one of worsening respiratory insufficiency that could be contributed by pneumothorax, pulmonary contusion, or atatlectasis. A change in his respiratory status at this time requires re-evaluation of the ABC, which indicates diminished breath sounds bilaterall, with less audible breath sounds on the left. A chest x-ray is very useful at this time to help determine the cause of his clinical deteriation. Endotracheal intubation and mechanical ventilation would be most appropriate if the patient's clinical picture is one of impending respiratory failure. Arterial blood gas (ABG) values are helpful in guiding treatment for patients with respiratory diseases, however the ABG results need to be considered within the proper clinical context.

23.5 **B.** This patient's findings are compatible with acute lung injury secondary to forced inspiration against a closed or narrow airway resulting in "negative-pressure pulmonary edema"; negative-pressure pulmonary edema is an unusual variant of acute lung injury and is often self-limiting with supportive care that include mechanical ventilation and IV fluids.

REFERENCES

Mendez-Tellez PA, Dorman T. Postoperative respiratory failure. In: Cameron JL, ed. *Current Surgical Therapy*. 9th ed. Philadelphia, PA: Mosby Elsevier; 2008:1196-1201.

Schuster DP, Iregui M, Blackmon M. Respiratory failure part II: the acute respiratory distress syndrome and pulmonary edema. In: Irwin RS, Rippe JM, eds. *Intensive Care Medicine*. 5th ed. Philadelphia, PA: Lippincott Williams & Wilkins; 2003:489-502.

Case 24

Following recovery from an exploratory laparotomy and repair of a colon injury caused by a gunshot wound to the abdomen, a 24-year-old man developed an infection in the superior portion of his wound that required local wound care. He was discharged from the hospital on postoperative day 10 and has returned approximately 2 weeks later for a follow-up visit to the outpatient clinic. The patient indicates that he has been doing well except for fluid drainage from his open midline abdominal wound. On physical examination, his temperature is 37.5°C (99.5°F), pulse rate 70 beats/min, blood pressure 130/80 mm Hg, and respiratory rate 18 breaths/min. The results of his cardiopulmonary examinations are within normal limits. Examination of the abdomen reveals a small amount of serosanguineous fluid from the superior aspect of his surgical incision. There is no redness, swelling, or tenderness around the incision. A 4-cm fascia defect in the superior aspect of the wound is present without signs of evisceration.

- ➤ What are the complications associated with this condition?
- ➤ What are the risk factors for this condition?
- ➤ What is the best treatment?

ANSWERS TO CASE 24:
Fascial Dehiscence and Incisional Hernia

Summary: A 24-year-old man presents with stable abdominal wound dehiscence 3 weeks following exploratory laparotomy for the treatment of traumatic injuries.

- **Complications:** Abdominal fascia dehiscence can lead to abdominal evisceration, the development of enterocutaneous fistulas, and the subsequent formation of incisional hernias.
- **Risk factors:** Contributing factors include technical failure of surgical techniques or anesthetic relaxation. The occurrence of a deep wound infection is contributory. Finally, patient factors include age more than 70 years, diabetes mellitus, malnutrition, and perioperative pulmonary disease.
- **Best treatment:** Local wound care, followed by elective repair of the fascia defect (incisional hernia) at a later time.

ANALYSIS

Objectives

1. Recognize the contributing factors and preventive measures for wound dehiscence and incisional hernias.
2. Learn the treatment of wound dehiscence and incisional hernias.

Considerations

Disruption of the fascia following an abdominal operation is referred to as *fascial dehiscence*. **Two factors guide the management of fascia dehiscence found in the early postoperative period: stability of the intra-abdominal contents and the presence or absence of ongoing infection.** In this patient's case, the dehiscence appears stable and without risk of evisceration. This opinion is based on the appearance of the wound and the event occurring 3 weeks after the initial surgery when fibrous scar formation should be sufficient to prevent abdominal evisceration. With the absence of symptoms, fever, and local infection, it is unlikely that an ongoing infectious process exists; however, the complete evaluation should include a leukocyte count with a differential. The treatment of stable wound dehiscence consists of local wound care. The patient needs to be advised that an incisional hernia will eventually develop and will require repair at a later time. **Early reoperation is indicated for patients at risk for evisceration, enterocutaneous fistula, or uncontrolled sepsis.**

APPROACH TO
Fascial Dehiscence and Incisional Hernias

DEFINITIONS

FASCIA DEHISCENCE: The disruption of fascia closure within days of an operation; this complication may occur with or without evisceration.

EVISCERATION: The presence of abdominal viscera (bowel or omentum) protruding through a fascial dehiscence or traumatic injury.

ENTEROCUTANEOUS FISTULA: A direct communication between the small bowel lumen and a skin opening. It can be the primary process leading to wound dehiscence, but this complication frequently develops from wound dehiscence and direct trauma to the underlying bowel. It can be a devastating complication leading to septic and metabolic derangements, long-term disability, and mortality.

INCISIONAL HERNIA: Delayed development of a fascia defect because of inadequate healing. For some patients this condition can remain undetectable for as long as 5 years after the operation.

CLINICAL APPROACH

Physiology of Wound Healing

Fascial dehiscence and incisional hernias generally develop as a result of inadequate healing of the fascia closure after surgery. **The phases of wound healing are the inflammatory, proliferation, and remodeling phases** (Table 24–1). Numerous environmental and host factors can affect the wound-healing

Table 24–1 PHASES OF WOUND HEALING

Inflammatory phase	Begins immediately and ends within a few days. Inflammatory cells function in sterilizing the wound and secreting growth factors stimulating fibroblasts and keratinocytes in the wound repair process.
Proliferation phase	Deposition of the fibrin-fibrinogen matrix and collagen, resulting in formation of the wound matrix and an increase in wound strength.
Remodeling phase	Capillary regression leads to a less vascularized wound, and with collagen cross-linking there is a gradual increase in wound tensile strength.

Table 24–2 CLINICAL FACTORS AFFECTING WOUND HEALING

Infections	Lead to delays in fibroblast proliferation, wound matrix synthesis, and deposition.
Nutrition	Vitamin C deficiency leads to inadequate collagen production/ vitamin A deficiency leads to impaired fibroplasias, collagen synthesis, cross-linking, and epithelialization. Vitamin B_6 deficiency causes impaired collagen cross-linking.
Oxygenation	Collagen synthesis is augmented with oxygen supplementation.
Corticosteroids	Reduce wound inflammation, collagen synthesis, and contraction.
Diabetes mellitus	Association with microvascular occlusive disease leading to poor wound perfusion; impair keratinocyte growth factor and platelet-derived growth factor functions in the wound.

process (Table 24-2). An understanding of the temporal occurrence and clinical implications of wound-healing events helps with the appropriate management of these complications (Figure 24–1).

TREATMENT

Approximately 2% to 20% of patients who undergo abdominal surgery develop fascial defects, with the incidence increased fourfold in patients with wound infections. Factors contributing to dehiscence and hernia formation include the patient factors listed in Table 24-2, the technical characteristics listed in Table 24-3, and environmental factors such as tobacco smoking, which causes a decrease in collagen strength. It is generally believed that a significant proportion of fascial defects arise as a result of technical problems.

Management

Fascial defects may be seen early in the postoperative course as drainage of serous or serosanguineous fluid from an otherwise normal wound or as development of a soft tissue mass beneath the incision. The discovery of significant fluid drainage from an abdominal incision should alarm the examiner to the possibility of fascia dehiscence. When this occurs in the early postoperative period, the initial management consists of opening of the skin incision and meticulously inspecting the wound and fascia. Depending on the precise timing and circumstances, the treatment may require an immediate return to the operating room for repair or initial local wound care with delayed repair of the hernia. **Immediate surgery is indicated for evisceration, impending evisceration, and bowel exposure with a concern for enterocutaneous fistula formation, and untreated intra-abdominal infections.** Factors favoring delayed

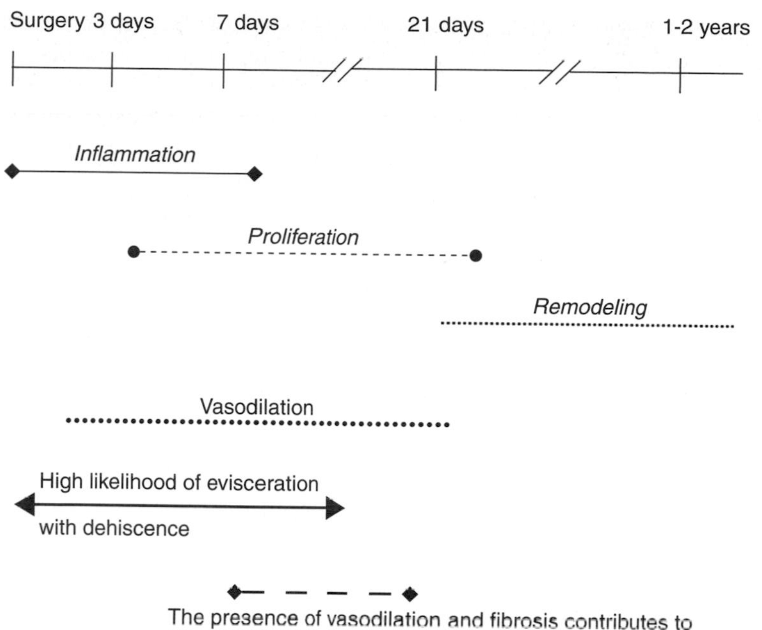

Figure 24–1. Temporal relationships of wound repair and implications in management. *Modified, with permission, from Norton JA, Bollinger RR, Chang AE, et al, eds.* Surgery: Basic Science and Clinical Evidence. *New York, NY: Springer; 2001:221-239.*

management include a stable dehiscence with no exposed bowel and the risk of a "hostile" abdominal environment associated with reoperation at this time.

Incisional Hernia Repair

Unlike the repair of a groin hernia, the repair of an incisional hernia is associated with a high-wound infection rate (7%-20%) and a high-recurrence rate (20%-50%). Contributing to a poor outcome are the coexisting conditions that may have originally led to development of the hernia (wound infection, patient factors, and fascia weakness). Primary repair of an incisional hernia is

Table 24–3 TECHNICAL FACTORS RELATED TO ABDOMINAL CLOSURE FAILURE
Inadequate tissue incorporation
Inappropriate sutures
Excessive tension
Inadequate patient relaxation
Inappropriate suture placement

performed infrequently because of the high rate of recurrence; therefore, whenever feasible, incisional hernias should be repaired with the placement of prosthetic material. The placement of polypropylene mesh in the peritoneal cavity can increase the risk of erosion into the hollow viscus and subsequent enterocutaneous fistula formation. Some of the newer products available include composite mesh containing expanded polytetrafluoroethylene (PTFE) on the inside and polypropylene on the outside. Most recently, biosynthetic prosthesis containing collagen harvested from cadavers or porcine sources have also become available for the repair of high-risk, contaminated wounds. Repair can be performed by an open or a laparoscopic approach, and currently no convincing evidence indicates a clear advantage for either repair technique.

Comprehension Questions

24.1 Which of the following conditions has been shown to have detrimental effects on wound healing?

A. Obesity
B. Hyperthyroidism
C. C-reactive protein deficiency
D. Diabetes mellitus

24.2 Five days following abdominal surgery, a patient is noted to have 30 to 40 mL of serosanguineous fluid draining from her midline laparotomy wound. Which of the following is the most appropriate management?

A. Reinforce the wound dressing and reassure the patient that it is a wound seroma that will resolve spontaneously.
B. Initiate antibiotic therapy.
C. Perform an immediate laparotomy.
D. Open the wound to evaluate the fascia.

24.3 A 36-year-old nursing student undergoes a laparotomy for appendicitis and asks about the possibility of incisional hernia formation. Which of the following statements is *true* regarding incisional hernias?

A. The incidence may reach upward of 20% in infected wounds.
B. Repairs are generally associated with < 2% recurrence.
C. Primary repair is associated with less infection and a lower recurrence rate.
D. Formation of a hernia is nearly always recognized within 3 months after surgery.

24.4 A 40-year-old man who underwent celiotomy and lysis of adhesions for small bowel obstruction 8 days ago. He was discharged home on post-operative day 6. He returns to the outpatient clinic for follow-up. On examination he is noted to have large amount of fluid drainage on his dressing. Which of the following would be helpful in differentiating abdominal wound dehiscence from enterocutaneous fistula?

A. Abdominal CT scan
B. Wound inspection for fascial defect
C. Blood sample for complete blood count analysis
D. Inspection of the drainage fluid

24.5 Which of the following statements is most accurate of incisional hernia?

A. Laparoscopic approach to the repair of incisional hernia repair has no proven advantage over open approaches
B. The result of incisional hernia repair is more favorable than the outcome of inguinal hernia repair
C. Incisional hernia recurrence is lower among patients who develop wound infections
D. Early occurrence of incisional hernia following celiotomy is commonly associated with the onset of small bowel obstruction

ANSWERS

24.1 **D.** Diabetes mellitus is associated with poor wound healing. Although obesity may predispose to wound separation and dehiscence, it does not lead to poor wound healing.

24.2 **D.** The drainage of a large amount of serosanguineous fluid is highly suggestive of fascia dehiscence; therefore, direct evaluation of the fascia should be performed.

24.3 **A.** The incidence of incisional hernia may approach 20% in infected wounds. Up to 20% to 50% of repairs may eventually fail. Primary repairs are seldom performed because of the high rate of hernia recurrence.

24.4 **D.** Inspection of the drainage fluid may be helpful in differentiating fascia dehiscence from enterocutaneous fistula. Dehiscences are usually associated with the drainage periotoneal fluid that is serous or serosanguinous, while patients with enterocutaneous fistulas generally have drainage of enteric contents that is either bilious or feculent. Inspection of the wound would most likely show fascial defect and would not reliably differentiate the two processes. A CBC is helpful to suggest the presence or absence of occult intraabdominal infection. CT scan in this setting could help identify undrained fluid collections that may represent abscesses but does not reliably differentiate the two processes.

24.5 **A.** Incisional hernias could be repaired by open or laparoscopic approaches, and there is no clinical evidence to indicate that one approach is superior over the other. The complications and recurrence rates of incisional hernia repair are higher than those associated with inguinal hernia repairs. Wound infections contribute to fascial destruction and dramatically increase the risk of incisional hernia development. While small bowel obstruction may increase abdominal pressure and contribute to incisional hernia development, this is a rare cause of incisional hernia.

Clinical Pearls

- The tensile strength of uncomplicated wounds steadily increases for approximately 8 weeks, when it reaches 75% to 80% of that of normal tissue; thereafter the wound continues to strengthen, but the strength never reaches that of uninjured tissue.
- The use of braided, nonabsorbable suture material is associated with the entrapment of infected debris within the suture material and may lead to an increased number of infections. Therefore, this type of suture material should be avoided in the closing of an infected abdomen.
- The 4:1 ratio refers to the optimal ratio of suture length to wound length that is required so that an adequate amount of tissue is incorporated into the fascia closure.
- Reclosure of a previously healed fascial incision is associated with lower strength of healing and increased wound breakdown.

REFERENCES

Barbul A. Wound healing. In: Brunicardi FC, Andersen DK, Billiar TR, et al, eds. *Schwartz's Principles of Surgery*. 8th ed. New York: McGraw-Hill; 2005:223-248.

Tufaro AP, Campbell KA. Incisional, epigastric, and umbilical hernias. In: Cameron JL, ed. *Current Surgical Therapy*. 9th ed. Philadelphia, PA: Elsevier Mosby; 2008:573-576.

Case 25

A 58-year-old man underwent an emergency laparotomy with sigmoid colectomy and colostomy for a perforated diverticulitis 7 days previously. Since the operation, the patient has had intermittent fevers to 39.0°C (102.2°F). He has been unable to eat since the surgery because of persistent abdominal distension. His indwelling urinary catheter was removed 2 days ago, and the patient denies any urinary symptoms. On examination, his temperature is 38.8°C (101.8°F), pulse rate 102 beats/min, and blood pressure 130/80 mm Hg. His skin is warm and moist. The lung examination reveals normal breath sounds in both lung fields, and his heart rate is regular without murmurs. His abdomen is distended and tender throughout, and the surgical incision is open without any evidence of infection. His current medications include maintenance intravenous fluids, morphine sulfate, and intravenous cefoxitin and metronidazole. A complete blood count reveals a white blood cell (WBC) count of 20,500/mm^3.

- What is the most likely diagnosis?
- What is the next step?

ANSWERS TO CASE 25:
Postoperative Fever (Intra-abdominal Infection)

Summary: A 58-year-old man has fever and ileus following sigmoid resection and colostomy for a perforated diverticulum. His physical examination does not reveal infection of the respiratory or urinary system or of the surgical site.

- **Most likely diagnosis:** Intra-abdominal infection.
- **Next step:** A thorough fever workup including an abdominal and a pelvic computed tomography (CT) scan.

ANALYSIS

Objectives

1. Recognize the sources of fever in postoperative patients and become familiar with strategies for fever evaluation.
2. Learn the principles of diagnosis and treatment of intra-abdominal infections.
3. Learn the pathogenesis of intra-abdominal infections.

Considerations

Persistent fever following definitive operative therapy for an intra-abdominal infection suggests the persistence of infection or the development of another infectious process. It is important to bear in mind that a hospitalized patient may have various sources of fever, including nosocomial infections and noninfectious causes. The possibility of urinary, respiratory, and blood-borne infections should be assessed with urinalysis, chest radiography, and blood cultures. A CT scan of the abdomen and pelvis is a useful diagnostic modality for intra-abdominal infections and is indicated in this setting. When identified, abscesses can be drained percutaneously under CT guidance (Figure 25-1). Inflammatory changes without abscesses are suggestive of persistent secondary peritonitis. Persistent secondary peritonitis may also be caused by inappropriate or inadequate antimicrobial therapy; in these cases, treatment consists of extending the course of therapy or modifying the antimicrobial regimen.

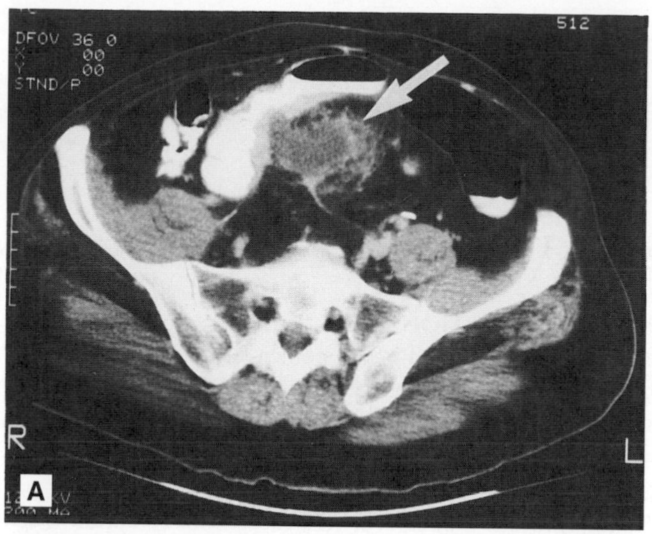

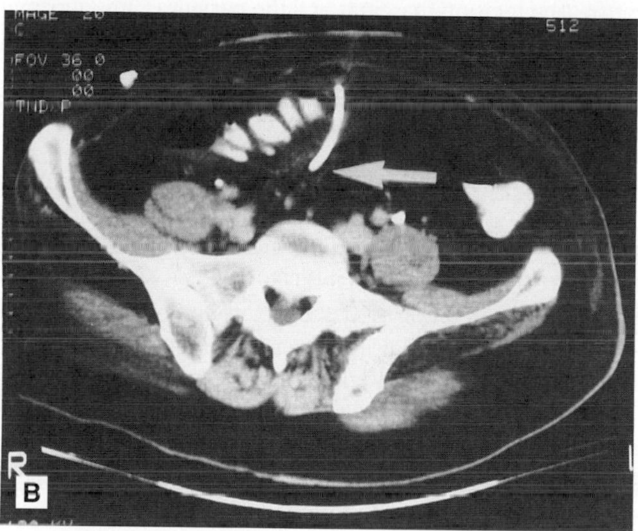

Figure 25–1. Diverticular abscess noted by arrow (**A**) and then evacuated by computer tomography–guided percutaneous drainage (**B**). *Reproduced, with permission, from Schwarz SI, Shires GT, Spencer FC, et al, eds.* Principles of Surgery. *7th ed. New York: McGraw-Hill, 1999:1041.*

APPROACH TO
Fever and Intra-abdominal Infection

DEFINITIONS

POSTOPERATIVE FEVER: Fever is arbitrarily defined by most clinicians as oral temperature higher than 38.0°C to 38.5°C (100.4°F to 101.3°F).

SURGICAL SITE INFECTIONS: Infections involving the skin and subcutaneous tissue, which are divided into superficial and deep categories depending on whether the fascia is involved. A CT imaging can be helpful when a deep surgical space infection is suspected.

SUPERFICIAL SURGICAL SITE INFECTIONS: Infectious processes above the fascia constitute superficial infections. These are treated primarily by wound exploration and drainage of the infected material, although systemic antibiotic therapy may be needed when there is extensive surrounding cellulitis (> 2 cm from the incision margins) or if the patient is immunocompromised.

DEEP SURGICAL SITE INFECTIONS: Infectious processes involving the fascia. The presence of deep surgical site infection mandates an evaluation for possible deep surgical space infection. A CT scan should be considered if deep surgical space infection is suspected.

DEEP SURGICAL SPACE INFECTIONS: Also referred to as *intra-abdominal infections* in the setting of postoperative abdominal surgery, they include secondary peritonitis, tertiary peritonitis, and intra-abdominal abscesses.

SECONDARY MICROBIAL PERITONITIS: Spillage of endogenous microbes into the peritoneal cavity following viscera perforation. The persistence of this infection is affected by microbial inoculum volume, the inhibitory and synergistic effects of the polymicrobial environment, and host response. Recurrent infections may result from insufficient antimicrobial therapy or inadequate control of the infectious source.

TERTIARY MICROBIAL PERITONITIS: This condition occurs in patients who fail to recover from intra-abdominal infections despite surgical and/or antimicrobial therapy because of diminished host peritoneal response. Frequently, low virulence or opportunistic pathogens such as *Staphylococcus epidermidis*, *Enterococcus faecalis*, and *Candida* species are identified.

INTRA-ABDOMINAL ABSCESS: A defined intraperitoneal collection of inflammatory fluid and microbes resulting from a host compartmentalizing process in which fibrin deposition, omental containment, and ileus of the small bowel localize the infectious material. This response produces loculated, infected inflammatory fluid that cannot be eliminated by the host translymphatic clearance process.

PREEMPTIVE ANTIBIOTIC THERAPY: Administration of antibiotics when a large microbial inoculum is thought to have occurred, such as with a perforated diverticulum with significant peritoneal spillage. Therapy should be directed toward gram-negative aerobes and anaerobes. The optimal therapeutic duration and endpoints are controversial.

CLINICAL APPROACH

Fever that occurs in a hospitalized surgical patient can have a number of causes. These include infections related to the original disease process, such as secondary peritonitis, intra-abdominal abscess, and wound infection. In addition, many hospital-acquired (nosocomial) infections can also occur, including urinary tract infection, pneumonia, bacteremia, intravenous catheter infection, and antibiotic-associated colitis. Noninfectious etiologics include systemic inflammatory response syndrome, endocrinopathies (adrenal insufficiency, thyrotoxicosis), drug reactions, and transfusion reactions. Generally, **a febrile postoperative patient who has had abdominal surgery for an infectious process is presumed to have an intra-abdominal infectious complication until proven otherwise.**

Pathophysiology of Intra-abdominal Infections

Perforation of the gastrointestinal tract results in microbial spillage into the peritoneal cavity. The severity of peritoneal contamination is related to the location of the perforation that determines the concentration and diversity of endogenous microbes (ie, colon contents with 10^{11}-10^{14} of aerobic and anaerobic microbes per gram of contents versus stomach contents containing 10^{2}-10^{3} aerobic microbes per gram of contents). A number of adaptive host responses occur following the inoculation of bacteria into the peritoneal cavity; these include peritoneal macrophage and polymorphonuclear (PMN) (leukocyte) recruitment and the development of ileus and fibropurulent peritonitis to localize the spillage. Normal peritoneal activity includes translymphatic clearance of sequestered microbes and inflammatory cells, leading to the resolution of peritonitis. Several factors influence the resolution or progression of secondary peritonitis: the size of the microbial inoculum; the timing of diagnosis and treatment; the inhibitory, synergistic, or cumulative effects of microbes on the growth of other microbes; and the status of the host peritoneal defenses.

The goals in the management of secondary peritonitis are directed toward eliminating the source of microbial spillage (an appendectomy for a perforated appendix or closure of a perforated duodenal ulcer) and early initiation of preemptive antibiotic therapy. With appropriate therapy, secondary peritonitis resolves in the majority of the patients; however, approximately 15% to 30% of individuals develop complications with recurrent secondary peritonitis, tertiary peritonitis, or intra-abdominal abscesses.

Factors contributing to the recurrence of secondary peritonitis include inappropriate and/or insufficient antimicrobial therapy and inadequate source control. Tertiary peritonitis, which is primarily caused by a failure of the host immune response, is treated with additional antimicrobial therapy and optimization of the host condition. **Patients with suspected deep surgical space infections following abdominal surgery should undergo CT imaging to search for intra-abdominal abscesses.** When identified, abscesses can be treated by percutaneous drainage. Patients with ongoing gastrointestinal tract spillage or abscesses that are inaccessible by percutaneous drainage should undergo open surgical drainage to control the primary source of infection. Initial systemic antibiotic therapy for the treatment of secondary peritonitis should be directed toward anaerobes and gram-negative aerobes, which can be accomplished with a single broad-spectrum agent or combination therapy (Table 25-1).

Table 25–1 ANTIMICROBIAL THERAPY FOR INTRA-ABDOMINAL INFECTIONS

Standard dual-agent therapy
- Aminoglycoside plus metronidazole or clindamycin
- This regimen should be used with extreme caution for older patients and those with renal insufficiency; aminoglycoside peak and trough levels should be monitored closely with prolonged use in most if not all patients

Nonstandard dual-agent therapy
- Second- or third-generation cephalosporin plus metronidazole or clindamycin
  For example, cefotetan, cefoxitin, ceftriaxone, cefotaxime, cefepime
- Fluoroquinolone plus metronidazole or clindamycin
  Ciprofloxacin, levofloxacin, gatifloxacin

Single-agent therapy
- For treatment of mild or moderate infections (eg, perforated appendix in otherwise healthy individuals)
  Cefoxitin, cefotetan, ceftriaxone, ampicillin–sulbactam
- For treatment of severe infections or infections in immunocompromised hosts
  Imipenem–cilastatin, meropenin, piperacillin–tazobactam, ticarcillin–clavulanate

Comprehension Questions

25.1 A 66-year-old woman undergoes exploratory laparotomy for suspected appendicitis. A ruptured appendix with purulent drainage into the peritoneal cavity is noted. Which of the following statements is most correct regarding this patient's condition?

A. The resulting infection is a difficult problem to resolve even with appropriate surgical and antimicrobial therapy.
B. The most common organisms involved are *Candida* and *Pseudomonas* species.
C. Treatment can be effectively accomplished with the use of first-generation cephalosporins.
D. Persistent secondary peritonitis may result because of inappropriate antibiotics selection or insufficient duration of therapy.

25.2 Which of the following is most accurate regarding patients who develop fever during the postoperative period?

A. They should receive broad-spectrum antibiotics until the fever resolves.
B. They require no specific therapy because fever is a physiologic response to surgical stress.
C. A thorough search for the fever source is required. Presumptive antibiotics should be given if the patient exhibits physiologic signs of sepsis or if the patient is immunocompromised.
D. The patients should undergo an immediate reoperation.

25.3 A 39-year-old man undergoes ileal resection and bowel anastomosis because of a perforation related to Crohn disease. Following surgery, he has persistent fever and abdominal pain despite the administration of intravenous cefoxitin and gentamicin. A CT scan reveals a 4 × 5 cm heterogeneous fluid collection in the pelvis. Which of the following is the best therapy for this patient?

A. Add vancomycin to the regimen.
B. Add fluconazole to the regimen.
C. Administer a thrombolytic to dissolve the pelvic hematoma.
D. Drain the fluid collection percutaneously.

25.4 Which of the following is the most accurate statement regarding secondary peritonitis?

A. Selection of appropriate antimicrobics regimen always produces successful treatment outcome.
B. Successful treatment cannot be accomplished with antimicrobial therapy alone.
C. Resection of the GI tract source producing the process will always result in the resolution of secondary peritonitis.
D. Antimicrobial therapy is not useful for treatment and would only lead to the selection of resistant organisms.

25.5 A 30-year-old man develops fever, abdominal distension, and leukocytosis 8 days following celiotomy and repair of 3 separate injuries to the small bowel produced by a gunshot wound to the abdomen. A CT scan reveals a single large fluid collection in the left upper quadrant with extensive surrounding inflammation. This collection is drained by CT-guided drainage and broad-spectrum antibiotic regimen is initiated. Despite these treatments, the patient has persistent fever and drainage of enteric contents from his drainage catheter, in addition, the patient develops drainage of purulent fluid from the inferior portion of his abdominal incision. Which of the following is the most appropriate treatment option?

A. Add empirical treatment to cover for fungal infection.
B. Repeat the CT scan.
C. Perform a celiotomy to address the intestinal leakage site.
D. Assess the patient for immunodeficiency, including skin anergy panel and CD4 cell count measurement.

ANSWERS

25.1 **D.** Inappropriate selection of and insufficient duration of antimicrobial therapy are the major causes of persistent secondary peritonitis. Gram-negative and anaerobic bacteria are the most commonly involved bacteria.

25.2 **C.** Routine antimicrobial therapy is not indicated for all febrile postoperative patients; however, patients with a poor physiologic reserve and a compromised immune system should be treated with broad-spectrum presumptive antimicrobial therapy prior to definitive diagnosis of the fever source.

25.3 **D.** This patient likely has an abscess, which is best treated by percutaneous drainage with CT guidance.

25.4 **B.** Successful treatment of secondary peritonitis cannot be accomplished by antibiotics alone. Since this form of peritonitis is generally the result of GI perforation such as perforated appendicitis, perforated diverticulitis, and intestinal anastamotic leakage, treatment must include control of leakage source, appropriate selection and duration of antibiotics, and appropriate host immunological response to infections.

25.5 **B.** Repeating the CT scan at this point may be helpful to determine if there are other collections of infected fluid that may need to be addressed with the placement of additional drains or if there are multiple collections or inaccessible collections, then operative drainage may be needed. The clinical presentation described here suggests the problem may be inadequate control of leakage rather than inadequate host response.

Clinical Pearls

- Prolonged dysfunction of the gastrointestinal tract following gastrointestinal surgery frequently indicates the presence of intra-abdominal infectious complications, whereas the prompt return of gastrointestinal function following surgery generally indicates the absence of intra-abdominal infections.
- Atelectasis is the most common cause of fever in a patient during the first 24 hours following surgery.
- With the availability of many effective antibiotics against gram-negative organisms, aminoglycosides are rarely used as first-line therapy.
- The colon has a very large number of bacteria (10^{11} to 10^{14} of aerobic and anaerobic microbes per gram of contents) versus the stomach (containing 10^2 to 10^3 aerobic microbes per gram of contents).
- CT imaging is often helpful in identifying intra-abdominal abscesses.

REFERENCES

Arnold MA, Barbul A. Surgical site infections. In: Cameron JL, ed. *Current Surgical Therapy*. 9th ed. Philadelphia, PA: Mosby Elsevier; 2008:1152-1160.

Dunn DL, Beilman GJ. Surgical infections. In: Brunicardi FC, Andersen DK, Billiar TR, et al, eds. *Schwartz's Principles of Surgery*. 8th ed. New York: McGraw-Hill; 2005:109-127.

Nenshi R, Marshall JC. Intraabdominal infections. In: Cameron JL, ed. *Current Surgical Therapy*. 9th ed. Philadelphia, PA: Mosby Elsevier; 2008:1160-1163.

Case 26

A 52-year-old woman presented with atrial fibrillation and an acute abdomen 8 days ago. She was taken to the operating room for exploratory laparotomy after the initial evaluation suggested the perforation of a hollow viscus. During the operation she was discovered to have a superior mesentery artery (SMA) embolism. She required resection of the infarcted bowel, and a jejunal-colonic anastomosis was performed. On postoperative day 8, the patient received enteral nutritional support with a polymeric formula diet through a nasogastric feeding tube. After the initiation of tube feeding, she began to produce a large amount of liquid stools. During the initial evaluation, the results of her physical examination are unremarkable except for postoperative changes. Her stool sample was analyzed and found negative for fecal leukocytes and *Clostridium difficile*.

- What is the most likely diagnosis?
- What is the best therapy?

ANSWERS TO CASE 26:
Short Bowel Syndrome

Summary: A 52-year-old patient with atrial fibrillation required right colon and extensive small bowel resection after an embolus was found in her SMA 8 days previously. She now has severe diarrhea with stool negative for fecal leukocytes or C. *difficile* toxin.

- **Diagnosis:** Malabsorption and diarrhea related to short bowel syndrome.
- **Best therapy:** Bowel rest and parenteral nutrition until bowel adaptation occurs.

ANALYSIS

Objectives

1. Learn the different routes of enteral nutritional support.
2. Know the advantages and disadvantages of enteral and parenteral nutrition.
3. Learn how small bowel adaptations occur following massive resection and the options for short- and long-term management of short gut syndrome.

Considerations

A patient presents with postenteral feeding diarrhea after a massive small bowel resection. The SMA supplies blood to most of the small bowel and proximal colon. Because an SMA embolus typically lodges in the distal artery, it causes necrosis of the right colon, ileum, and distal jejunum. In this case, the absence of fecal leukocytes and C. *difficile* toxin makes an infectious cause of the diarrhea unlikely. Her surgical history and negative laboratory test results indicate malabsorption related to short bowel syndrome. The most important therapeutic objective for this patient is maintenance of nutritional status.

APPROACH TO
Short Bowel Syndrome and Malnutrition

DEFINITIONS

SMALL BOWEL SYNDROME: Malabsorption and maldigestion due to extensive resection of small bowel.

NECROTIZING ENTEROCOLITIS: Extensive ulceration and necrosis of the ileum and colon in premature infants in the neonatal period; possibly due to perinatal intestinal ischemia and bacterial invasion

TOTAL PARENTERAL NUTRITION (TPN): Nutrition maintained entirely by central intravenous injection or other nongastrointestinal route.

CLINICAL APPROACH

Pathophysiology

Short bowel syndrome, which results from either extensive bowel resection or a functional defect such as radiation enteritis or severe inflammatory bowel disease, is characterized by diarrhea, dehydration, electrolyte disturbance, malabsorption, and progressive malnutrition. The ileum and jejunum of the small intestine are the most important organs in dietary nutrient digestion and absorption. Nutrients are digested in the small intestinal lumen and absorbed by intestinal epithelia lining along the lumen. The normal small bowel length is approximately 300 to 500 cm. **An individual with 90 to 180 cm of small bowel** (or approximately a third of the normal intestinal length) **may develop transient diarrhea and malabsorption; whereas, individuals with less than 60 cm of small bowel may require permanent parenteral nutrition.** The **most common causes of short bowel syndrome are Crohn disease and mesenteric infarction in adults and necrotizing enterocolitis and small bowel volvulus in infants.**

After an extensive small bowel resection, the remaining intestine undergoes both structural and functional adaptations. Structural changes include elongation, increase in villous height, mucosal surface area, bowel luminal circumference, and wall thickness. Functionally, there is usually an increase in nutrient absorption and a decrease in diarrhea and malabsorption. The adaptive process begins within 12 to 24 hours and continues for 1 to 2 years. The degree of intestinal adaptation depends on many variables including the length and site of intestinal loss, the functional status of the remaining bowel, and the elapsed time from the insult. Intestinal failure associated with short bowel syndrome may be temporary or permanent.

Recent scientific and clinical evidence suggest that the colon is involved in nutrient absorption and restoration of intestinal continuity in patients with short bowel syndrome may have some advantages, including the absorption of short-chain fatty acids and the reduction in infectious complication. Some potential disadvantages with the restoration of intestinal continuity include increase diarrhea (from bile acid malabsorption) and increase in calcium oxalate kidney stone formation.

TREATMENT

Nutritional Support

Nutritional support is the cornerstone of short bowel syndrome management; this management is used to provide the caloric requirements and promote gut adaptation, so that the patient may eventually survive on an oral diet.

ROUTES OF NUTRITIONAL SUPPORT: Enteral feeding via mouth, nasogastric or nasojejunal tube, gastrostomy, or jejunostomy; total parenteral nutrition; or a combination of both.

ENTERAL NUTRITION: The advantages of enteral nutrition are that it is more physiologic and more economical, and it promotes intestinal mucosal hyperplasia and gut adaptation. The disadvantage is that it requires enough healthy intestine to absorb sufficient nutrients.

TOTAL PARENTERAL NUTRITION (TPN): The advantages of total parenteral nutrition are that it provides sufficient nutrition to support growth and development in children and weight gain and positive nitrogen balance in adults regardless of the length of the bowel. The disadvantages of parenteral nutrition include intestinal atrophy, intravenous line sepsis, high cost, high morbidity and mortality (liver dysfunction), and poor quality of life. The initial decision between enteral and parenteral nutrition is based on whether the patient is able to maintain a healthy nutritional status via enteral feeding alone. With patients receiving only parenteral nutrition, a period of transition is usually needed before full enteral feedings are tolerated. Specific intestinal nutrients, such as the amino acids ornithine and glutamine, triglycerides, and soluble and short-chain fatty acids, are important in promoting adaptation.

Medical Therapy

The use of medications to reduce gastrointestinal motility and secretion are helpful to reduce diarrhea and improve absorption. The medications include loperamide and codeine phosphate, proton pump inhibitors (PPIs), and octreotide. Clonidine (an alpha-2 adrenergic agonist) may also be helpful in reducing fluid secretion. For some individuals with diarrhea related to bile acid malabsorption (generally, those with ileal resections), cholestyramine can be helpful. Glutamine and recombinant human growth hormone in combination with dietary regimen are potential pharmacological interventions that are currently under investigation.

Surgical Therapy

Surgical intervention may be useful in carefully selected patients with either temporary or permanent short bowel syndrome. Small bowel transplantation holds potential future promise. One study noted that transplantation recipients had a 1-year overall survival of 69%, with three-quarters of the patients surviving without TPN. Other operative procedures, used with the goal of promoting absorption and/or delaying intestinal emptying, include lengthening of the intestine, implantation of artificial intestinal valves, and the use of reversed intestinal segments or a recirculating loop.

Comprehension Questions

26.1 A 2-month-old preterm infant is noted by a neonatologist to have probable short bowel syndrome. Which of the following is the most likely cause?

A. Crohn disease
B. Hirschsprung disease
C. Necrotizing enterocolitis
D. Radiation enteritis

26.2 A 40-year-old man underwent massive bowel resection (from the ligament of Treitz to the midtransverse colon) secondary to SMA thrombosis. Which of the following therapies is most appropriate?

A. Oral diet
B. Feeding gastrostomy
C. Short-term TPN and progressive advance to an oral diet
D. Small bowel transplantation

26.3 A 50-year-old woman has undergone multiple small bowel resections for severe Crohn disease. She notices weight loss and disturbances in electrolyte levels while on an oral diet. Which of the following therapies is most appropriate?

A. Complete bowel rest and long-term TPN.
B. Small bowel transplantation.
C. Continued limited oral diet with short-term TPN support and progress toward a total oral diet.
D. Continued observation and no intervention at this time.

26.4 Which of the following is most accurate regarding the role of the colon in nutritional absorption in patients with short bowel syndrome?

A. The colon interferes with the absorption of nutrients.
B. The colon does not play a role in the absorption of nutrients.
C. Short chain fatty acid absorption occurs in the colon.
D. Colonic functions become modified to resume the role of small bowel.

26.5 Which of the following is a beneficial effect of TPN in the treatment of short bowel syndrome?

A. TPN provides nutritional support and fluid hydration when GI absorptive properties are inadequate.
B. TPN provides nutritional support and promotes GI adaption.
C. TPN is associated with lower rates of infectious complications.
D. TPN improves liver functions.

ANSWERS

26.1 **C.** Necrotizing enterocolitis is the most common cause of short bowel syndrome in an infant of this age, particularly a preterm infant.

26.2 **D.** The loss of the entire absorptive surface of the bowel in this patient is incompatible with enteral nutritional tolerance because there is no ileum or jejunum left. Therefore, small bowel transplantation is an appropriate consideration.

26.3 **C.** Initial TPN and a subsequent slow reintroduction of enteral feeding are appropriate for this patient to allow for adaptive changes in the intestine.

26.4 **C.** Until recently, the colon was considered to be of no nutritional benefits in patients with short bowel syndrome; however, it is now known that benefits of the colon include short-chain fatty acid absorption and delay in intestinal transit time. Disadvantages of the colon in these patients include the absorption of oxalate leading to increased risk of calcium oxalate kidney stones, and patients with their colons in continuity are prone to the development of secretory diarrhea from bile acid exposure to the colonic mucosa.

26.5 **A.** TPN is an important element in the early phase of nutritional support of patients with short bowel. TPN use provides a source of nutritional and fluid intake when patients are incapable of receiving adequate enteric nutrients. TPN use have a number of drawbacks including increase in infectious complications (from hyperglycemia and central venous access) and the promotion of cholestatic changes in the liver. In addition, the exclusive use of TPN does not allow for the continued enteral stimulation that is needed for intestinal adaptation.

Clinical Pearls

- Individuals with < 200 cm (a third) of small bowel are at risk for diarrhea and malabsorption.
- The most common causes of short bowel syndrome in adults are Crohn disease and mesenteric infarction.
- Selected patients with short bowel syndrome may be candidates for small bowel transplantation.

REFERENCES

Platell CFE, Coster J, McCauley RD, et al. The management of patients with the short bowel syndrome. *World J Gastroenterol.* 2002;8(1):113-120.

Thompson JS. Management of short bowel syndrome. In: Cameron JL, ed. *Current Surgical Therapy*. 9th ed. Philadelphia, PA: Mosby Elsevier; 2008:145-151.

Case 27

A 43-year-old woman presents with a sudden onset of abdominal pain approximately 1-hour prior to coming to the emergency center. She denies previous abdominal complaints. Her systolic blood pressure is 88 mm Hg on evaluation and becomes stable at 120 mm Hg after the infusion of 2 L of intravenous fluid. The abdominal examination demonstrates no peritoneal signs, her bowel sounds are hypoactive, and there is mild right upper quadrant tenderness. The hematocrit value is 22%. A computed tomography (CT) scan is performed and demonstrates free intra-abdominal blood and a 5-cm solid mass in the right hepatic lobe with evidence of recent bleeding into the mass. By history, the patient denies recent trauma, weight loss, a change in bowel habits, hematemesis, or hematochezia. The only medication she takes is an oral contraceptive agent, which she has been using without problems for approximately 20 years.

- What are your next steps?
- What is the most likely diagnosis?

ANSWERS TO CASE 27: Liver Tumor

Summary: A 43-year old woman who uses an oral contraceptive presents with acute abdominal pain, hypotension, anemia, and recent intra-abdominal hemorrhage. A CT imaging shows a right hepatic tumor.

- **Next steps:** Hemodynamic monitoring and admission to the intensive care unit with serial hematocrit determinations are indicated. Once the patient is stable, the etiology of the liver mass should be sought.
- **Most likely diagnosis:** Hepatic adenoma with hemorrhage.

ANALYSIS

Objectives

1. Learn to develop appropriate differential diagnoses for hepatic masses based on patient characteristics and risk factors.
2. Know the pertinent differences in the management of primary and secondary liver masses.
3. Know the natural history and imaging characteristics of liver tumors to avoid unnecessary investigations and operations.

Considerations

Most patients with liver tumors are asymptomatic or may have only vague symptoms. This patient's dramatic presentation is unusual when compared to that of all patients with liver tumors but represents a classic presentation of hepatic adenoma complicated by hemorrhage. Hepatic adenomas were quite uncommon prior to the introduction of oral contraceptives, but this disease process is now recognized as being associated with exposure to estrogenic compounds. Benign focal liver masses are present in 9% to 10% of the general population, and most of these individuals are asymptomatic and can be treated with observation. Hepatic adenoma is an exception to this rule. Because of the propensity of these tumors to produce symptoms, cause hemorrhage, and undergo malignant transformation, most patients with hepatic adenomas should be advised to undergo tumor resection. Hepatic adenomas are hormonally stimulated; therefore, some patients with small asymptomatic adenomas can be initially treated with cessation of the use of oral contraceptives and close surveillance at 3- to 6-month intervals.

APPROACH TO
Hepatic Tumors

DEFINITIONS

PRIMARY LIVER TUMOR: A tumor originating from hepatocyte, bile duct epithelial, or mesenchymal tissue within the liver. This tumor may be benign, have a potential for malignant transformation, or be frankly malignant. The most common primary malignant tumors in adults are hepatocellular carcinoma and cholangiocarcinoma; the most common benign tumors are hemangioma, adenoma, and focal nodular hyperplasia.

SECONDARY LIVER TUMOR: A tumor that arises from tissue outside the liver and spreads to the liver by a metastatic process. This tumor is by definition malignant. The most common metastatic tumors found in the liver are colorectal carcinomas.

BENIGN TUMOR: A tumor that does not have the biologic ability to spread via the lymphatic or vascular system. This type of tumor may cause significant symptoms or may be locally aggressive.

MALIGNANT TUMOR: A tumor with the potential to spread by either a lymphatic or a hematogenous route.

FOCAL NODULAR HYPERPLASIA (FNH): The second most common benign liver tumor occurring most commonly in reproductive-age women. Most FNH is asymptomatic and discovered incidentally. An FNH is a truly benign tumor without malignant potential. Some FNH may be difficult to distinguish from adenomas on the basis of radiographic criteria, and typical appearance is a "central scar" pattern on a CT scan. Biopsy may be needed if the tumor cannot be differentiated from hepatic adenoma. Surgery is indicated when malignancy cannot be excluded or when FNH produces severe symptoms.

HEMANGIOMA: The most common benign liver tumor. This lesion may produce vague abdominal pain but frequently is asymptomatic. **Spontaneous rupture is rare.** The diagnosis may be made on the basis of contrast CT imaging, magnetic resonance imaging, or tagged red blood cell scan. **Biopsy is contraindicated because it may result in life-threatening hemorrhage.** Indications for surgery are severe symptoms, inability to rule out the possibility of malignancy, and rupture.

CLINICAL APPROACH

Liver tumors may be found incidentally or during the evaluation of nonspecific abdominal symptoms; however, more frequently, they are identified in patients at risk for primary or secondary liver tumors (e.g., a patient with cirrhosis or with a history of advanced breast carcinoma who develops upper abdominal pain). The approach to a hepatic mass in a patient begins with a thorough history and physical examination, imaging studies, measurement of serum tumor markers, and in some cases tissue biopsy. **The primary goals of the evaluation** are to determine whether the lesion in question is **a primary versus a secondary liver tumor, characterize the nature of the tumor, and define the location and local extent of the mass.**

Imaging Liver Tumors

Selection of the imaging modality is perhaps the most crucial aspect of the evaluation. Proper selection of imaging studies may help establish the diagnosis of many liver tumors, thus avoiding unnecessary biopsies and/or operations for some patients. Although liver tumors are readily visualized by ultrasonography and CT scans, these images generally provide insufficient information for patient treatment. CT with angioportography, magnetic resonance imaging (MRI), angiography, and laparoscopic ultrasonography are the modalities available for the further characterization of liver tumors. Table 27–1 lists the imaging selection criteria for primary and secondary liver tumors.

Secondary Liver Tumors

The liver is a frequent site of malignant metastasis, most commonly involving colorectal carcinoma. Listed here are the characteristics associated with secondary liver tumors.

1. Resection of a primary tumor with known metastatic potential within the previous 5 years (e.g., a history of stage III adenocarcinoma 2 years previously).
2. Current signs and symptoms of an untreated primary tumor with known metastatic potential (e.g., a large left breast mass and multiple hepatic lesions in a 74-year-old woman).
3. Miliary or diffuse distribution of hepatic lesions.
4. Significant elevation of tumor marker levels (> 10-fold) in the setting of a new liver mass.

When a secondary liver tumor of unknown primary origin is identified, an investigation to identify the primary malignancy should be undertaken. Important in this evaluation are the history and physical examination. Weight loss, a history of new narrow-caliber stools, and a rectal examination with Hemocceltpositive results should prompt further gastrointestinal tract evaluation. A history of long-time smoking in a man older than 50 years with hematemesis and a new hilar mass seen on chest radiography should prompt further evaluation of the respiratory tract, including a cytologic examination

Table 27–1 IMAGING MODALITIES FOR LIVER TUMORS

MODALITY	HEMANGIOMA	FOCAL HYPERPLASIA	ADENOMA	HEPATOCELLULAR CARCINOMA	METASTATIC ADENOCARCINOMA
Computed tomography angioportography	High sensitivity and specificity, early contrast enhancement with peripheral outlining of tumor	Low specificity (central scar is characteristic finding)	Low specificity	Low specificity	High sensitivity and specificity; gold standard
Magnetic resonance imaging	High sensitivity and specificity	Low specificity (central scar is characteristic finding)	Low specificity	Low specificity	High sensitivity and specificity
Angiography	Gold standard test with high sensitivity and specificity, but invasive	High sensitivity and specificity, but invasive	Low specificity	Low specificity	Infrequently used
Laparoscopic ultrasound	Poor	Poor	Helpful when combined with laparoscopic biopsy	Gold standard test	Highly sensitive when combined with laparoscopic biopsy
Biopsy	Contraindicated because of high risk for bleeding	Rarely useful	Helpful	Mandatory	Mandatory

Table 27–2 5-POINT SCORING SYSTEM* FOR PATIENTS UNDERGOING LIVER RESECTION FOR METASTATIC COLORECTAL CANCER

		3-YEAR SURVIVAL (%)	5-YEAR SURVIVAL (%)	MEDIAN SURVIVAL (MO)
0		72	60	74
1	Node-positive primary tumor	66	44	51
2	Disease-free interval < 12 months	60	40	47
3	> 1 Liver Metastasis	42	20	33
4	Metastasis > 5cm	38	25	20
5	CEA > 200	27	14	22

* Each category contributes 1 point and survival is predicted based on the total score.

Fong Y, Fortner J, Sun RL, et al. Clinical score for predicting recurrence after hepatic resection for metastatic colorectal cancer: Analysis of 1001 consecutive cases. *Ann Surg.* 1999;230:309-318

of the sputum, bronchoscopy, and subsequent CT-guided biopsy. The search for the primary tumor is important not only in treating the primary site but also in considering treatment of the liver metastasis. Although the presence of liver metastasis frequently indicates an advanced tumor stage and may preclude the possibility of cure, certain tumor types and distribution in carefully selected patients are amenable to curative resection or ablative therapy. A 5-point clinical prognostic scoring system is generally applied to predict survival for patients undergoing liver resection for colorectal metastasis (see Table 27–2). Liver transplantation has no role in the treatment of patients with secondary liver tumors.

Primary Liver Tumors

Tumor markers are invaluable tools in the evaluation of both secondary and primary liver masses. Although the specificity of most tumor markers for a given primary cancer is not high, these assays are sensitive in most cases and are an important part of the workup for liver masses. Table 27–3 lists some of the primary tumor markers that are helpful in the diagnosis of liver masses.

Many liver tumors are either cancerous or have significant premalignant potential or significant morbidity such as bleeding or the production of

Table 27–3 TUMOR MARKERS POTENTIALLY USEFUL FOR IDENTIFYING THE ORIGIN OF SECONDARY LIVER TUMORS

TUMOR MARKER	TYPE OF CANCER
CEA	Colon cancer
AFP	Hepatocellular carcinoma
CA 19-9	Pancreatic cancer
CA 125	Ovarian cancer
β-hCG	Testicular cancer
PSA	Prostate cancer
CA 50	Pancreatic cancer
Neuron-specific enolase	Small cell lung cancer
CA 15-3	Breast cancer
Ferritin	Hepatocellular carcinoma

Abbreviations: CEA, carcinoembryonic antigen; AFP, α-fetoprotein; CA 19-9, carbohydrate antigen 19-9; CA 125, carbohydrate antigen 125; β-hCG, β-human chorionic gonadotropin; PSA, prostate-specific antigen; CA 50, carbohydrate antigen 50; CA 15-3, carbohydrate antigen 15-3.

abdominal pain. For this reason, early surgical consultation is recommended to facilitate the appropriate workup and diagnosis. When appropriate imaging studies are unable to verify the lesion as a tumor without malignant potential, biopsy of the mass or masses may be needed to determine the tumor type and subsequent therapy. Liver resection is both safe and in many cases may provide either a cure or long-term survival benefits. **The cornerstone of workup for a liver mass is the development of an appropriate differential diagnosis based on history and physical examination and appropriate imaging to facilitate diagnosis.**

Comprehension Questions

27.1 A 30-year-old woman is noted to have a hepatic mass on laparoscopy for a sterilization procedure. She undergoes a liver biopsy that reveals focal nodular hyperplasia. Which of the following is the most accurate statement regarding this condition?

A. These tumors have malignant potential over 10 to 20 years.
B. Surgical excision is often the best therapy.
C. Angiography has high sensitivity and specificity for the diagnosis of this tumor.
D. Oral contraceptive use is a risk factor.

27.2 A 65-year-old man is found to have a 6-cm mass of his liver on sonography of his gallbladder. He has a history of hepatitis B surface antigen present on serology, but his liver transaminase levels are within normal limits. Which of the following is the most appropriate therapy for this patient?

A. Superior mesenteric artery embolization procedure
B. Surgical resection
C. Intravenous interferon therapy
D. Prolonged antibiotic therapy for probable amebic abscess

27.3 A 75-year-old icteric woman is noted to have multiple lesions in her liver that on CT imaging are suspicious for metastatic cancer. Which of the following is the most likely source of the primary cancer?

A. Stomach
B. Lung
C. Colon
D. Cervix

27.4 A 47-year-old man with colon cancer undergoes right colectomy for adenocarcinoma of the cecum. At the time of the operation, the 10-cm tumor appears to be confined to the cecum, several 2-3 cm lymph nodes are seen in the mesentery of the right colon, 2 metastic deposits measuring 3-cm are noted on the right lobe of the liver and 3 metastatic deposits measuring 2-cm are found in the left lobe. Which of the following is the most appropriate treatment option?

A. Biopsy the cecal mass, lymph nodes, liver tumors, and terminate the procedure.
B. Remove the right colon including the enlarged mesenteric lymph nodes, biopsy the liver tumors, and refer patient for chemotherapy.
C. Remove the right colon including the enlarged mesenteric lymph nodes, biopsy the liver, and refer the patient for liver transplantation.
D. Remove the right colon including the enlarged mesenteric lymph nodes, biopsy the liver, and refer the patient for chemotherapy and radiation therapy to target the liver metastases.

27.5 A 46-year-old woman who underwent an abdominal CT scan for evaluation of nephrolithiasis was noted to have a 5-cm mass in the right lobe of the liver. A CT scan with contrast was done that revealed early contrast enhancement with peripheral outlining of the mass. The patient is asymptomatic from the standpoint of the liver mass. Which of the following is the most appropriate management?

A. Obtain serum alpha-fetal protein measurement and obtain a CT-guided biopsy to rule out hepatocellular carcinoma.
B. Perform colonoscopy to evaluate for a possible colorectal primary cancer.
C. Observe the patient clinically and repeat the imaging if the patient becomes symptomatic.
D. Refer the patient for liver transplantation.

ANSWERS

27.1 **C.** Focal nodular hyperplasia is the second most common hepatic tumor. It is not associated with oral contraceptive use and is usually asymptomatic. It has no malignant potential and rarely needs biopsy for diagnosis because angiography is an excellent diagnostic tool for this disorder.

27.2 **B.** This patient is at risk for hepatocellular carcinoma because he has a large hepatic mass and a likely chronic hepatitis B infection (surface antigen positive). Surgical resection is the best therapy for early stage disease and the only hope for cure in this condition. Interferon therapy is used for hepatitis C disease.

27.3 **C.** The colon is the most common primary site when metastatic disease is found in the liver.

27.4 **B.** Resection of the right colon, biopsy of the liver tumors, and chemotherapy are appropriate for this individual with apparent stage IV colon cancer. Resection of the liver tumor at this time is probably of limited benefit and may pose unnecessary morbidity for the patient. Liver transplantation is not an option for patients with metastatic liver tumors. Radiation therapy directed toward the liver produces unacceptable liver toxicity and is generally not done.

27.5 **C.** The description of her presentation and CT findings are consistent with an asymptomatic liver hemagioma, which is benign tumor with no malignant potential. Treatment in asymptomatic patient is not indicated. Biopsy of hemagiomas should not be obtained because of the risk of bleeding; furthermore, CT findings are generally highly specific for diagnosis.

Clinical Pearls

- Hemangiomas are the most common benign tumors of the liver and usually asymptomatic.
- Hepatic adenomas are associated with estrogen use and should be excised because of the risk of hemorrhage or malignant transformation.
- The most common metastatic disease to the liver is colorectal cancer. Because of the risk of hemorrhage, hepatic hemangiomas should be ruled out prior to needle biopsy.

REFERENCES

Fong Y, Fortner J, Sun RL, et al. Clinical score for predicting recurrence after hepatic resection for metastatic colorectal cancer: Analysis of 1001 consecutive cases. *Ann Surg*. 1999;230:309-318.

Gray KD, Ribero D, Vauthey JN. Malignant liver tumors. In: Cameron JL. *Current Surgical Therapy*. 9th ed. Philadelphia, PA: Mosby Elsevier; 2008:346-351.

Liaw JM, Chapman WC. Benign liver tumors. In: Cameron JL. *Current Surgical Therapy*. 9th ed. Philadelphia, PA: Mosby Elsevier; 2008:335-341.

Case 28

A 62-year-old man presents to the emergency department with a 1-week history of left lower quadrant abdominal pain. He complains of increased pain, nausea, and fever. He has had one prior episodes of similar left lower quadrant pain that resolved with antibiotic treatment alone. He has no cardiac or pulmonary risk factors. On examination, his blood pressure is 140/80 mm Hg, heart rate 110 beats/min, and temperature 101.5°F. His abdomen is soft and mildly distended, with left lower quadrant tenderness to palpation. He does not have evidence of generalized peritonitis. His white blood cell (WBC) count is 20,000/mm^3.

- What is the most likely diagnosis?
- How would you confirm the diagnosis?
- What are the complications associated with this disease process?

ANSWERS TO CASE 28: Diverticulitis

Summary: A 62-year-old man presents with signs and symptoms compatible with recurrent sigmoid diverticulitis.

- **Most likely diagnosis:** Acute sigmoid diverticulitis with an abscess.
- **Confirmation of diagnosis:** A CT imaging demonstrating sigmoid diverticula, colonic wall thickening, and mesenteric fat stranding.
- **Associated complications:** Perforation, abscess formation, bowel obstruction, and development of fistulas.

ANALYSIS

Objectives

1. Learn the etiology of diverticular disease and the pathophysiology of diverticulitis.
2. Learn the workup and management of diverticulitis and its complications.

Considerations

This patient's clinical history of left lower quadrant pain and fever are suggestive of acute sigmoid diverticulitis. Although he has no evidence of generalized peritonitis; however, this fever, leukocytosis, and tachycardia are causes for concern at this time. **A CT scan in this case is very helpful in assessing for complications of diverticulitis, particularly an abscess.** Small mesenteric abscesses associated with diverticulitis usually resolve with antibiotic therapy alone, whereas large abscesses may require CT-guided drainage in addition to antibiotic therapy, and multiple abscesses and abscesses in inaccessible locations may require operative drainage. If the patient fails to improve clinically after 72 hours with nonoperative treatment, surgical intervention is usually warranted. Once this bout of diverticulitis is resolved with nonoperative management, a discussion regarding long-term care should be carried out with the patient. In generally, nonopeartive treatment has become more widely applied for the treatment of patients with recurrent uncomplicated diverticulitis. In the past, patients with a second bout of diverticulitis and young patients below the age of 40 were recommended to undergo elective colon resections. Given the advances in antimicrobial therapy and supportive care, the recent clinical observations suggest that most uncomplicated recurrent diverticulitis patients can be safely and cost-effectively managed with nonoperative management for 4 bouts of attacks.

APPROACH TO Diverticulitis

DEFINITIONS

DIVERTICULOSIS: Outpouchings of the colon that do not contain all layers of the colon wall, most commonly in the sigmoid colon in Western societies. Right-sided or cecal diverticulosis tends to occur in Asian populations.

DIVERTICULITIS: Inflammation of a diverticulum caused by obstruction of the neck of the diverticulum and microperforation.

CLINICAL APPROACH

The clinical diagnosis of diverticulitis often can be made on the basis of history and a physical examination. However, when the diagnosis is uncertain, there are signs of systemic toxicity, or there is a lack of improvement, further diagnostic studies are indicated. An abdominal CT scan is the radiologic examination of choice. A barium enema is generally deferred because of concerns for intraperitoneal leakage of barium, and colonoscopy should be used with caution. However, after the acute episode is resolved, these tests can be used to document the presence of diverticulosis or fistulas and to assess for other pathologic conditions such as malignancies.

Uncomplicated Diverticulitis

Patients can be successfully managed nonoperatively, with more than 70% of the patients expected to remain free of recurrences. Mild cases of diverticulitis can be treated on an outpatient basis. Patients with signs of systemic toxicity (fever, tachycardia, and peritonitis) should be hospitalized for hydration, treatment with intravenous antibiotics, bowel rest, and close observation. After the clinical resolution of acute diverticulitis, patients with their first, second, or third episodes and who are not immunocompromised may not require treatment other than dietary and life style modifications. However, patients who are **immunocompromised tend be unresponsive to medical treatment alone and usually require surgical intervention.** Patients who have had four or more episodes of diverticulitis or have significantly compromised quality of life due to diverticulitis should be advised to undergo elective resection.

Complicated Diverticulitis

Complicated diverticulitis typically requires surgical management. Perforated diverticulitis with generalized peritonitis should be treated with surgical exploration. If the patient is hemodynamically unstable or fecal peritonitis is present, surgical resection, colostomy, and closure of the rectal stump (Hartmann procedure) are recommended. Reanastomosis should then be performed at a later date. In the absence of significant contamination, primary anastomosis can be performed with or without proximal diversion.

Perforation that results in localized fluid collection or a diverticular abscess can be initially managed with nonoperative therapy in the absence of peritoneal signs or systemic toxicity. Mesenteric abscesses typically are treated with antibiotic therapy, and pelvic abscesses can be initially managed with percutaneous drainage. An elective one-stage procedure should then be performed at a later date. Intestinal obstruction can occur either at the time that acute diverticulitis occurs secondary to inflammation or at a later date due to a stricture. If the patient has a partial bowel obstruction, resection with anastomosis may be feasible after bowel preparation. However, patients with complete bowel obstruction should undergo urgent surgical intervention.

Diverticular fistulas can occur between the sigmoid colon and the bladder, vagina, skin, or another segment of bowel. A barium enema, a CT scan,

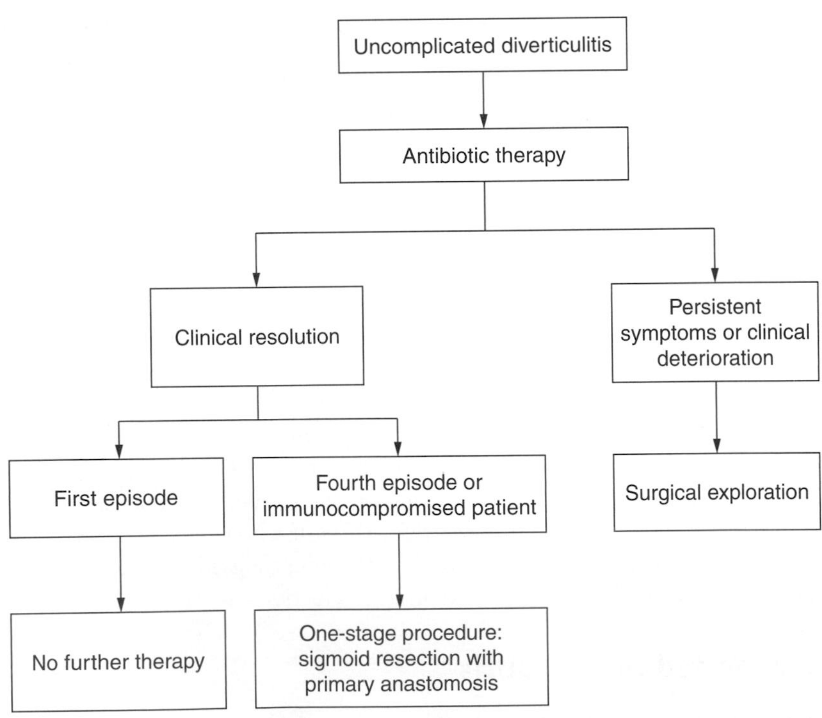

Figure 28–1. Algorithm for the management of uncomplicated diverticulitis.

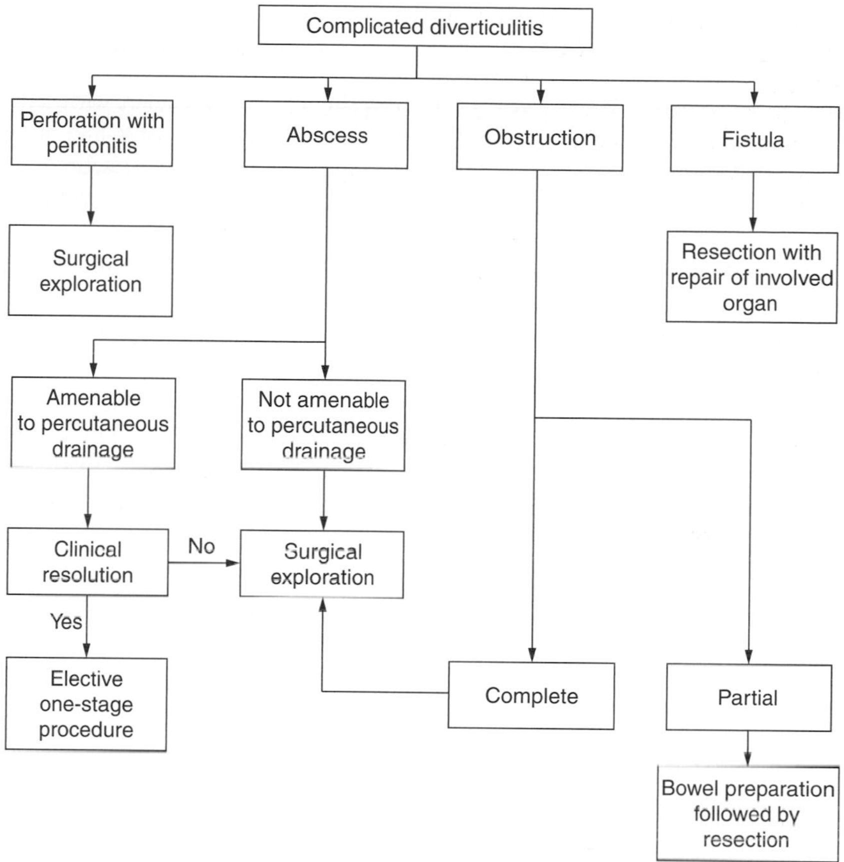

Figure 28–2. Algorithm for the management of complicated diverticulitis—early complications.

and sigmoidoscopy can be used to visualize a fistula. Cystoscopy or a vaginal speculum examination may help identify a colovesical or a colovaginal fistula, respectively. **Treatment consists of resection of the sigmoid colon, excision of the fistulous tract, and repair or resection of the other involved organ.** See Figures 28–1 and 28–2 for management schemes.

Comprehension Questions

28.1 A 57-year-old man presents to his primary care physician with left-sided abdominal pain of 5 days' duration, nausea, vomiting, and diarrhea. He is unable to maintain his oral intake at home. On presentation, he has mild tenderness to palpation in the left lower quadrant without peritoneal signs. His WBC count is 14,000/mm^3. He has never had a similar episode in the past. What is the appropriate treatment for this patient?

A. Hospitalize for bowel rest, administration of intravenous fluids and antibiotics, and close observation.
B. Prescribe a course of outpatient antibiotics with appropriate follow-up.
C. Obtain an emergent barium enema to diagnose diverticulitis.
D. Consult the surgery department regarding future elective sigmoid resection.

28.2 A 61-year-old woman presents to the emergency department with left-sided abdominal pain of 10 days' duration. She has had constipation and states that her last bowel movement was 2 days ago. She also complains of fever to 38.9°C (102°F) and nausea and vomiting. On examination, she is diffusely tender to palpation. Plain films demonstrate dilated loops of small bowel and a paucity of gas in the rectum. Her WBC count is 26,000/mm^3. What is the appropriate next step in the treatment of this patient?

A. Barium enema to confirm the diagnosis of diverticulitis
B. Urgent sigmoidoscopy to evaluate for diverticulitis versus colonic neoplasm
C. Urgent surgical exploration
D. Admission for nasogastric decompression and administration of intravenous antibiotics

28.3 A 59-year-old woman presents to her primary care physician with complaints of pneumaturia or air in the urine and recurrent urinary tract infections. She has a prior history of diverticulitis occurring 6 months ago. Which of the following tests would most likely lead to the diagnosis?

A. Order a CT scan of the abdomen to look for a colovesical fistula.
B. Urinalysis
C. Intravenous pyelogram
D. Colonoscopy

28.4 Which of the following is the most common cause of gastrointestinal tract fistulas?

A. Peptic ulcer disease
B. Inadvertent enterotomy
C. Crohn disease
D. Ulcerative colitis
E. Diverticulitis

28.5 For which of the following patients is sigmoid colectomy an appropriate treatment option?

A. 30-year-old man who developed a bout of sigmoid diverticulitis that resolved with antibiotics therapy
B. A 55-year-old man with a bout of sigmoid diverticulitis that resolved with antibiotics. His follow-up colonoscopy confirmed diverticuli in the colon. The patient is significantly concerned that he has occult colon cancer because his brother died of colon cancer recently
C. A 57-year-old man with three bouts of diverticulitis that have resolved with antibiotics; however, he has now developed pain and distension associated with narrowing of the lumen in the sigmoid colon
D. A 66-year-old woman with 5 prior episodes of diverticulitis managed successfully with bowel rest and antibiotics

ANSWERS

28.1 **A.** The patient clinically has diverticulitis and is unable to maintain oral hydration. He should be admitted to the hospital. Surgery is not indicated at this point for a patient his age with his first episode of uncomplicated diverticulitis.

28.2 **C.** The patient clinically has evidence of a complete bowel obstruction, and the tenderness and leukocytosis are worrisome. Surgical exploration is therefore warranted. A barium enema and colonoscopy are contraindicated in this situation.

28.3 **D.** The CT scan can be used to confirm the diagnosis of a colovesical fistula and to localize the fistulous tract. Urinalysis will be unhelpful, since there will be bacteria in the bladder. The IVP will not likely be helpful since there is no ureteral injury.

28.4 **E.** The most common cause of gastrointestinal tract fistulas is diverticulitis, usually causing a colovesical (colon-to-bladder) fistula. Air or stool in the urine or frequent urinary tract infections are typical.

28.5 **D.** Risk-benefit analysis has demonstrated that surgery benefits outweigh the risks when colectomy is performed after the 4th bout of diverticulitis; however, any decision for surgery also must take into account of the patient's life expectancy and overall fitness to undergo operative intervention. Young age is no longer considered an indication for colectomy in diverticulitis treatment. Follow-up of patients with uncomplicated diverticulitis suggest that only 13% of patients would ultimately require surgery, therefore medical treatment is highly successful in these patients.

Clinical Pearls

- CT imaging is often helpful in identifying and guiding percutaneous drainage of abscesses related to diverticulitis.
- Diverticulitis is the most common cause of gastrointestinal tract fistulas.
- Surgical intervention for uncomplicated diverticulitis is safe and cost-effective when applied in patients with 4 or more episodes of uncomplicated diverticulitis.
- Complicated diverticulitis such as perforation or fistula is usually treated surgically.

REFERENCES

Dixon MR, Trudel JL. Diverticular disease of the colon. In: Cameron JL, ed. *Current Surgical Therapy*, 9th ed. Philadelphia: Mosby Elsevier, 2008:166-170.

Fry RD, Mahmoud N, Maron DJ, Ross HM, Rombeau J. Colon and rectum. In: Townsend CM, Beauchamp RD, Evers BM, Mattox KL, eds. *Textbook of Surgery*. 18th ed. Philadelphia, PA: Saunders Elsevier; 2008:1348-1432.

Case 29

During a routine physical examination, a family physician identifies an asymptomatic pulsatile abdominal mass in a 62-year-old man. The ultrasound evaluation that followed demonstrated a 4.2-cm aneurysm in the infrarenal aorta. This patient is subsequently referred to you for evaluation and management. His past medical history is significant for hypertension and stable angina. He has a history of 40 pack-year of cigarette smoking. His current medications include aspirin, a β-blocker, and nitrates. The patient describes himself as an active man who is retired and plays 18 holes of golf twice a week. On examination, the carotid pulses and upper extremity pulses are found to be normal. The abdomen is nontender with a prominent aortic pulsation. Pulses in the femoral and popliteal regions are easily palpated and appear more prominent than usual.

- What are the complications associated with this disease process?
- What is the best treatment?

ANSWERS TO CASE 29:
Abdominal Aortic Aneurysm

Summary: A 62-year-old reasonably healthy man presents with an asymptomatic 4.2-cm abdominal aortic aneurysm (AAA).

- **Complications:** Rupture, thrombosis, distal embolism, and other peripheral aneurysms.
- **Best treatment:** The best treatment for this patient is debatable. The risk of complications from the aneurysm must be weighed against the risk of surgical or endovascular intervention.

ANALYSIS

Objectives

1. Learn the presentation, evaluation, treatment, and follow-up of patients with aneurysms.
2. Learn the risks and outcomes associated with elective open aneurysm repair, elective endovascular repair, and the repair of ruptured aneurysms.

Considerations

A relatively healthy 62-year-old man presenting with a 4.2-cm AAA can be observed with serial examinations and repeated ultrasonography or undergo elective aneurysm repair. The risks and benefits of the options must be discussed with the patient. If the patient wishes to undergo elective repair, a thorough evaluation to assess other comorbidities should be undertaken. Two large randomized controlled clinical trials have been compared surveillance versus prophylactic surgery for patients with asymptomatic AAA less than 5.5 cm, and both trials demonstrated no advantages to prophylactic repairs; the only limitation to these trials was that relatively few women were included in these trials.

APPROACH TO
Abdominal Aortic Aneurysm

CLINICAL APPROACH

More than 95% of AAAs develop as complications of atherosclerosis, and more than 90% are infrarenal. Many are found asymptomatically, but some can cause distal emboli or pain. Others are found in association with other peripheral (ie, popliteal and femoral) aneurysms. The majority of AAAs are detected asymptomatically. An AAA is a disease where size matters. Because of the relationship between AAA size and the risk of rupture, the maximal diameter is an important discriminant in assessment and management. The law of Laplace (wall tension is proportional to the square of the radius and the inverse of wall thickness) provides the physics behind the pathophysiology of AAA rupture. **The rupture rate for asymptomatic aneurysms less than 5 cm is 0.6% per year. Once an AAA reaches 5 cm in diameter, the risk of rupture is 5% to 10% per year.** At 6 cm it rises to 10% to 20% per year, and at 7 cm the rupture risk is 20% to 30% per year.

Surgical risk of patients for aneurysm repair can be stratified based on patient age, functional status, cardiac risk, pulmonary risk, renal risk, and other systemic illnesses (liver disease, malignancies, diabetes). Patients can be stratified as low, intermediate, or high risk based on these factors. Risk modification strategies including the initiation of perioperative β-blocker and statin therapy may be considered appropriate in addition to lifestyle modifications, such as smoking cessation. High-risk individuals with AAAs should be referred to a vascular surgery specialist for consideration of endovascular repair.

Repair of a ruptured AAA can be attempted in only half of patients because others never reach the hospital alive. Even today, 40% to 60% of patients with a ruptured AAA do not survive emergency surgery. Because good-risk patients have a mortality rate of 1% to 3% when undergoing elective surgery, the **usual criterion for recommending repair is when an AAA reaches 5.5 cm in men and 5.0 cm in women.** However, as AAAs arise in patients with atherosclerosis, there is a significant association with other risks and comorbidities that can complicate repair. **Cardiac complications remain the most common cause of perioperative morbidity and mortality.**

AAAs found on routine examination should have their size confirmed by an imaging study. Ultrasound is inexpensive and safe but not as reproducible over time. Computed tomography scanning requires radiation exposure but can give enough information to assess suitability for endovascular aneurysm repair (EVAR) or conventional open surgery. Arteriography cannot diagnose an AAA because it only delineates the lumen of a vessel. However, a preoperative angiogram helps in operative planning for both EVAR and open repairs. Open repair has withstood the test of time and remains the standard of care. However, patients with a higher risk for open repair complications (severe coronary artery disease, chronic obstructive pulmonary disease, obesity, malignancy, adhesions, and others) can be offered protection from rupture with EVAR. One must realize that EVAR currently has a risk of rupture of 0.7% to 1.0% per year (according to the EUROSTAR Registry). In addition, because of technical issues in EVAR, following EVAR the patient requires intensive imaging follow-up every 3 to 6 months. Because of associated risk profiles, the ultimate perioperative patient mortality for EVAR is still in the 2% to 3% range. **The actual recommendation for EVAR versus open AAA repair should be made by a trained vascular specialist well versed in both techniques.**

For a patient who presents with AAA rupture (back pain, hypotension, and a pulsatile epigastric mass), operative open repair is the most available and most potentially life-saving therapy. If AAA rupture is clinically suspected, the patient should undergo emergent operative repair. There is no role for radiologic imaging if the clinical impression is a ruptured AAA—the delay involved in obtaining imaging is too risky for the patient as compared to a potentially negative exploration.

Comprehension Questions

29.1 A 58-year-old man is found on physical examination to have an AAA. He has no symptoms. Ultrasound reveals that it is 4 cm in diameter. Which of the following is considered appropriate surveillance for this patient?

A. Observation with yearly ultrasound
B. Percutaneous graft replacement
C. Angiography every 6 months
D. Aortofemoral bypass surgery

29.2 In which of the following conditions is conservative management indicated in the patient described at the beginning of the case?

A. Presenting 11 months later with an AAA that is 5.5 cm in size
B. Unexplained back pain in a 4.2-cm aneurysm and normotensive
C. Bilateral embolization to all his toes
D. Presenting 3 years later with shock and severe abdominal pain
E. AAA is 4.3 cm on ultrasound 2 years later

29.3 Which of the following is a complication associated with abdominal aortic aneurysms?

A. Early satiety
B. Colonic obstruction
C. Painful discoloration of the great toe
D. Hematuria

29.4 Which of the following statement is most accurate regarding endosvascular aneurysm repair (EVAR)?

A. EVAR requires more intensive postprocedural follow-up than open repairs.
B. Perioperative complications associated with EVAR and open repairs are identical.
C. EVAR is an inferior approach for patients with prior intra-abdominal operations.
D. EVAR application is no longer indicated based on its complication profile.

29.5 For which of the following patients is nonoperative management most appropriate?

A. A 63-year-old petite woman with an asymptomatic 5.2 cm AAA

B. A 96-year-old man with severe dementia and an 6-cm AAA. The patient has been a long-term resident of a chronic care facility due to the inability to ambulate or perform activities of daily living

C. A 63-year-old man with a 5.3-cm AAA who has developed unexplainable back pain and abdominal pain over the past several days

D. A 61-year-old man with a 5.3 cm AAA and recent onset of pain and echemosis in the tips of several of his toes on both feet

ANSWERS

29.1 **D.** Yearly ultrasound is part of conservative protocol for the follow-up of patients with AAA. The choice of ultrasound or CT for the imaging depends on which is more available in one's practice environment.

29.2 **E.** The patient in D is presenting with a rupture. The patient in B is the most controversial candidate for operative repair; however, if a complete workup cannot find another cause of back pain, the AAA must be implicated and strong recommendations for repair should be made.

29.3. **D.** Most AAAs are asymptomatic. Patients may have abdominal discomfort or back pain. Rarely, aneurysmal erosion into a ureter may be seen, leading to gross hematuria. Rupture should be suspected with increasing abdominal or back pain with hypotension. Mortality exceeds 50% with AAA rupture. Ischemia of the lower extremity may occur, but will involve more than the great toe.

29.4 **A.** EVAR is an approach that is associated with lower perioperative cardiopulmonary complications in comparison to open aneurysm repairs; however, as the result of continued enlargement of the aorta and migration of the device, leakage around the device can occur following EVAR. With appropriate surveillance, endoleaks are often successfully managed with minimal risk of mortality from rupture. EVAR offers advantages over open repair especially in patients with potential "hostile abdomen" from prior abdominal operations or other unrelated intra-abdominal pathology.

29.5 **B.** The risk of rupture with his 6-cm AAA is approximately 10-20% per year and EVAR may offer protection against rupture and may improve the longevity of this patient. However, in this individual with advanced age and an extremely poor quality of life, a prophylactic operation to extend his life presents a difficult ethical dilemma. Performing an expensive intervention to prolong the life of this individual also constitutes poor allocation of medical resources. The patient described in choice "A" fits the size criteria for elective repair. The presentation of patient in choice "C" suggests symptoms related to his aneurysm which could indicate increased risk of rupture. The patient presentation in choice "D" is consistent with embolic disease associated with AAA, or the "blue toe syndrome".

Clinical Pearls

- Patient diagnosed with an AAA should have a thorough pulse examination to look for associated aneurysms in the periphery and/or concomitant occlusive disease.
- AAAs are palpated in the epigastrium; iliac aneurysms, in the infraumbilical position.
- A AAA $\geq$5.5 cm in a man and $\geq$5.0 cm in a woman are at increased risk for rupture and should be considered for elective repair.
- In the case of a suspected rupture, negative laparotomy findings are much better than delay in control of the AAA in the operating room.

REFERENCES

Curi MA, Rubin BG. Abdominal aortic aneurysm: open repair. In: Cameron JL, ed. *Current Surgical Therapy*. 9th ed. Philadelphia, PA: Mosby Elsevier; 2008;731-736.

Malas MB. Endovascular treatment of abdominal aortic aneurysm. In: Cameron JL, ed. *Current Surgical Therapy*. 9th ed. Philadelphia, PA: Mosby Elsevier; 2008;736-742.

Case 30

A 44-year-old woman is admitted to the ICU 1 hour after having undergone a 3-hour abdominal operation for the debridement of infected necrotizing pancreatitis. The operation apparently resulted in 3500 mL of blood loss. She received approximately 4000 mL of crystalloid and 2 U packed red blood cell (PRBC) replacement during the operation. Prior to the procedure, the patient had been receiving Imipenem and fluconazole for gram-negative bacteremia and fungemia. The patient's skin appears cool and mottled. She is intubated and ventilated. Her vital signs are pulse 115 beats/min, blood pressure 85/60 mm Hg, and temperature 35.5°C (95.9°F). Her breath sounds are present bilaterally and her abdomen is soft and distended. A chest radiograph reveals bibasilar atelectasis. Electrocardiogram (ECG) reveals sinus tachycardia. Complete blood count reveals WBC 24,000/mm^3, hemoglobin 12 g/dL, and hematocrit 40%.

➤ What are the likely causes of this patient's low blood pressure?

➤ What should be the next steps in this patient's management?

➤ What are the best methods to provide ongoing assessment of this patient's condition?

ANSWERS TO CASE 30:
The hypotensive patient

Summary: A 44-year-old woman has recently undergone a 3-hour abdominal operation for the debridement of infected necrotizing pancreatitis and lost 3500 mL of blood. She received 4000 mL of crystalloid and 2 U PRBC during the operation. The patient had been receiving Imipenem and fluconazole for gram-negative bacteremia and fungemia. She has poor skin perfusion, tachycardia, and hypotension.

- **Likely causes of low blood pressure**: Combined effects of inadequate resuscitation of blood loss and sepsis.
- **Next steps in management:** Fluid resuscitation. Consider blood transfusion if patient is a transient responder.
- **Best methods to provide ongoing assessment:** Place central venous pressure (CVP) monitor and arterial catheter for continuous blood pressure monitoring; consider echo/pulmonary artery (PA) catheter placement to assess ventricular function or cardiac output; consider uncontrolled ongoing surgical blood loss if the patient fails to respond to resuscitation.

ANALYSIS

Objectives

1. Recognize the presence and severity of hemorrhagic shock and understand the principles of early treatment.
2. Be able to describe the causes and treatment of postoperative hypotension.
3. Understand the principles of resuscitation, infection source control, and metabolic support for patients with sepsis.

Considerations

This patient is exhibiting concerning signs of inadequate tissue perfusion with mottling and coolness of her extremities. Given her current situation, she likely has underresuscitation of volume. In general, each unit of PRBC contains 250 to 300 mL in volume. One of the deceptive factors that can lead to underreplacement of blood loss is that because of the Starling forces dictated by osmotic and hydraulic pressures in the microvascular circulation, only a fraction of crystalloid fluids infused remains in the intravascular space, and in this patient, the so-called normal amount of fluid egress is further accentuated by pathological microvascular leakage associated with systemic inflammation and infection. A concerning factor in this patient's case is the extremely bloody nature of her procedure that raises our clinical suspicion for potential inadequate control of intra-abdominal bleeding sources. To make matters even more complex, this patient has symptoms consistent with systemic infection such as leukocytosis, hypothermia, and a known history of gram-negative bacteremia and fungemia, therefore implicating sepsis as another potential cause of shock.

The initial approach is to begin resuscitation with crystalloid fluids and simultaneously begin close monitoring of response to resuscitative efforts. The patient's clinical picture, including mentation, urine output, and peripheral circulation, should be assessed. In addition, CVP monitoring would be helpful to guide our endpoint of intravascular volume replacement. Because the primary therapeutic goals are to minimize the degree and duration of shock and correct the underlying cause, aggressive resuscitation should accompany diagnostic workup. In most cases, the initial approach to resuscitation for hypotension is to give crystalloid fluids (eg, normal saline, lactated Ringer's). This will begin to stabilize the patient as the workup proceeds. Because this patient is clearly compromised physiologically and has a known history of systemic infection, it is important to bear in mind that uncontrolled infection could be a cause of the clinical picture; therefore, it would not be unreasonable to broaden her antimicrobial coverage after having obtained blood cultures. In this case, vancomycin should be considered preemptive coverage for resistant strains of gram-positive microbes.

APPROACH TO The Hypotensive Patient

DEFINITIONS

SHOCK: An acute clinical syndrome initiated by ineffective perfusion, resulting in injury and dysfunction in various organs systemically.

CENTRAL VENOUS CATHETER: An intravenous catheter of adequate length to measure pressures in the superior vena cava when placed via internal jugular vein or subclavian vein.

ECHOCARDIOGRAPHY: Ultrasonography that evaluates ventricular function, distension (or collapse) of the vena cava, and right heart. An experienced echocardiographer can also often accurately estimate the presence of pulmonary hypertension.

LACTATE: When this end product of anaerobic metabolism is elevated, it suggests a global deficit in oxygen delivery.

PA CATHETER: A catheter capable of measuring venous pressures that is placed in the pulmonary artery. The pressure measured when inflow is blocked (by an inflated balloon) is extrapolated to be equal to the right atrial pressures because normally pulmonary vascular resistance is very low. This catheter can also measure cardiac output by the thermodilution method, thus permitting the clinician to track cardiac performance and response to interventions. Despite the theoretical advantages of PA catheter for the direction of perioperative care in the high-risk population, observations from the Canadian randomized controlled trial did not demonstrate benefits related to PA catheter-directed therapy.

Note: This extrapolated number and unsure nature of intravascular/intrathoracic pressures are two of the many drawbacks to routine use of the PA catheter.

CLINICAL APPROACH

Hypotension leading to shock can result from decreased intravascular volume, intrinsic cardiac pump dysfunction, and/or acute vasodilation without a concomitant increase of intravascular volume. **Persistent hypotension** results in lack of perfusion to organ systems and can lead to **multiorgan system dysfunction and organ failure.** A systematic approach is mandatory to minimize the length of time of the patient who is in shock. Consider the hemodynamic system as an arrangement of pump, pipes, and fluid. All components of this system must be intact to maintain perfusion. Malfunction of individual components or a mixture of components may contribute to hypotension. Evaluation of a patient with postoperative hypotension should include a review of the pertinent history, a careful physical examination, vital signs and urine output, and review of administered medications.

Table 30–1 lists the differential diagnoses of common causes of hypotension in the perioperative period.

Diagnosis

Central venous monitoring or **cardiac echocardiogram** can provide valuable information concerning hypotension and help guide efforts at fluid resuscitation when the clinical picture is unclear; however, these diagnostic maneuvers should not be used to replace one's clinical judgment. In a patient with previously normal renal function, urine output is often a reliable indicator of adequate resuscitation. Potential drawbacks of using urine output as the major endpoint of resuscitation may occur in hyperglycemic patients with falsely high urine output caused by glucose spillage in the urine, and the patient who may develop low urine output from acute renal insufficiency following severe or prolonged shock.

Table 30–1 CLASSIFICATION OF SHOCK

CLASSIFICATION OF SHOCK	ETIOLOGIES
Hypovolemic	Hemorrhage Dehydration
Distributive	Sepsis Neurogenic Anaphylaxis Medications
Cardiac: Intrinsic	Acute coronary syndrome Cardiomyopathy
Cardiac: Extrinsic	Cardiac tamponade Tension pneumothorax Massive pulmonary embolus
Mixed	Any combination of one or more of the above

Monitoring and measurements of resuscitation endpoints include

- Foley catheter
- Central venous catheter for frequent CVP measurements
- Arterial catheter for continuous blood pressure monitoring (preferred) or *frequent* noninvasive blood pressure measurements
- Serial hemoglobin measurements
- Serial arterial blood gases (ABGs) for trends in lactate level or base deficit

Note: Early hemoglobin levels may not reflect active hemorrhage prior to the dilutional effect of crystalloid resuscitation.

Hypovolemia

Patients who respond initially to crystalloid resuscitation but then have a subsequent drop in arterial blood pressure may have **ongoing surgical bleeding.** An alternative cause is microvascular leak from systemic inflammatory mediators. In comparison to actively bleeding patients, those with microvascular leak syndrome show a more gradual decrease in blood pressure. In the setting in which hemorrhage is suspected and crystalloid only stabilizes the patient transiently, transfusion with PRBC is advised. In patients suspected of hemorrhage, a **coagulation profile** consisting of international normalized ratio (INR), partial thromboplastin time (PTT), and platelets should be checked to rule out nonsurgical sources of bleeding. Once the coagulopathies are corrected, reexploration may be necessary to address persistent surgical bleeding.

Distributive

Often the patient's recent medical history suggests possible etiologies of hypotension. A thorough history and clinical examination will direct appropriate workups. **Distributive causes** for hypotension include any condition that causes **acute vasodilation** of the vascular space. This increase in the capacity of this vast network of vessels without a concomitant increase in intravascular fluid results in hypotension. The initial treatment for distributive shock involves fluid resuscitation to fill the increased volume of the vascular pool. Once this has begun, application of vasoconstrictive agents may be necessary to maintain a balance of normovolemia and pharmacologic vascular tone. If the etiology of the distributive shock is sepsis, treatment of the underlying infection with "source control" should accompany aggressive resuscitation. This may include broad-spectrum antimicrobial therapy and operative intervention to stabilize the systemic repercussions of infection.

Medications may also induce vasodilation. In a patient with mild to moderate hypovolemia, iatrogenic vasodilation with vasodilatory drugs can result in profound hypotension. It is important to remember that some drugs used for sedation, analgesia, and induction of anesthesia are vasodilators. Less commonly, anaphylaxis can accompany medication or blood product infusions. Hemodynamic support with epinephrine is often needed in acute anaphylactic shock.

Acute injury to the cervical or upper thoracic spinal cord can result in the loss of autonomic tone and produce acute hypotension (neurogenic shock). A hallmark of this type of hypotension is a normal or low heart rate in someone who is not on β-blockers.

Cardiogenic: Intrinsic and Extrinsic

Intrinsic conditions may include **cardiogenic shock** related to acute coronary syndrome in someone with preexisting cardiac disease. Conversely, classic extrinsic causes of cardiac function include tension pneumothorax that results in compression of the vena cava and right heart by a unilateral increasing intrathoracic pressure and shifting of the mediastinum away from the affected side. Another extrinsic cause is cardiac tamponade that limits right heart filling by compressing the thin-walled right ventricle and shifting the septum toward the more robust left ventricle, thus decreasing left ventricular end diastolic volume.

Mixed

A patient's history and physical examination often suggest a primary diagnosis for hypotension and shock. There are patients, however, who present with combinations of causes for their hypotension. These patients can be a diagnostic dilemma and require more invasive methods for determining the source and management of their shock.

The PA catheter is an instrument that can give additional information in situations in which pump dysfunction is contributing to hypovolemic or septic shock. It may also prove beneficial in patients with acute renal failure where urine output cannot be used as an indication of normovolemia.

Therapy

Restore oxygen delivery! This can be approached from the basic pump, pipes, fluid algorithm. First, there has to be adequate fluid in the system for perfusion. If vasodilation is contributing to a perceived hypovolemia in the presence of adequate fluid resuscitation, then and only then should vasoconstrictive agents (eg, norepinephrine, dopamine, Neo-Synephrine, epinephrine, vasopressin) be considered. The specific etiology of the vasodilation will help determine which agent is most appropriate. If the primary problem is an intrinsic pump problem, augmentation of preload with gentle fluid resuscitation and addition of an inotrope may be the first step to stabilization. If there is an external pump problem such as tension pneumothorax or cardiac tamponade, these should be quickly decompressed with thoracostomy tube for the former and pericardiocentesis for the latter. If the etiology is mixed, a combination of the modalities just described may be needed. For these complex patients, a PA catheter may give the additional information needed to fine-tune diagnosis and management (see Table 30–2).

Table 30–2 HEMODYNAMIC VARIABLES IN DIFFERENT SHOCK STATES

SHOCK STATE	CARDIAC INDEX	SYSTEMIC VASCULAR RESISTANCE	PULMONARY CAPILLARY WEDGE PRESSURE	PRIME MOVER*
Normal	2.4-3.0 L/min/m^2	800-1200 dyne-s *or* dyne-s/cm^5	8-12 mm Hg	Not applicable
Distributive (sepsis, neurogenic, anaphylaxis)	Elevated	Decreased (because of decreased vascular tone)	Low to normal	Decreased vascular tone
Cardiogenic (myocardial infarction, cardiomyopathy)	Decreased	Increased	Increased	Decreased cardiac contractility
Hypovolemic (hemorrhage, dehydration)	Decreased (because of decreased volume)	Increased (to attempt to maintain blood pressure)	Decreased	Decreased preload
Obstructive (tamponade, tension pneumothorax, pulmonary embolus)	Decreased	Increased	Normal to increased flow	Obstruction of blood flow

*The prime mover is the initial pathophysiologic change; this change then causes compensatory changes in other variables.

Comprehension Questions

30.1 A 65-year-old man is noted to have a blood pressure of 90/62 mm Hg on the evening after an uncomplicated small bowel resection of obstruction. His heart rate is 110 beats/min, respiratory rate 24 breaths/min, and temperature 37.4°C (99.3°F); urine output only 20 mL over 2 hours and oxygen saturation by pulse oximetry 95%. His preoperative hemoglobin level was 12.6 g/dL. Which of the following statements is most accurate regarding this patient?

A. A hemoglobin level performed in the recovery room after surgery of 12.4 g/dL is good evidence against active hemorrhage.
B. Intravenous furosemide (Lasix) should be administered.
C. This patient is most likely affected by anxiety and a mild anxiolytic and careful observation should be initiated.
D. Initial therapy should be intravenous crystalloid fluid bolus.

30.2 A 56-year-old woman is admitted to the intensive care unit (ICU) for ventilator management after an AAA repair. The patient is noted to have a urine output of 20 mL over 3 hours. Her blood pressure is 100/55 mm Hg, heart rate 110 beats/min, and temperature 35.6°C (96.1°F). Her serum troponin levels are elevated. Which of the following is the most likely diagnosis?

A. Intra-abdominal hemorrhage
B. Renal insufficiency
C. Myocardial infarction
D. Postsurgical hypothermia

30.3 A 51-year-old woman has undergone an open elective cholecystectomy 5 days previously. She has fever of 1-day duration and complains of shortness of breath and cough. Her pulse rate is 120 beats/min, temperature 39.5°C (103.1°F), respiratory rate 46 breaths/min, blood pressure 110/70 mm Hg, and O_2 saturation level 89% on 60% O_2 by face mask. She has crackles in the left lung base and her leukocyte count is 17,000 cells/mm^3. Her chest radiograph shows left lower lobe subsegmental infiltrate. Which of the following is correct regarding this patient's care?

A. A higher FIO_2 should be avoided so oxygen toxicity is avoided.
B. Intravenous streptokinase for pulmonary embolus should be initiated.
C. Mechanical ventilation and transfer to the ICU is indicated.
D. A perinephric abscess is the most likely diagnosis.

30.4 Which of the following statements regarding fluid resuscitation is most accurate regarding volume repletion?

A. PRBC should be transfused when hemoglobin values are less than 12 g/dL.
B. Colloid resuscitation is preferable to crystalloid resuscitation in patients with acute blood loss.
C. At equilibrium, approximately a third of administered crystalloid remains in the intravascular space.
D. Hetastarch distributes to the extracellular space at equilibrium.

30.5 Which of the following statements best describes the difference between distributive shock and hemorrhagic shock?

A. Distributive shock requires treatment with vasoconstrictive agents only while hemorrhagic shock is treated with volume repletion.
B. The transfusion of blood products improves hemorrhagic shock but is not indicated in distributive shock.
C. Both processes produce low urine output, but only hemorrhagic shock produces prerenal azotemia.
D. Central venous pressure measurement allows for the differentiation between distributive shock and hemorrhagic shock.

ANSWERS

30.1 **D.** This patient has hypotension, tachycardia, tachypnea, and low urine output following surgery. These are indicators of volume depletion. A normal hemoglobin level acutely does not accurately reflect volume status. The initial treatment should be intravenous cystalloid fluid resuscitation.

30.2 **C.** Other causes are possible, however. The serum troponin elevation is highly suggestive of myocardial infarction. A 12-lead ECG and echocardiography should be obtained as adjunctive studies, which may provide valuable information to help direct subsequent fluid and pharmacologic therapy.

30.3 **C.** This patient has significant hypoxemia and tachypnea despite high levels of oxygen; this portends the possible need for mechanical ventilation. The differential diagnosis includes subphrenic abscess, postoperative pneumonia, and pulmonary embolism. Intravenous heparin (and not intravenous streptokinase) would be the treatment in pulmonary embolism.

30.4 **C.** At equilibrium, only a third of isotonic crystalloid remains in the intravascular space; thus, 3 mL of crystalloids is usually infused for every 1 mL of blood lost. No clinical or laboratory evidence indicates an advantage of colloid over crystalloid for acute blood loss resuscitation. Hetastarch is a colloid solution and tends to remain in the intravascular space at equilibrium.

30.5 **B.** Transfusion of blood products helps replace the loss of volume, oxygen-carrying capacity, and clotting capacity associated with the blood loss due to hemorrhagic shock. Blood products administration may help improve the vital signs in patients with distributive shock based on the volume of the blood product, but in general, this is not the best method of addressing the volume depletion; intravenous crystalloid and/or vasopressor agents are the best treatment for distributive shock. Blood products should not be administered only for the purpose of volume resuscitation.

Clinical Pearls

- The **initial therapy** for hypotension in most patients in whom sepsis is suspected should be aggressive fluid resuscitation—**not vasopressors!**
- Source control in patients with a surgical infection frequently requires appropriate procedures to control infection (eg, drainage, debridement, bowel resection). For these types of patients, antibiotics alone **are not** usually adequate for source control.
- Clinical measures of perfusion status are adequate in most patients for determination of the adequacy of resuscitation.
- Invasive monitoring using pulmonary artery catheterization should be considered when patients do not respond appropriately to initial therapy with stabilization of organ function and vital signs.
- Do not be falsely reassured by a normal hemoglobin value in hypotensive surgical patients: They bleed whole blood!
- Patients under 30 years of age with a good cardiac reserve and patients on β-blockers may not exhibit the expected tachycardia response to hemorrhage until late in the course of shock.

REFERENCES

Dunn DL, Beilman GJ. Surgical infections. In: Brunicardi FC, Andersen DK, Billiar TR, et al, eds. *Schwartz's Principles of Surgery*. 8th ed. New York, NY: McGraw-Hill; 2005:109-127.

Peitzman AB, Harbrecht BG, Billiar TR. Shock. In: Brunicardi FC, Andersen DK, Billiar TR, et al, eds. *Schwartz's Principles of Surgery*. 8th ed. New York, NY: McGraw-Hill; 2005:85-107.

Sandham JD, Hull RD, Brant RF, et al. A Randomized, Controlled trial of the use of pulmonary-artery catheters in high-risk surgical patients. *N Eng J Med* 2003;348:5-14.

Case 31

A 26-year-old man is seen in the emergency department for abdominal pain that began after returning home from a party where he consumed pizza and eight beers. The pain is constant, located in the upper part of his abdomen, and radiates to his back. Approximately 3 to 4 hours after onset of the pain, the patient vomited a large amount of undigested food, but the emesis did not resolve his pain. His past medical history is unremarkable, and he consumes alcohol only during the weekends when he attends parties with his friends. On examination, the patient appears uncomfortable. His temperature is 38.8°C (101.8°F), heart rate 110 beats/min, blood pressure 110/60 mm Hg, and respiratory rate 28 breaths/min. The abdomen is distended and tender to palpation in the epigastric and periumbilical areas. Laboratory studies reveal a WBC count of 18,000/mm^3, hemoglobin 17 g/dL, hematocrit 47%, glucose 210 mg/dL, total bilirubin 3.2 mg/dL, AST 380 U/L, ALT 435 U/L, lactose dehydrogenase (LDH) 300 U/L, serum amylase 6800 IU/L. Arterial blood gas studies (room air) reveal pH 7.38, $Paco_2$ 33 mm Hg, Pao_2 68 mm Hg, and HCO_3 21 mEq/L. Chest radiography reveals the presence of a small pleural effusion.

- What is the most likely diagnosis?
- What are your next steps?
- What are the complications associated with this disease process?

ANSWERS TO CASE 31:
Pancreatitis (Acute)

Summary: A 26-year-old man presents with acute nausea and vomiting and abdominal pain radiating to the back following binge drinking. The clinical presentation of fever, leukocytosis, hemoconcentration, elevated amylase level, and hypoxemia suggests severe acute pancreatitis.

- **Most likely diagnosis:** Acute pancreatitis.
- **Next steps:** Resuscitative measures including administration of supplemental oxygen and intravenous fluids.
- **Complications of the disease:** Acute pancreatitis can cause local complications including hemorrhage, necrosis, fluid collection, and infection. Pancreatitis may also lead to systemic complications such as pulmonary, cardiac, and renal dysfunction.

ANALYSIS

Objectives

1. Be familiar with the diagnosis and initial treatment of patients with acute pancreatitis.
2. Recognize the value and limitations of clinical prognosticators and CT scans in evaluating patients with acute pancreatitis.
3. Understand the diagnosis and management of the regional and systemic complications of acute pancreatitis.

Considerations

This patient, with a history of alcohol consumption and the sudden onset of abdominal and back pain, likely has acute alcoholic pancreatitis. This diagnosis is further supported by findings from the patient's physical examination and the elevated serum amylase level. **The amylase level is helpful for diagnosis but does not correlate with the severity of the disease.** The patient's fever, tachypnea, and hyperdynamic state are caused by the systemic inflammation related to acute pancreatitis. The presence of three of the Ranson criteria (WBC, LDH, and AST measurements) and initial radiographic evidence of pleural effusion indicate a severe process. Based on these initial findings, close monitoring of the patient's cardiopulmonary status in an ICU and a CT scan of his abdomen to assess the pancreas for evidence of necrosis may be appropriate. During the ICU stay, the patient is monitored for signs of distant organ dysfunction, including respiratory insufficiency (PaO_2/FIO_2), renal insufficiency (urine output and serum creatinine), cardiac dysfunction (blood pressure, pressor requirement), and neurologic dysfunction (GCS). Patients with severe pancreatitis experience severe catabolism leading to rapid loss of lean body mass, therefore nutritional support should be considered and initiated early to counterbalance this effect. For most patients, intragastric or enteral nutritional support can be initiated as soon as initial resuscitation for shock is completed.

APPROACH TO Acute Pancreatitis

DEFINITIONS

INFECTED PANCREATIC NECROSIS: An infectious complication with necrotic pancreas and peripancreatic tissue, which is most frequently caused by secondary infection by bowel-derived microorganisms within the first few weeks of onset. Antibiotic prophylaxis may be beneficial in preventing this complication, and operative debridement is indicated in managing this process.

PANCREATIC ABSCESS: Secondary infection of the pancreas and peripancreatic fluid collection. This condition is usually encountered at 3 to 6 weeks after the onset of severe pancreatitis and is recognized by the accumulation of thick, purulent fluid and infected debris. Surgical drainage is generally indicated in treating this condition.

INFECTED PANCREATIC PSEUDOCYST: Usually a late process that occurs several weeks or months after the onset of severe pancreatitis. This process usually occurs ≥6 weeks following the onset of severe pancreatitis and can be adequately treated by percutaneous drainage.

CLINICAL APPROACH

In North America and Europe, **the most common etiologies of acute pancreatitis are gallstones and alcohol consumption.** Acute pancreatitis should be diagnosed early because it may alter the management of the disease. The diagnosis is based on the history and typical clinical presentation of severe epigastric pain that radiates to the back, nausea, vomiting, and fever. Serum amylase and lipase levels confirm the diagnosis in patients with the symptoms just listed, but by themselves they are not diagnostic because they can be elevated in other pathologic conditions.

The severity of acute pancreatitis ranges from mild and self-limited (85% of cases) to severe and complicated (15% of cases). Mild pancreatitis is characterized by edema of the pancreas and rarely proceeds to necrosis or infection. Severe pancreatitis is characterized by necrosis of the pancreas and may be complicated by infection in approximately 50% of cases. Furthermore, severe pancreatitis is associated with increased microvascular permeability, leading to large volume losses of intravascular fluid into the tissues, thereby decreasing perfusion of the lungs, kidneys, and other organs. **The most important element in preventing multiple organ failure is fluid resuscitation and intensive monitoring.** Much current investigation has focused on the systemic inflammatory response syndrome and multiple organ failure during pancreatitis.

Prognostic Criteria

Several prognostic systems have been developed to differentiate between mild and severe pancreatitis. The most widely used system is the Ranson criteria (Table 31–1), which include five parameters determined at the time of admission and six parameters determined during the subsequent 48 hours. The Ranson criteria attempt to reflect the severity of the retroperitoneal inflammatory process, and the original purpose was to help predict patient outcome. **Patients with three or more Ranson criteria have more severe disease and an increased risk of complications and death; however, with current improvements in patient care, the high-mortality rates identified by the investigators are no longer applicable.** Although helpful in the diagnosis, serum amylase and lipase levels do not correlate with the severity of pancreatitis. Other prognostic systems such as APACHE II and C-reactive protein levels have similar sensitivity and specificity compared to the Ranson criteria.

Computed Tomography Imaging of the Abdomen

Contrast-enhanced CT imaging of the pancreas should be performed when the diagnosis of pancreatitis is in question. In addition, patients who do not improve clinically in 3 to 5 days or who have severe pancreatitis based on the Ranson score should undergo contrast-enhanced CT scanning of the pancreas to determine the presence of necrosis. Two or more extrapancreatic fluid

Table 31–1 RANSON CRITERIA

ON ADMISSION	SUBSEQUENT 48 HOURS
White blood cell count > 16,000/mm^3	Hematocrit fall of 10%
Glucose > 200 mg/dL	Calcium < 8 mg/dL
Age > 55 y	Serum urea nitrogen increase of 5 mg/dL
Aspartate aminotransferase > 250 U/L	Fluid requirement of > 6 L
Lactate dehydrogenase > 350 U/L	Base excess of > 4 mEq/L
	Po_2 < 60 mm Hg

collections or necrosis (nonenhancement) of more than 50% of the pancreas indicates severe disease and an increased risk of complications. **Necrotizing pancreatitis is complicated by infection approximately 50% of the time, and prophylactic antibiotics should be administered when necrosis is confirmed by a CT scan.** Severe pancreatitis can lead to other complications such as hemorrhage and splenic vein thrombosis. Pancreatic abscesses and pseudocyst formation are other possible complications of acute pancreatitis.

The diagnosis of acute pancreatitis is initially a presumptive one. Patients presenting with acute abdominal symptoms require careful clinical, biochemical, and radiologic evaluations to exclude other intra-abdominal processes such as bowel obstruction, perforated viscus, and mesenteric ischemia. It is also important to determine the severity of the disease. The presence or absence of gallstones should be determined as early as possible, usually with ultrasonography. **Patients with gallstone pancreatitis require cholecystectomy once the pancreatitis has resolved.**

Treatment

The **initial treatment of acute pancreatitis is nonoperative and focuses on fluid resuscitation, pain management, maintenance of ventilation, adequate oxygenation, and renal perfusion.** Patients with severe pancreatitis should be monitored in an intensive care unit. **Gastric decompression** is indicated for patients with nausea and vomiting. Approximately **85% of patients improve** with these supportive measures. In the 15% of patients who do not improve within 3 to 5 days, a **contrast-enhanced CT scan** of the pancreas should be obtained to determine the presence of **pancreatic necrosis.** Broad-spectrum antibiotics against enteric pathogens are indicated in treating necrotizing pancreatitis. One very effective **antibiotic in penetrating** the pancreatic tissue is imipenem/cilastatin. Aggressive nutritional support and proper electrolyte replacement are also important in the successful management of patients with severe pancreatitis.

Percutaneous needle aspiration of fluid collections or necrotic areas found on CT imaging can be performed to identify the presence of infection and guide therapeutic decisions about the need for drainage. When infected pancreatic necrosis or infected fluid is present, operative debridement and drainage are indicated. Patients with sterile necrosis generally improve with nonoperative therapy including antibiotics and intensive support; however, **surgical exploration may be indicated in patients showing clinical deterioration despite appropriate nonoperative therapy.**

Patients with gallstone pancreatitis (confirmed by ultrasound) may require **endoscopic retrograde cholangiopancreatography (ERCP) if evidence of biliary obstruction persists.** The patient described in this case should undergo abdominal ultrasonography on admission, and daily serum liver function test values should be measured. If the total bilirubin level does not decrease, the patient should undergo ERCP to clear the duct of stones and to prevent biliary complications. Patients with **gallstone pancreatitis usually undergo**

cholecystectomy before discharge to prevent recurrent attacks, which occur in up to a third of patients who do not undergo cholecystectomy.

The initial nutritional support for patients with acute pancreatitis has been extensively studied. The traditional concept of acute pancreatitis was that pancreatic injury and destruction associated with the process was secondary to overstimulated acinar cell functions; therefore, resting of the pancreas was considered the mainstay of therapy. Recent evidences have shown that acinar cell stimulation does not appear to exacerbate the injury associated with pancreatitis, and that the pain that some patients with pancreatitis experience with food ingestion is not associated with worsening of the pancreatitis. Based on these recent evidences, it is appropriate to attempt oral feeding in patients with acute pancreatitis, and if the patient should develop pain, an alternate route of nutritional support (eg: postpyloric tube feeding) can be attempted.

Comprehension Questions

31.1 A 28-year-old man with a 5-day history of progressively worsening abdominal pain and nausea and vomiting is diagnosed with acute pancreatitis. Which of the following is the best treatment for this patient?

A. Observation and monitoring
B. Restriction of fluids to 80 mL/h
C. Intravenous antibiotic therapy to prevent pancreatic abscess formation
D. Hypertonic glucose solution to prevent hypoglycemia

31.2 A 42-year-old man with alcoholism has chronic pancreatitis and presents with a palpable abdominal mass. He is noted to have a slightly elevated serum amylase level. Which of the following is the most likely diagnosis?

A. Pancreatic cancer
B. Pancreatic abscess
C. Hepatic hemangioma
D. Pancreatic pseudocyst

31.3 A 65-year-old woman is hospitalized with gallstone pancreatitis and noted to have significant abdominal pain, emesis, tachycardia, and tachypnea. Her amylase level is 3100 IU/L, glucose is 120 mg/dL, and calcium level is 13 mg/dL. Which of the following is most likely to correlate with poor prognosis in disease severity?

A. The patient's age
B. The high amylase level
C. A glucose level less than 140 mg/dL
D. Hypercalcemia

31.4 A 43-year-old woman has been hospitalized for 7 days due to worsening pancreatitis. She now has developed fever and leukocytosis and is diagnosed with an infected necrotic pancreatitis. Which of the following is the most appropriate treatment option for this patient?

A. Antibiotic therapy alone
B. Percutaneous drainage
C. Surgical pancreatic debridement and drainage
D. Endoscopic drainage

ANSWERS

31.1 **A.** Observation and monitoring to determine the severity of pancreatitis, identification and treatment of local and systemic complications, fluid hydration, and parenteral analgesia are the mainstay of therapy. Antibiotic therapy does not decrease the incidence of pancreatic complications unless significant pancreas necrosis is present. Strict gycemic control is important for patients with pancreatitis to help prevent infectious complications.

31.2 **D.** Pancreatic pseudocysts are collections of fluid and necrotic tissue around the pancreas and usually resolve over several weeks to months, but they occasionally persist, necessitating surgery.

31.3 **A.** The level of the amylase or lipase does not correlate with disease severity. Hypoxemia, hypocalcemia, age more than 55 years are some of the poor prognostic factors based on Ranson criteria.

31.4 **C.** Surgical debridement and drainage are indicated in the treatment of infected pancreatic necrosis. In addition to surgical debridement, antimicrobial therapy, enteral nutritional support, and glycemic control are important adjuncts for the treatment of patients with infected pancreas necrosis. Percutaneous drainage is best reserved for the management of infected pseudocysts and some pancreatic abscesses.

Clinical Pearls

- The most important element in preventing multiple organ failure is fluid resuscitation with intensive monitoring.
- Serum amylase and lipase levels are useful in diagnosing acute pancreatitis, but these values correlate poorly with disease severity.
- Infected pancreatic necrosis and clinical deterioration in sterile necrosis are indications for operative debridement and drainage.
- The primary indications for surgery in chronic pancreatitis include intractable pain, bowel or biliary obstruction, and persistent pseudocysts.

REFERENCES

Clancy TE, Benoit EP, Ashley SW. Current management of acute pancreatitis. *J Gastrointest Surg*. 2005;9:440-452.

Eatcock FC, Chong P, Mendez N, et al. A randomized study of early nasogastric versus nasojejunal feeding in severe acute pancreatitis. *Am J Gastroenterol*. 2005;100:432-439.

Mayerle J, Simon P, Lerch MM. Medical management of acute pancreatitis. *Gastroenterol Clin N Am*. 2004;33:855-869.

Case 32

A 43-year-old woman presents with blood-tinged discharge from her right nipple. She indicates that this problem has been occurring intermittently over the past several weeks. Her past medical history is significant for hypothyroidism. She has no prior history of breast complaints. The patient is premenopausal and currently not lactating. Her medications consist of oral contraceptives and levothyroxine. On physical examination, she is found to have minimal fibrocystic changes in both breasts. There is evidence of thickening in the right retroareolar region. Small amounts of serosanguineous fluid can be expressed from the right nipple. There is no evidence of nipple discharge or a dominant mass in the left breast.

- ➤ What should be your next step?
- ➤ What is the most likley diagnosis?

ANSWERS TO CASE 32:
Nipple Discharge (Serosanguineous)

Summary: A 43-year-old premenopausal, nonlactating woman presents with unilateral nipple discharge that is serosanguineous.

- **Next step:** The examination should begin with bilateral mammography to evaluate for suspicious lesions and ultrasonography to evaluate the retroareolar thickening; a ductogram or biopsy should also be considered.
- **Most likely diagnosis:** Intraductal papilloma.

ANALYSIS

Objectives

1. Become familiar with an approach to the evaluation of nipple discharge by categorizing the condition as physiologic, pathologic, or galactorrheic.
2. Appreciate the relative cancer risks of patients presenting with nipple discharge.

Considerations

This patient's history indicates that a pathologic etiology for nipple discharge should be investigated. **Characteristics of concern include** being **spontaneous** (not produced by manipulation—patients often find the discharge on their clothing), being **bloody or blood tinged** (as opposed to milky, purulent or—as is characteristic of fibrocystic changes—yellow, brown, or green), and being **unilateral** (see Table 32–1). Although the **most common pathologic cause of bloody nipple discharge is intraductal papilloma,** prompt evaluation of this patient must be performed to exclude carcinoma. Solitary papillomas are benign and do not increase the risk of cancer; in half of all cases, they are characterized by a serous rather than a bloody discharge. **Duct ectasia (also benign) is the next most common cause of bloody nipple discharge. Carcinoma** and infection follow, with the former being one of the main reasons to pursue a diagnosis. After the history is obtained and a physical examination is completed, bilateral mammography should be performed to evaluate for suspicious lesions, and ultrasonography to evaluate the patient's retroareolar thickening. Ultrasonography can diagnose duct ectasia or further characterize the thickening and fibrocystic changes. Mammography is indicated in women older than 40 years. In this case, it can be used for both screening and diagnostic purposes. When nipple disease is suspected, such as squamous carcinoma (Bowen disease) or ductal carcinoma (Paget disease) or when a solitary mass is present, these lesions should be biopsied.

Table 32–1 DIFFERENTIAL DIAGNOSIS FOR NIPPLE DISCHARGE

DIAGNOSIS	HISTORY	TESTS*	TREATMENT
Pregnancy	Reproductive age and female. This diagnosis is the most common reason for nipple discharge. Milk can be secreted intermittently for as long as 2 y after breastfeeding, particularly with stimulation.	Pregnancy test.	Remember to consider this diagnosis in all women of reproductive age.
Infection and or mastitis or abscess	Purulent discharge; nipple is erythematous and tender.	Gram stain and culture of discharge. Complete blood count (CBC).	Antibiotics and/or drainage Antibiotics and/or drainage.
Galactorrhea secondary to pituitary adenoma	Galactorrhea of all causes is usually characterized by bilateral milky white discharge.	Prolactin level to rule out pituitary adenoma (if pregnancy is excluded). If pregnancy test results are negative, magnetic resonance imaging. (Tumors usually seen only for levels ~ 100 ng/mL†).	Treatment as per pituitary adenomas.
Galactorrhea secondary to medications	Patient taking phenothiazines, metoclopramide, oral contraceptives, α-methyldiphenylalanine, reserpine, or tricyclic antidepressants.		Change medications if possible and exclude other causes.

(*Continued*)

Table 32–1 DIFFERENTIAL DIAGNOSIS FOR NIPPLE DISCHARGE (*CONT.*)

DIAGNOSIS	HISTORY	TESTS*	TREATMENT
Galactorrhea secondary to hypothyroid	May have symptoms of hypothyroidism, but may exclude with testing.	Thyroxine and thyroid-stimulating hormone levels.	If hypothyroid, treat with appropriate medications.
Fibrocystic changes	Nodularity of breasts, often varying with menstrual cycle. May have mastodynia. Discharge can be yellow, brown, or green.	Hemoccult test. Ultrasound is helpful in delineating cystic lesions and fibroglandular tissue. Mammogram may be appropriate.	If discharge is from fibrocystic changes, observe and reassure. Consider abstention from methylxanthines (caffeine) for mastodynia. If lesion is suspicious, perform a biopsy, but otherwise, there is no increased risk of breast cancer for fibrocystic changes.
Intraductal papilloma	Usually unilateral serous or bloody discharge.	Consider ductogram. Ultrasound may be helpful during workup.	Subareolar duct excision to confirm diagnosis. No increased risk of breast cancer.
Diffuse papillomatosis	Serous rather than bloody discharge, often involves multiple ducts more distant from the nipple, and can be bilateral. Discharge can recur if entire portion of ductal system is not removed.	Ductogram to identify duct system. Needle localization following ductogram may assist in excision. Ultrasound may be helpful during workup.	Excision of involved ducts. This diagnosis is associated with an increased risk of breast cancer.

Table 32–1 DIFFERENTIAL DIAGNOSIS FOR NIPPLE DISCHARGE (*CONT.*)

DIAGNOSIS	HISTORY	TESTS*	TREATMENT
Carcinoma	Bloody or serous nipple discharge (or none), newly inverted nipple, abnormal skin changes, suspicious mass on examination or mammogram.	Prior to diagnosis, consider ductogram and ultrasound in workup, or needle localization if not palpable.	Biopsy and then treatment as per breast cancer.

*Bilateral mammograms should be obtained for the evaluation of all these diagnoses except for milky discharge related to pregnancy.

†Minor elevations in prolactin without a tumor can be caused by polycystic ovary or Cushing syndrome or can be idiopathic.

APPROACH TO Bloody Nipple Discharge

DEFINITIONS

DUCTOGRAM: A radiologic test with contrast injected into the duct causing the discharge.

INTRADUCTAL PAPILLOMA: A benign breast mass that is usually microscopic but may grow to 2 to 3 mm, often associated with spontaneous discharge from one nipple.

GALACTORRHEA: Milky breast discharge that is often related to hyperprolactinemia.

CLINICAL APPROACH

Nipple discharges are broadly categorized as physiologic and pathologic, with physiologic discharge typically being bilateral, clear, involving multiple duct orifices and occurring nonspontaneously (in other words, with stimulation or massaging of breast or nipple). Occasionally the discharge of fibrocystic changes can be difficult to delineate from old blood; however, this drainage is rarely spontaneous. A Hemoccult test can help differentiate the two. Although some advocate cytologic examination of the discharge, false-negative and false-positive results are common. Awaiting results can produce further delay and cost without providing data that would change the evaluation process. Therefore, it is reasonable to forgo cytological testing and proceed to a **ductogram.** A patient must have ongoing discharge for this test to be performed. It requires a skilled radiologist, and the patient may experience discomfort during the examination. A lesion can be identified by the presence of a filling defect (a "cutoff"), an abrupt end to the duct rather than normal confluent arborization. **An abnormal ductogram generally mandates surgical biopsy.** A ductogram can also help localize the lesion for the surgeon performing the biopsy. If the ductogram is normal, the patient can be judiciously observed for the possibility of underlying carcinoma. A dominant mass, a newly inverted nipple, skin changes, or mammographic abnormalities generally necessitate surgical biopsy.

Surgery is performed by either a partial or a complete duct excision, recognizing that complete excision will affect the patient's ability to breast-feed in the future. Undergoing the procedure in the operating room will help in the planning of the excision. The duct is cannulated with a fine lacrimal probe, which is used as a guide for excision. The injection of methylene blue dye into the duct with a fine angiocatheter may also serve as a guide in directing the excision, which is done through a circumareolar incision.

Comprehension Questions

32.1 A 35-year-old woman with two children and no previous operations has noticed increased fatigue and a whitish nipple discharge. Which of the following is the best next step?

A. Determination of the thyroid releasing hormone level
B. Imaging of the sella turcica
C. Measurement of the human chorionic gonadotropin level
D. Ultrasonography of the breasts

32.2 A 32-year-old woman is noted to have nipple discharge. She is concerned about the possible association with breast cancer. Which of the following etiologies of nipple discharge most likely increases the risk of breast cancer?

A. Fibrocystic changes
B. Diffuse papillomatosis
C. Intraductal papilloma
D. Pregnancy

32.3 A 44-year-old woman is seen by her physician for breast discharge. Blood tests and imaging tests are performed. Which of the following findings in a workup for nipple discharge must be further evaluated?

A. An ultrasonogram of the nipple showing duct ectasia
B. A ductogram with no filling defects or abnormalities
C. An ultrasonogram with fibrocystic changes and a 2-mm simple cyst
D. A prolactin level of 100 ng/mL

32.4 A 65-year-old woman who takes tricyclic antidepressants and metoclopramide has a serosanguineous discharge from her right nipple. She has no palpable masses, normal bilateral mammograms, and a right breast ultrasonogram that does not demonstrate any masses. Her ductogram shows a cutoff in an inferior lateral duct 2 cm from the right nipple. Of the following choices, which is the most appropriate approach?

A. Observation and instructions not to manipulate the nipple during self-examination
B. Changing her medications
C. Checking the prolactin level
D. Duct excisional biopsy

ANSWERS

32.1 **C.** This patient likely has galactorrhea. Although these can also be symptoms of hypothyroidism, the first step is to exclude pregnancy as an etiology.

32.2 **B.** Diffuse papillomatosis increases the risk of cancer.

32.3 **D.** A prolactin level in the range of 100 ng/mL or more is suggestive of a pituitary adenoma, whereas the other findings are benign and can be observed.

32.4 **D.** Abrupt cut-off of the ductogram is associated with breast cancer, and necessitates biopsy. Other features of ductography that are suspicious for breast cancer include multiple irregular filling defects or external compression of the duct. A ductogram that shows a well filled duct except for a solitary lobulated filling defect is more consistent with intraductal papilloma.

Clinical Pearls

- The causes of nipple discharge can be grouped as pathologic or physiologic. This grouping may be useful in directing evaluation and therapy. Patients that require surgical evaluation have spontaneous, unilateral, and recurrent discharges.
- Nipple discharge is a disturbing complaint for the patient; notably, only 4%-6% of patients with nipple discharge without an associated breast mass are found to have a breast cancer. The risk for cancer is increased if the patient is postmenopausal or if a mass is found.
- The most common cause of unilateral serosanguineous nipple discharge in the absence of a mass is an intraductal papilloma. Nevertheless, breast cancer must be considered.

REFERENCES

Bland KI, Beenken SW, Copeland III EM. The breast. In: Brunicardi FC, Andersen DK, Billiar TR, Dunn DL, Hunter JG, Pollock RE, eds. *Schwartz's Principles of Surgery*. New York, NY: McGraw-Hill; 2005:453-499.

Lange JR. Benign breast disease. In: Cameron JL, ed. Current Surgical Therapy, 9th ed. Philadelphia, PA: Mosby Elsevier; 2008: 644-647.

Case 33

During an office visit, a 66-year-old man tells you that several weeks ago he experienced weakness in his right hand at work that resulted in a temporary inability to write or hold a pen. These symptoms persisted for approximately 45 minutes and resolved without further recurrence. The patient's past history is significant for hypertension and coronary artery disease with stable angina. He has a history of 45 pack-year smoking. His medications include aspirin, nitrates, and a β-blocker. On examination, bruits can be heard over both carotid arteries. The results from the cardiopulmonary examination and the remainder of the physical examination are unremarkable. You obtain a duplex ultrasonogram of the carotid arteries that reveals an 80% narrowing of the left carotid artery and a 95% narrowing of the right carotid artery.

- What is the most likely diagnosis?
- What is the best therapy?

ANSWERS TO CASE 33: Carotid Artery Disease

Summary: A 66-year-old man presents with signs and symptoms suggestive of a recent transient ischemic attack (TIA) involving the left cerebral hemisphere. He has evidence of severe bilateral carotid stenoses as confirmed by a duplex scan.

- **Most likely diagnosis:** Bilateral carotid artery stenoses with a history of a left hemispheric TIA.
- **Best therapy:** The patient should undergo staged bilateral carotid endarterectomies, beginning with the left carotid artery.

ANALYSIS

Objectives

1. Understand the natural history and evaluation of asymptomatic carotid bruits.
2. Be familiar with the medical and surgical treatment of patients with asymptomatic carotid stenosis and symptomatic carotid stenosis.
3. Understand the current role of endovascular management of carotid stenosis.

Considerations

This patient provides a history that is fairly classic for TIA; however, TIA symptoms are not always easy for patients or physicians to recognize. Because the disability is frequently minor and short lived, patients frequently attribute the symptoms to fatigue or other reasons and fail to bring them to the physician's attention. **Neurologic events arising from carotid disease are almost always unilateral, with the exception of speech impediment.** After reviewing the initial history and physical examination, it is also important to look for evidence of coronary artery disease and atherosclerotic disease involving other parts of the vascular system. This particular patient has bilateral carotid disease. Surgical treatment should be directed toward the symptomatic side first. Once he has recovered from his left carotid endarterectomy (CEA), he should undergo an asymptomatic right CEA. Both sides meet operative stenosis criteria, but the symptomatic side is addressed first because it is the higher risk lesion to leave on conservative therapy.

APPROACH TO Carotid Artery Disease

CLINICAL APPROACH

Stroke is the third leading cause of death in the United States and the leading cause of disability in adults. Cerebrovascular disease involves a classic state of balancing the risks of intervention with the risks of conservative treatment. The conundrum is that the main complication of both modes of management is the same: stroke. As a general rule, the more severe the stenosis in a given situation, the higher the incidence of symptoms. **A bruit represents turbulent blood flow that resonates at an audible frequency.** Duplex ultrasonography can be very accurate in confirming the presence of significant carotid disease. However, this is an operator-dependent procedure. The accuracy of stenosis grading should be at the highest level if a surgeon plans to recommend treatment based on duplex ultrasonography alone. If there is question of stenosis grade on ultrasonography, other tests are needed to help guide the therapy. This could be a magnetic resonance angiogram, a conventional carotid angiogram, or a CT reconstruction angiogram. **An additional workup for a patient with carotid disease should include a thorough assessment of cardiopulmonary risks.**

The North American Symptomatic Carotid Endarterectomy Trial (NASCET) and the Asymptomatic Carotid Atherosclerosis Study (ACAS) have categorized the stroke-preventing potential of CEA. For high degrees of stenosis in an internal carotid artery, surgery is better at reducing the risk of stroke when compared to risk modification and antiplatelet therapy alone (Table 33–1).

Table 33–1 SURGICAL VERSUS MEDICAL THERAPY IN CAROTID DISEASE

TRIAL	STENOSIS GRADE (%)	CAROTID ENDARTERECTOMY 5-Y EVENT RATE (%)	CONSERVATIVE THERAPY 5-Y EVENT RATE (%)
NASCET (symptomatic)	> 70	7	24
ACAS (asymptomatic)	> 60	5.5	11.1

Abbreviations: ACAS, Asymptomatic Carotid Atherosclerosis Study; NASCET, North American Symptomatic Endarterectomy Trial.

The important issues in applying NASCET or ACAS data to decisions on recommending CEA are a solid knowledge of the operator's risk rate and profile. If the particular surgeon and hospital have a safety record equal to or better than the perioperative complication rates observed during the trials, recommendations based on trial stenosis grades are fair and reasonable. However, if a surgeon or hospital has a complication rate greater than 5% with symptomatic patients or greater than 2% with asymptomatic patients, CEA should not be recommended aggressively. Many adjuncts are available to reduce the risk of perioperative stroke. The use of an intraluminal shunt, cerebral monitoring, and a patch angioplasty closure all can make CEA safer. The majority of patients who undergo CEA are home from the hospital in less than 24 hours.

Current Status of Carotid Angioplasty/Stenting

The short-term safety of carotid artery stenting (CAS) has been improved with the recent introduction of cerebral protection devices that are deployed during the procedure to trap embolic debris. Despite these advances surgeons can offer even lower complication rates in patients who would belong to higher risk profiles than those studied in controlled, randomized trials. However, there are a few subsets of patients who are at high risk for an open CEA and instead might be considered for CAS. Patients with previous neck radiation or recurrent stenosis are currently two reasonable populations for possible CAS. The Stenting and Angioplasty with Protection in Patients at High Risk for Endarterectomy (SAPPHIRE) trial result was reported in 2002, in which patients with more than 80% asymptomatic stenosis and more than 50% symptomatic stenosis and high-risk operative profiles were randomized to stenting versus endarterectomy. This trial reported 30-day death and major complication rates favoring stenting. In 2008, the 3-year follow-up results from the SAPPHIRE trial suggest no significant differences in long-term outcome between the treatment groups, thus suggesting that CAS may be a reasonable approach for appropriately selected high-risk patients.

Comprehension Questions

33.1 A patient has a 4-minute period of documented expressive aphasia that completely resolves. A workup reveals an 80% to 85% left internal carotid stenosis. A 50% right internal carotid stenosis is present. Which of the following is the most appropriate care?

A. Right CEA
B. Left CEA
C. Aspirin therapy at 81 mg/day
D. Aspirin therapy at 325 mg/day

33.2 An 84-year-old female patient with diabetes and class IV congestive heart failure presents in the office with a right neck bruit. Duplex sonography reveals a 50% to 75% stenosis in the right carotid artery. Which of the following is the most appropriate treatment?

A. Right CEA
B. Aspirin at 325 mg/day
C. Aspirin at 325 mg/day and repeated studies in 6 months
D. Confirmatory imaging with magnetic resonance angiography

33.3 A 71-year-old man suffers a moderately dense cerebrovascular accident (CVA) affecting his right arm and leg. He initially was hemiplegic. However, over the last 3 weeks he has recovered 80% of the strength in his right leg and 80% of the strength in his right arm. It has been 8 weeks since his stroke. A workup reveals a 95% stenosis in his left internal carotid artery; his right internal carotid artery is occluded. Which of the following is the most appropriate treatment?

A. Aspirin at 325 mg/day
B. Right CEA
C. Left CEA with intraluminal shunting
D. Warfarin anticoagulation therapy

33.4 A 66-year-old woman underwent right CEA for symptoms of cerebrovascular insufficiency (right eye visual loss and left arm weakness that resolved) confirmed by a bruit and 90% stenosis on angiography. On postoperative day 1, the patient expired. Which of the following was the most likely cause of her death?

A. Myocardial infarction
B. Vascular surgical failure leading to exsanguination
C. Pulmonary embolism
D. Electrolyte imbalances

33.5 Which of the following statements regarding carotid artery stenting is most accurate?

A. In high-risk patients, carotid stenting resulted in better early outcome than CEA.
B. Cerebral protection devices have not reduced operative stroke rate related to carotid stent placement.
C. The three-year outcome comparing CEA to stent placement has favored CEA.
D. The success of carotid stenting with cerebral protection has extended operative indications to include asymptomatic patients with 50% carotid stenosis.

ANSWERS

33.1 **B.** Left CEA. The patient has a high-grade (exceeding 70%) stenosis in the appropriate artery distribution for his symptomatic TIA. Although aspirin therapy is essential for both operative and nonoperative patients with cerebrovascular disease, this patient meets the operative criteria. The definitive dose of aspirin is still debatable.

33.2 **D.** Confirmatory magnetic resonance angiography. This is a medically high-risk patient who has an equivocal duplex stenosis. If the stenosis actually turns out to be 75%, a careful discussion of the risks and benefits can be held with the patient. However, it still would be prudent to continue conservative management in this high-risk asymptomatic individual.

33.3 **C.** Left CEA using an intraluminal shunt. This is a symptomatic patient with significant recovery from a CVA. His highest risk of recurrent stroke is during the first 6 months following the first event. As such, his contralateral occlusion is not a contraindication to CEA. Based on his presentation, most surgeons would use an intraluminal shunt for his CEA.

33.4 **A.** Acute myocardial infarction and perioperative stroke are the two most common severe complications following carotid CEA. This knowledge should encourage preoperative evaluation for cardiovascular disease, and also monitoring for early symptoms and signs postoperatively.

33.5 **A.** The Stenting and Angioplasty with Protection in Patients at High Risk for Endarterectomy (SAPPHIRE) trial showed that high-risk patients with asymptomatic stenoses >80% and symptomatic stenoses >50% had lower 30-day morbidity and mortality associated with stenting in comparison to CEA. In the 2008 report of the 3-year follow-up of SAPPHIRE patients, no significant difference in outcome was reported between CEA and stenting patients, suggesting the intermediate duration outcome of stenting is perhaps equivalent to CEA.

Clinical Pearls

- The success and complication rates associated with CEA and carotid stenting are highly operator dependent; therefore, it is important to consider these factors prior to recommending therapy.
- Embolization is the most common cause of a cerebral ischemic event related to carotid stenosis.
- Dizziness, syncope, and confusion are almost never caused by carotid artery stenoses.

REFERENCES

Kelley L, Becquemin JP. Balloon angioplasty and stents in carotid occlusive disease. In: Cameron JL, ed. *Current Surgical Therapy*, 9th ed. Philadelphia: Elsevier Mosby Elsevier, 2008:791-795.

Nguyen LL, Conte MS. Carotid endarterectomy. In: Cameron JL, ed. Current Surgical Therapy, 9th ed. Philadelphia: Elsevier Mosby, 2008:779-783.

Gurm HS, Yadav JS, Fayad P, et al. Long-term results of carotid stenting versus endarectomy in high-risk patients. N Eng J Med 2008; 358: 1572-1579.

Case 34

A 57-year-old man has a 2-month history of a nonproductive cough. He denies weight loss or hemoptysis. His past medical history is significant for hypertension that is treated with a β-blocker. The patient has had no known exposure to asbestos. He has a 30-pack-year history of tobacco use. On examination, the patient is afebrile and has no significant abnormalities. A chest radiograph (CXR) reveals a 2-cm soft tissue mass in the perihilar region of the left lung field, which appears to be a new lesion that was not present on a CXR obtained 2 years previously.

➤ What should be your next steps?

ANSWER TO CASE 34:

Pulmonary Nodule

Summary: A 57-year-old male smoker presents with a left lung mass that is highly suggestive of a malignancy.

- **Next steps:** A contrast-enhanced computed tomography (CT) scan of the chest that includes the liver and adrenal gland should be obtained to better define the mass and narrow the differential diagnosis. Based on the findings, the most efficient diagnostic technique can be selected. Examples that could be offered to this patient include sputum cytology studies, bronchoscopy with or without a transbronchial biopsy, a transthoracic biopsy, or thoracotomy.

ANALYSIS

Objectives

1. Be familiar with the strategy for the evaluation and management of a lung mass in patients with and without a known history of malignancy.
2. Be familiar with the staging and treatment of non–small cell and small cell lung cancer.
3. Understand the role of surgery in the management of pulmonary metastasis.

Considerations

This solitary pulmonary nodule most likely represents non–small cell lung cancer. The presence of a **cough, although nonspecific and common in smokers, should prompt further evaluation when it is new and persistent.** With typical tumor doubling time, a 2-cm lung cancer would have been present for nearly one year; therefore, the identification of a lesion on chest radiographs not present 2 years earlier helps narrow the differential diagnosis to either an infectious or a malignant process. The absence of clinical evidence of an infection based on history or physical examination further increases the likelihood of a malignancy. A CT scan of the chest should be obtained to further delineate the mass. The presence or absence of calcifications and their radiographic pattern can assist in narrowing the differential diagnosis, and inclusion of the liver and adrenals, common sites of metastatic lung cancer involvement, can provide staging information. A tissue diagnosis will likely be required; the CT can help define the anatomic location of the mass and will assist in choosing the method of tissue procurement with the highest chance of success.

APPROACH TO Lung Masses

DEFINITION

POSITRON EMISSION TOMOGRAPHY (PET) SCAN: Detects the increased rates of glucose metabolism (positron-emitting glucose analogue) that occur commonly in malignant tumors. It can detect primary lung cancers, metastases to the lung, and mediastinal lymph nodes but may lack anatomic details.

CLINICAL APPROACH

A thorough history and physical examination allow the clinician to generate a differential diagnosis. A patient's cigarette use, known prior or concurrent neoplasms, family history of cancer, exposure to *Mycobacterium*, and symptoms of ongoing infection as well as symptoms of metastatic disease are important and may help establish the diagnosis. **Patients with a history of prior malignancies who develop a new lung mass should be assumed to have metastatic disease until proven otherwise.** Similarly, multiple primary lung cancers occur in less than 2% of patients with lung cancer; therefore, the presence of multiple pulmonary tumors results in a greater likelihood of metastasis or a benign condition. **New nodules in smokers as revealed by CXR have a very high risk of malignancy, as high as 70% in some series, and should be approached with a high degree of suspicion.**

The initial evaluation should begin with a review of prior chest radiographs. With serial films the radiologist can determine the rate of growth, allowing a differentiation between benign and malignant disease. **If the clinical and radiographic presentations suggest pneumonia, a 10- to 14-day course of antibiotics can be attempted with a mandatory radiographic examination on completion. Persistence of the mass demands further evaluation.** The next stage in evaluation is a contrast-enhanced CT scan of the chest. The presence of specific patterns of calcifications can be pathognomonic of a benign process; however, some calcified lesions and all noncalcified lesions require further investigation (see Figure 34–1).

The options, in order of increasing aggressiveness, include repeated radiographic evaluation, PET imaging, sputum cytologic studies, transthoracic fine-needle aspiration (FNA), bronchoscopic biopsy, and surgical resection.

The decision concerning which method to use is based on a wide variety of patient variables (age, smoking history, prior granulomatous disease, prior or concurrent cancers, and family history of cancers) and tumor variables (size and location). As a general rule, patients with a high risk of malignancy are

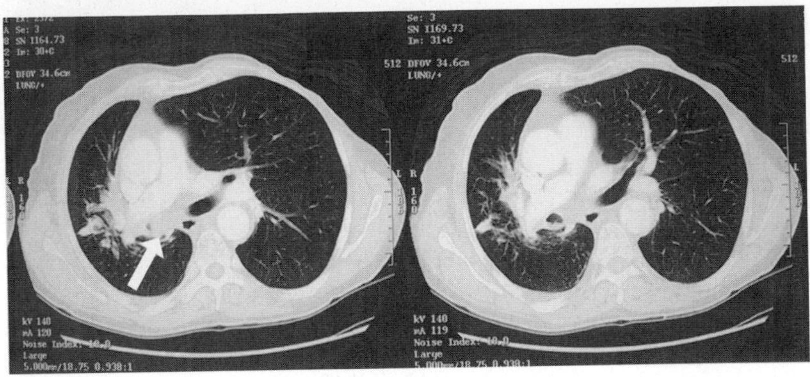

Figure 34–1. Chest CT of an obstructed right main stem lung tumor. Arrow indicates location of right main stem bronchus. *Reproduced with permission from Brunicardi FC, et al. Schwartz' Principles of Surgery, 8th ed., p 569.*

evaluated with more invasive methods providing more information (ie, some form of biopsy or surgical resection), whereas those with a low risk of cancer or significant concomitant medical problems are evaluated initially with less invasive methods. PET scanning combined with CT imaging can effectively diagnose a malignancy (sensitivity, 82%-100%; specificity, 75%-100%) but is less effective with smaller lesions (< 1 cm) or when concomitant infection is present. The use of sputum cytologic studies can assist in obtaining a tissue diagnosis in 10% to 15% of cases, with higher rates of detection for centrally located lesions. Transthoracic FNA and bronchoscopic biopsies are highly effective when applied to appropriately positioned lesions (peripheral and central, respectively). Finally, surgical resection can be used for patients with a high risk of malignancy and a peripherally based lesion. Although it is the most aggressive method, it does have the greatest accuracy and can simultaneously diagnose and treat an early stage lung cancer. This advantage actually makes it relatively cost effective in patients with a high risk of lung cancer (eg, a 65-year-old heavy smoker with hemoptysis but otherwise asymptomatic who has a new lung mass).

Once cancer is diagnosed, every effort should be made to obtain accurate clinical staging of the disease. Staging of non–small cell lung cancer uses the tumor-node-metastasis (TNM) system and is outlined in Tables 34–1 and 34–2. The T status is determined using CT scanning as well as any information obtained on bronchoscopy. Magnetic resonance imaging of the chest may help with lesions involving the brachial plexus and the spine. The N status is determined by physical examination, CT imaging, the results of any biopsies (FNA of palpable nodes, transbronchial FNA of mediastinal nodes, scalene node

Table 34–1 DEFINITIONS OF T, N, AND M CATEGORIES FOR CARCINOMA OF THE LUNG

CATEGORY	DESCRIPTION
T: Primary tumor	
TX	Tumor proven by the presence of malignant cells in bronchopulmonary secretions but not visualized
T0	No evidence of a primary tumor.
Tis	Carcinoma in situ
T1	A tumor that is ≤ 3.0 cm in greatest dimension, surrounded by lung or visceral pleura, and without evidence of invasion proximal to a lobar bronchus on bronchoscopy*
T2	A tumor > 3.0 cm in greatest dimension, or a tumor of any size that either invades the visceral pleura or has associated atelectasis or obstructive pneumonitis extending to the hilar region. On bronchoscopy, involves the lobar bronchus or at least 2.0 cm distal to the carina. Any associated atelectasis or obstructive pneumonitis must involve less than the entire lung
T3	A tumor of any size with direct extension into the chest wall (including superior sulcus tumors), diaphragm, or mediastinal pleura or pericardium without involving the heart, great vessels, trachea, esophagus or vertebral body, or a tumor in the main bronchus within 2 cm of the carina without involving the carina, or associated atelectasis or obstructive pneumonitis of the entire lung
T4	A tumor of any size with invasion of the mediastinum or involving the heart, great vessels, trachea, esophagus, vertebral body, or carina, or with the presence of malignant pleural or pericardial effusion† or with satellite tumor nodules within the ipsilateral, primary tumor lobe of the lung
N: Nodal involvement	
N0	No demonstrable metastasis to regional lymph nodes
N1	Metastasis to lymph nodes in the peribronchial or the ipsilateral hilar region or both, including direct extension
N2	Metastasis to ipsilateral mediastinal lymph nodes and subcarinal lymph nodes
N3	Metastasis to contralateral mediastinal lymph nodes, contralateral hilar lymph nodes, ipsilateral or contralateral scalene, or supraclavicular lymph nodes
M: Distant metastasis	
M0	No (known) distant metastasis
M1	Distant metastasis present. ‡Specify site(s)

*An uncommon superficial tumor of any size with its invasive component limited to the bronchial wall that may extend proximal to the main bronchus is classified as T1.

†Most pleural effusions associated with lung cancer are due to tumor. There are, however, a few patients in whom cytopathologic examination of pleural fluid (on more than one specimen) is for tumor; the fluid is nonbloody and is not an exudate. In such cases where these elements and clinical judgment dictate that the effusion is not related to the tumor, the patient should be staged T1, T2, or T3 excluding effusion as a staging element.

‡Separate metastatic tumor nodules in the ipsilateral nonprimary tumor lobe(s) of the lung also classified M1.

Table 34–2 STAGE GROUPING OF TNM SUBSETS

Stage 0	Carcinoma in situ		
Stage IA	T1 NO MO		
Stage IB	T2 NO M0		
Stage IIA	T1 N1 M0		
Stage IIB	T2 N1 MO		
	T3 NO MO		
Stage IIIA	T3 N1 M0		
	T1 N2 M0	T2 N2 M0	T3 N2 M0
Stage IIIB	T4 NO M0	T4 N1 M0	T4 N2 M0
	T1 N3 M0	T2 N3 M0	T3 N3 M0
	T4 N3 M0		
Stage IV	Any T	Any N	M1

biopsy, or mediastinoscopy), and, most recently, PET scanning. The M status is determined by physical examination, radiographic techniques (magnetic resonance imaging of the brain, CT scanning of the chest with inclusion of the liver and adrenals), and nuclear medicine techniques (bone scanning and PET scanning). **The five most common sites of metastasis should be examined, namely, the contralateral and noninvolved ipsilateral lung, liver, adrenals, bone, and brain.** For very early stage lesions, evaluation of the bone and brain can be reserved for patients exhibiting symptoms of metastatic involvement of these organs. However, these techniques should not preclude a thorough physical examination because lung cancer can metastasize to any location.

Small Cell Carcinoma

Staging of small cell lung cancer is much less involved because of the advanced nature of this disease at presentation. Patients have limited disease (confined entirely within the chest), extensive disease, or extrathoracic metastasis. Small cell carcinoma is associated with paraneoplastic syndromes, which are effects not related per se to the cancer itself, but due to the immunological or other endocrine effect. These include EatonLambert masthenias gravis like effect, hypercalcemia, Cushings syndrome, SIADH, and paraneoplastic cerebellar degeneration. Very rarely, small cell lung cancer is incidentally discovered at an early stage, and in these situations it can be treated using the staging system for non–small cell lung cancer.

Lung Cancer Treatment

The treatment of lung cancer depends on the histology (small cell versus non–small cell) and the stage of the disease. For non–small cell lung cancer, early stage disease is primarily treated with surgery, whereas later stages are managed with chemotherapy with or without radiotherapy. However, all treatments depend on the physiologic reserve of the patient. Therefore, concurrent with evaluation of the tumor, a thorough examination of the pulmonary and cardiac systems should be performed. This consists of complete pulmonary function testing and in selected cases a more extensive evaluation including exercise oxygen consumption studies. Smoking cessation for at least 2 weeks is mandatory, and pulmonary function can be improved dramatically with this single intervention. Patients at risk of cardiac disease should undergo evaluation by a cardiologist, with aggressive examination and treatment of any signs or symptoms of coronary artery disease. For small cell lung cancer, limited disease is treated with combination chemotherapy and radiotherapy, whereas patients with extensive disease are offered palliative chemotherapy with radiation reserved for symptomatic relief only. Figure 34–2 outlines the treatment of small cell and non–small cell lung cancer.

Management of Pulmonary Metastasis

Patients with metastatic lung disease who primarily receive chemotherapy usually have very poor outcomes. However, in very specific cases, surgical extirpation can lead to a reasonable chance of cure. The minimal necessary criteria include local control of the primary tumor, metastatic disease confined to the lung parenchyma, disease that is resectable, and adequate pulmonary reserve to tolerate the planned resection. When these criteria are used, 5-year survival rates approximate 30%. Other criteria that can be considered before surgical resection is recommended include tumor doubling time, disease-free intervals, and the number of metastases.

Lung Cancer Screening

The screening of high-risk patients with sputum cytology or by CXR is not sensitive enough to reliably identify lung cancers at the resectable stages. A current trial involving the screening of high-risk patients using CT scans is ongoing.

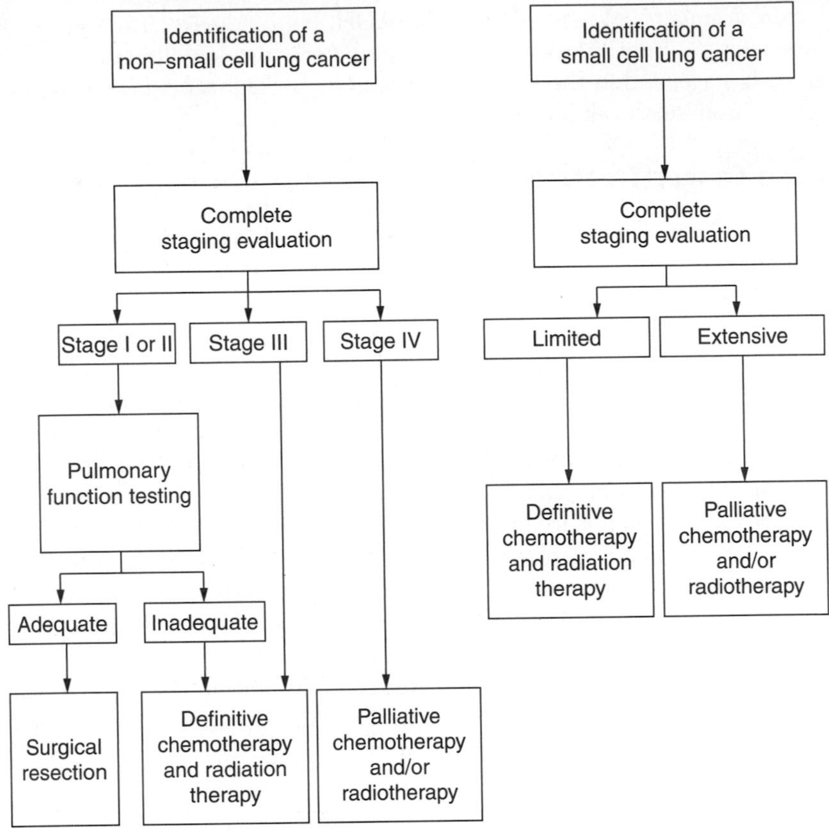

Figure 34–2. Simplified treatment approach for non–small cell and small cell lung cancer.

Comprehension Questions

34.1 A 45-year-old nonsmoker is found to have a 2-cm soft tissue mass in the left lung. Which of the following is the most appropriate next step?

A. Perform a CT-guided biopsy of the mass.
B. Obtain sputum samples.
C. Evaluate all previously obtained CXRs.
D. Obtain a repeated CXR in 6 months.

34.2 A 45-year-old man with a persistent cough was noted to have a suspicious lesion on a chest radiograph. The physician orders a CT scan of the chest. Which of the following describes the main purpose of CT imaging of chest masses?

A. Discern between a pleural effusion and transudate.
B. Differentiate between malignant and benign neoplasm.
C. Determine the anatomic location of the mass.
D. Differentiate between primary and metastatic masses.

34.3 Which of the following patients is the best candidate to undergo resection of pulmonary metastases?

A. A 33-year-old woman, who is a non-smoker presenting with 2 isolate left lung nodules measuring 3 cm in diameter. Biopsy of one of the lesions has revealed adenocarinoma of unknown primary source.
B. A 46-year-old man with a history of left thigh soft tissue sarcoma, who underwent complete resection of the primary tumor. He has remained without evidence of disease recurrence for 3 years. Recently developed a 2-cm mass in the left lung that has been confirmed at sarcoma by FNA.
C. An 86-year-old woman with history of COPD who underwent treatment of rectal cancer (T3N1) three years ago, and she presents with a newly discovered 5-cm mass in the left lung that is in the left lower lobe.
D. A 23-year-old man with a pigmented skin lesion on the left shoulder. Biopsy has revealed malignant melanoma, and imaging studies have identified 1-cm suspicious mass in the left frontal lobe of his brain and a 2-cm mass in his right lung.

34.4 A 53-year-old man with 20 pack-year smoking history presents with 2-week history of productive cough. The chest X-ray reveals a right middle lobe infiltrate. Which of the following is the most appropriate management?

A. CT scan of the chest, pulmonary function test, and thoracoscopic wedge biopsy of the right middle lobe
B. Antibiotic therapy for 2 weeks, followed by repeat chest X-ray. If infiltrates persists, proceed with CT of chest and bronchoscopy
C. CT scan with CT-guided biopsy
D. Right thoracotomy and right middle lobe resection

34.5 Which of the following tumor characteristics of non-small cell lung cancer contraindicate pulmonary resection?

A. Involvement of the parietal pleura by a 3-cm tumor
B. 2.5-cm tumor with a single 1.5-cm peribronchial node on the ipsilateral side
C. 3-cm left lower lobe tumor with left pleural effusion that contains malignant cells
D. 5-cm tumor involving the right upper and middle lobe

ANSWERS

34.1 **C.** Evaluation of all available CXRs is a reasonable first step in treating any patient with a newly identified lung mass. A new mass will most likely suggest malignancy, whereas a mass that was present and unchanged on numerous prior radiographs is perhaps infectious. Further evaluation would still be required.

34.2 **C.** The primary purpose of CT imaging of chest masses is to determine the anatomic location of the lesion, not whether it is benign or malignant.

34.3 **B.** This is a 40-year-old man who apparently had complete resection of extremity soft tissue sarcoma 3 years ago, who now presents with a single pulmonary metastasis. Resection of the metastasis is reasonable if no other site of metastasis is identified. The patient in choice "A" has a pulmonary metastasis without location or treatment of the primary site, therefore resection of the metastasis is not indicated. Patient in "C" has a lesion that may be treatable by surgery, but because of her advanced age and comorbid conditions, the risk-benefit analysis makes surgery less desirable. The patient presented in "D" has multiple sites of metastases, therefore is unlikely to benefit from the resection of these lesions.

34.4 **B.** Initial antibiotic treatment with follow-up of CXR is appropriate for a smoker who presents with a cough. More aggressive follow-up is appropriate, if the infiltrate persists after treatment because the infiltrate and infection can be produces by partial airway obstruction by a tumor.

34.5 **C.** Pleura effusion associated with lung cancer is common and is not always produced by the tumor, however in this case the presence of malignant cell indicates extension of the tumor into the pleural space that precludes operative treatment. Isolated parietal pleura involvement by tumor extension can be treated with en-bloc resection of the lung, involved pleura and chest wall. A 2.5-cm primary lung cancer with peribronchial or ipsilateral hilar nodal involvement constitutes stage IIA non-small cell carcinoma, which is best treated by pulmonary resection with chemotherapy + radiation therapy. A patient with tumor involvement of the right upper and middle lobe can still be successfully treated by lung resection if his/her pulmonary reserve is adequate.

Clinical Pearls

- Approximately 95% of patients with lung cancer present with symptoms related to the disease, whereas only 5% present with asymptomatic chest findings.
- Cough is the initial presenting symptom in 75% of patients with lung cancer, and this cough is produced by endobronchial tumor growth causing inflammation or irritation of the airway.
- Approximately 10% to 20% of lung cancer patients are affected by paraneoplastic syndromes, and these syndromes are most commonly associated with small cell and squamous carcinoma.

REFERENCE

Maddaus MA, Luketich JD. Chest wall, lung, mediastinum, and pleura. In: Brunicardi FC, Andersen DK, Billiar TR, Dunn DL, Hunter JG, Pollock RE, eds. *Schwartz's Principles of Surgery*. New York: McGraw-Hill; 2005:545-610.

Smythe WR, Reznik SI, Putnum Jr JB. Lung (including pulmonary embolism and thoracic outlet syndrome). In: Townsend Jr CM, Beauchamp RD, Evers BM, et al, eds. *Sabiston Textbook of Surgery*. 18th ed. Philadelphia, PA: Saunders Elsevier; 2008:1698-1748.

Case 35

A 58-year-old woman presents to your office complaining of generalized itching. On examination, she appears jaundiced. During your interview, you learn that she has experienced a 10-lb (4.5-kg) weight loss over the past several months and recently has noted the passage of tea-colored urine. Her past medical history is significant for type II diabetes mellitus that was diagnosed 5 months previously, and she denies any history of hepatitis. She smokes one pack of cigarettes a day but does not consume alcohol. Her temperature and the remainder of her vital signs are within normal limits. The abdomen is soft and nontender. The gallbladder is palpable but without tenderness. Her stool is Hemoccult negative. The laboratory evaluation reveals a normal complete blood count. Other laboratory findings are total bilirubin 12.5 mg/dL, direct bilirubin 10.8 mg/dL, AST 120 U/L, ALT 109 U/L, alkaline phosphatase 348 mg/dL, and serum amylase 85 IU/L.

- ➤ What is the most likely diagnosis?
- ➤ How would you confirm the diagnosis?

ANSWERS TO CASE 35: Periampullary Tumor

Summary: A 58-year-old woman presents with painless obstructive jaundice, weight loss, and recent-onset diabetes mellitus.

- **Diagnosis:** Obstructive jaundice caused by a periampullary tumor.
- **Confirmation of diagnosis:** Begin with ultrasonography to rule out biliary stones as the source of obstruction and assess the anatomic location of the biliary obstruction. A CT scan should be obtained subsequently to evaluate the periampullary region if indicated by ultrasonography findings.

ANALYSIS

Objectives

1. Be familiar with the diagnostic approach to suspected periampullary tumors.
2. Be familiar with the roles and outcomes of surgical and palliative therapies in the treatment of periampullary tumors.

Considerations

Mechanisms contributing to jaundice can be broadly categorized as disorders of bilirubin metabolism, liver disease, and biliary tract obstruction. This patient's predominance of **direct bilirubinemia** suggests **biliary obstruction** as the cause. Her clinical presentation strongly suggests **malignant extrahepatic biliary obstruction because she has painless jaundice with a palpable, nontender gallbladder (Courvoisier sign),** weight loss, and recent-onset type II diabetes mellitus. Ultrasonography of the right upper quadrant is an inexpensive and noninvasive imaging modality that should be used initially in this patient's evaluation. The study may reveal cholelithiasis, thus suggesting choledocholithiasis (common bile duct stone) as the cause of biliary obstruction. Ultrasonography may also help identify the anatomic location of the biliary obstruction (eg, the presence of dilated intrahepatic ducts and a nondilated distal common bile duct implies obstruction of the midportion of the common bile duct). If the ultrasound findings suggest obstruction not related to gallstone disease, a CT (computed tomography) scan would be useful to further differentiate between extrinsic compression and stricture and to stage the tumor. A periampullary tumor that invades the superior mesenteric artery (SMA) is considered unresectable; similarly, the presence of distant metastasis indicates disseminated disease and precludes the possibility of a surgical cure. Involvement of the superior mesenteric vein (SMV) or portal vein by tumor was traditionally considered a sign of unresectability and a contraindication to pancreaticoduodenectomy (PD); however, this is considered by many as a relative contraindication to surgery because a number of centers have now achieved acceptable complication rates and long-term survival following PD with portal vein and/or SMV resection and reconstruction. It has been shown **that patients have delayed disease recurrences when they are treated with adjuvant chemotherapy over those patients treated with surgery alone.** It is unclear at this time whether patients receiving chemoradiation therapy prior to surgery (neoadjuvant therapy) have additional survival benefits compared to those receiving postoperative therapy.

APPROACH TO Periampullary Tumors

DEFINITIONS

PERIAMPULLARY CANCERS: Commonly cancers of the pancreas, distal bile duct (cholangiocarcinoma), duodenum, and ampulla of Vater. Some of the less common periampullary tumors are mucinous cystic tumors of the pancreas and pancreatic lymphoma.

PANCREATICODUODENECTOMY: An operation involving resection of the duodenum, the head of the pancreas, the common bile duct, and sometimes the distal stomach. PD is indicated for the treatment of patients with tumors and benign disease localized in the area surrounding the ampulla of Vater. The classic form of the operation is called a **Whipple resection.** The operative mortality of PD has improved significantly over the past decade (approaching 0%-2%), but the complication rates are still quite high (20%-40%).

GEMCITABINE: A relatively new chemotherapy agent (a deoxycytidine analogue) that appears to prolong the survival of patients with pancreatic carcinoma and other periampullary carcinomas. Gemcitabine is an effective radiation sensitizer; therefore, it is sometimes given in conjunction with external beam radiation therapy.

CLINICAL APPROACH

Carcinoma of the Pancreas

Pancreatic cancer is the most common periampullary cancer, but it carries the **worst prognosis.** Overall, carcinoma of the pancreas is an uncommon tumor, consisting of only 2% of newly diagnosed cancers in the United States. This cancer, however, is the fourth leading cause of cancer death in men and the fifth leading cause of cancer death in women; it is responsible for 5% of all cancer deaths. Tumor staging is performed according to the tumor-

Table 35–1 TNM STAGING OF ADENOCARCINOMA OF THE PANCREAS

Tumor status (T)	
TX:	Primary tumor cannot be assessed
T0:	No evidence of primary tumor
T1:	Primary tumor limited to the pancreas and measures < 2 cm in diameter
T2:	Primary tumor limited to the pancreas and measures > 2 cm in diameter
T3:	Primary tumor involves the duodenum, bile duct, or peripancreatic tissue
T4:	Primary tumor involves the stomach, colon, or adjacent vessels
Nodal status (N)	
NX:	Regional lymph nodes cannot be assessed
N0:	No regional lymph node involvement
N1:	Regional lymph node involvement
Metastasis (M)	
MX:	Distant metastasis cannot be assessed
M0:	Absence of distant metastasis
MI:	Presence of distant metastasis
Stage 1:	T1-T2, N0, M0
Stage 2:	T3, N0, M0
Stage 3:	T1-T3, N1, M0
Stage 4A:	T4, N0-N1, M0
Stage 4B:	Any T, any N, M1

node-metastasis (TNM) classification (Table 35–1), which also predicts patient survival. Roughly 70% of the carcinomas are located in the head of the pancreas. **Common clinical manifestations of carcinoma in the head of the pancreas include obstructive jaundice, weight loss, diabetes mellitus, abdominal pain, and gastric outlet obstruction.** Patients with tumors located in the body and tail of the pancreas typically present only after tumor growth has caused obstruction or chronic pain from splanchnic nerve invasion. In terms of prognosis, a patient who has significant weight loss and chronic abdominal and/or back pain tends to have more advanced disease and a worse prognosis.

Patient Treatment

Figure 35–1 illustrates the initial evaluation of a patient presenting with biliary obstruction. When CT imaging demonstrates a mass in the head of the pancreas without evidence of liver or intraperitoneal metastases, or a CXR reveals pulmonary metastases, some groups have advocated CT-guided biopsy to confirm the diagnosis and initiate induction of chemoradiation therapy. Other investigators believe that patients with potentially resectable cancers should proceed directly to laparoscopy, followed by open exploration and resection. Proponents of neoadjuvant therapy think that chemoradiation given preoperatively is better tolerated so that patients are more likely to complete the course of therapy. It is possible that the additional benefits of neoadjuvant therapy may be in selecting out those patients whose disease rapidly progresses or undergoes clinical deterioration during therapy and therefore would not benefit from surgical resection (only a third to a half of patients ultimately undergo resection). Issues regarding preoperative versus postoperative systemic therapy remain unresolved at this time.

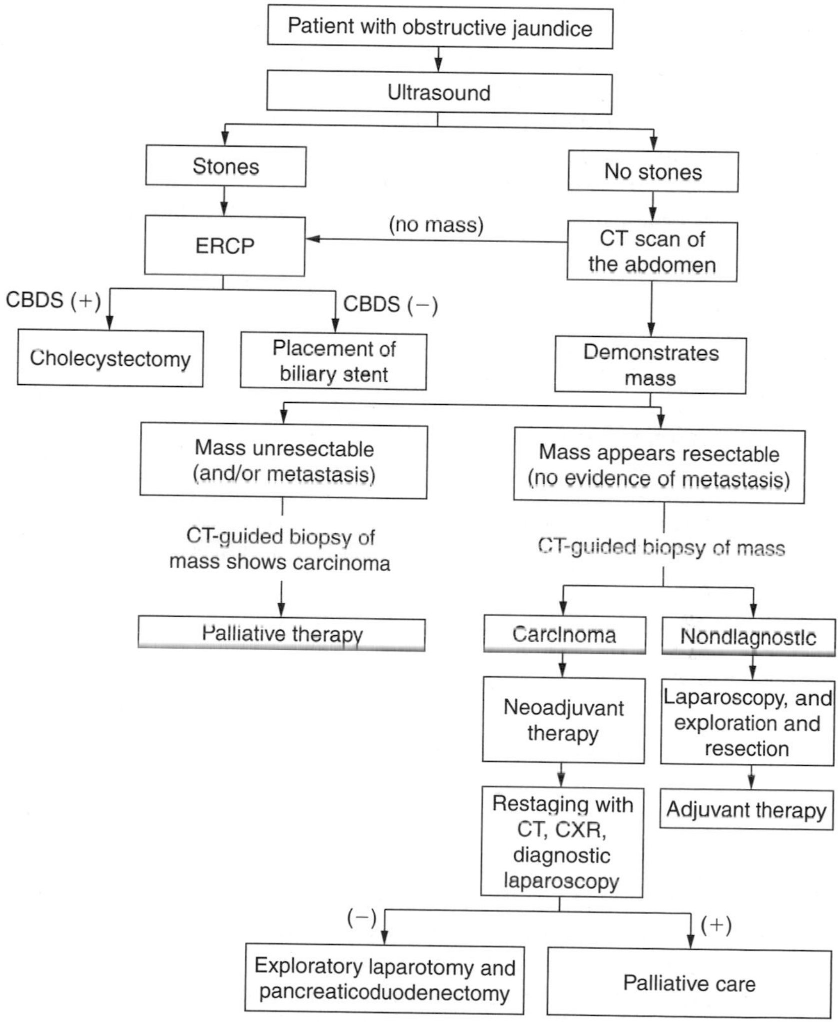

Figure 35–1. Algorithm for the treatment of a patient with obstructive jaundice. ERCP, endoscopic retrograde cholangiopancreatography; CT, computed tomography; CBDS, common bile duct stone; CXR, chest radiograph.

Palliative Therapy

The majority of patients with pancreatic carcinoma have unresectable disease at the time of diagnosis, and these patients have limited survival ranging from months to 1 to 2 years. Surgical and/or other interventions are frequently indicated to relieve biliary obstruction, gastric outlet obstruction, and pain. For patients with **locally advanced and/or metastatic disease, endoscopic placement of a biliary stent is often feasible to provide effective relief of biliary obstruction** and improves the quality of life by relieving the itching and the metabolic and cosmetic effects of the obstructive jaundice. When endoscopic approach is not feasible, percutaneous and/or operative approaches can be used to facilitate biliary drainage. Approximately 10% to 20% of the patients may develop gastric outlet obstruction and may benefit from the creation of an internal bypass (gastrojejunostomy). The development of severe, persistent abdominal and back pain is frequently seen in patients with tumor infiltration of the splanchnic nerves. This is a difficult problem to resolve. Some surgeons have reported good results with the injection of alcohol into the celiac plexus during abdominal exploration, whereas others have obtained only limited success. Alternatively, percutaneous celiac injections have been used with less effective results for nonoperative patients.

Comprehension Questions

35.1 A 42-year-old woman is evaluated and diagnosed with probable adenocarcinoma of the pancreas. Which of the following is most accurate regarding this condition?

A. A majority of patients have unresectable tumors at presentation.
B. Anemia is a common presenting symptom.
C. Patients with isolated liver metastasis can often be cured with surgical resection.
D. It is usually associated with a predominantly elevated indirect serum bilirubin level.

35.2 Pancreaticoduodenectomy is indicated for which one of the following patients?

A. A 55-year-old man with a history of alcoholism who presents with jaundice and an isolated mass in the head of the pancreas. Biopsy of the mass has been nondiagnostic.
B. A 60-year-old man with cirrhosis and cancer of the head of the pancreas. A CT scan indicates the presence of ascites.
C. A 40-year-old man with carcinoma of the head of the pancreas with tumor invasion of the superior mesenteric vein and artery.
D. A 50-year-old man with Gardner syndrome and an adenoma of the second portion of the duodenum.

35.3 A 33-year-old man has been diagnosed with widely metastatic pancreatic cancer. He has severe itching and hyperbilirubinemia. Which of the following is the best therapy?

A. Administration of cholestyramine
B. Radiation therapy directed to the head of the pancreas
C. Pancreaticoduodenectomy (Whipple procedure)
D. Placement of an endoscopic stent

35.4 A 45-year old woman is noted to be diagnosed with pancreatic cancer, and the histology appears to be adenocarcinoma. Which of the following is most accurate regarding this type of malignancy?

A. Most of these cancers are located in the head of the pancreas.
B. Right upper quadrant pain, fever, and jaundice are commonly seen.
C. Most of these cancers are located in the tail of the pancreas.
D. Curative surgery is typically obtained when the malignancy is located in body of the pancreas.

35.5 A 50-year-old man is noted to have painless jaundice which on CT scan reveals a periampullary tumor. Which of the following is most common periampullary cancer?

A. Pancreatic adenocarcinoma
B. Cholangiocarcinoma
C. Ampullary carcinoma
D. Duodenal adenocarcinoma

ANSWERS

35.1 **A.** Weight loss and the presence of back pain are generally indicative of disseminated and locally advanced tumors, respectively. Unlike colon cancer, pancreatic cancer is not commonly associated with anemia. Resection is not indicated for any patient with metastatic disease.

35.2 **A.** Pancreaticoduodenectomy can be performed when reasonable attempts at tissue biopsy have not revealed cancer and the clinical suspicion of cancer is high. Benign adenomas may be treated with local resection. The presence of ascites is a contraindication to surgery, as the ascites likely indicate poor hepatic reserve or disseminated cancer. Invasion of the SMA by tumor is a contraindication to surgery, as the risks associated with arterial reconstruction have not been demonstrated to be acceptable. An adenoma of the duodenum is a benign lesion that may be amendable by local resection.

35.3 **D.** A patient with widely metastatic disease will not benefit from a pancreaticoduodenectomy (Whipple procedure). The placement of an endoscopic biliary stent will bring relief with minimum morbidity and thus ameliorate the symptoms.

35.4 **A.** 70% of pancreatic cancers are located in the head of the pancreas. Some patients with tumors involvement of the SMV or portal vein are candidates for pancreaticoduodenectomy with en-bloc resection of the venous structures, followed by venous reconstruction. Adjuvant chemotherapy following resection is associated with increased length of survival. Right upper quadrant pain, fever, and jaundice are associated with cholangitis, whereas painless jaundice is more likely to be associated with pancreatic cancer. Adenocarcinomas of the body or tail of the pancreas typically will have spread by the time of diagnosis.

35.5 **A.** Pancreatic adenocarcinoma is the most common of the periampullary tumors. These tumors can give rise to painless jaundice, which is a common sign of pancreatic cancer, specifically the head of the pancreas.

Clinical Pearls

- ➤ The classic presentation of malignant extrahepatic biliary obstruction is painless jaundice and a palpable nontender gall bladder.
- ➤ Pancreatic cancers typically are not diagnosed until late and are usually unresectable.
- ➤ In general, pancreaticoduodenectomy should be reserved for patients with localized malignancies near the ampulla of Vater.

REFERENCES

Hines OJ, Reber HA. Periampullary cancer. In: Cameron JL, ed. *Current Surgical Therapy*. 9th ed. Philadelphia, PA: Elsevier Mosby; 2008:506-13.

Oettle H, Post S, Neuhaus P, et al. Adjuvant chemotherapy with gemcitabine vs observation in patients undergoing curative-intent resection of pancreatic cancer. A randomized controlled trial. *JAMA*. 2007;297:267-277.

Steer ML. Exocrine pancreas. In: Townsend CM Jr, Beauchamp RD, Evers BM, et al, eds. *Sabiston Textbook of Surgery*. 18th ed. Philadelphia, PA: Elsevier Saunders; 2008:1589-1623.

Case 36

A 47-year-old woman underwent a comprehensive health evaluation as part of an application for a life insurance policy. She was noted to have a history of hypertension that was controlled with dietary modification. She was otherwise healthy, and no problems were identified. The results of her physical examination were unremarkable. Routine screening blood work was obtained, and she was noted to have a serum calcium level of 11.8 mg/dL (8.4-10.4 mg/dL), phosphate level of 1.9 mg/dL (2.5-4.8 mg/dL), and chloride level of 104 mmol/L (95-109 mmol/L). The other electrolyte levels determined, a complete blood count, urinalysis, chest radiograph, and 12-lead electrocardiogram were all normal.

- ➤ What is the most likely cause of this patient's hypercalcemia?
- ➤ How would you confirm the diagnosis?
- ➤ What is the most appropriate therapy?

ANSWERS TO CASE 36: Hyperparathyroidism

Summary: A 47-year-old woman is found to have incidental hypercalcemia and hypophosphatemia.

- **Cause of hypercalcemia:** Primary hyperparathyroidism.
- **Confirmation of diagnosis:** An elevated serum parathyroid hormone (PTH) level and the absence of a familial pattern of hypercalcemia.
- **Treatment:** The treatment for primary hyperparathyroidism is surgery.

ANALYSIS

Objectives

1. Formulate a differential diagnosis for hypercalcemia.
2. Describe the diagnosis and treatment of primary hyperparathyroidism.
3. Appreciate the natural history and long-term consequences of untreated primary hyperparathyroidism.

Considerations

Primary hyperparathyroidism and malignancy account for 90% of all cases of hypercalcemia. In the **ambulatory setting, primary hyperparathyroidism is by far the most common cause of hypercalcemia.** In this patient, the chloride/phosphate ratio is greater than 33:1, suggesting hyperparathyroidism. The diagnosis can be confirmed by elevation of serum PTH and urinary calcium measurement demonstrating normal or increased calcium excretion in the urine. For this 47-year-old woman, if the serum PTH and urinary calcium levels confirm hyperparathyroidism, parathyroid localization and surgical exploration are indicated.

APPROACH TO Hypercalcemia and Hyperparathyroidism

CLINICAL APPROACH

The differential diagnosis for hypercalcemia is extensive (Table 36–1). **Primary hyperparathyroidism and malignancies** account for 90% of all causes of hypercalcemia. **In the ambulatory setting, primary hyperparathyroidism is the most common cause of hypercalcemia, accounting for 50% to 60% of all cases.** Hypercalcemia is the hallmark of primary hyperparathyroidism. Patients may also have a low or low-normal serum phosphorus level, a high or high-normal serum chloride level, and mild metabolic acidosis. This is a result of the inhibitory effects of PTH on the reabsorption of phosphorus and bicarbonate in the renal tubule. Because of the increased amount of bicarbonate excreted, more chloride is reabsorbed with sodium to maintain electroneutrality. **A chloride-to-phosphorus ratio of greater than 33:1 is consistent with a diagnosis of primary hyperparathyroidism.** In malignancy related hypercalcemia, phosphate may also be low or normal, but the chloride will generally be normal. Other causes of hypercalcemia are usually associated with normal to elevated phosphate levels.

Table 36–1 DIFFERENTIAL DIAGNOSIS FOR HYPERCALCEMIA

Hyperparathyroidism
- Primary
- Tertiary (occurs as a result of autonomous parathyroid function that develops in patients with long-standing secondary hyperparathyroidism, usually from chronic renal failure; also refers to hyperparathyroidism that develops after renal transplantation)

Malignancy
- Tumor metastases to bone
- Pseudo-hyperparathyroidism (secretion of parathyroid hormone–related peptide by renal cell carcinoma, squamous cell carcinoma of the lung, carcinoma of the urinary bladder)
- Hematologic malignancies (multiple myeloma, lymphoma, leukemia)

Other endocrine disorders
- Hyperthyroidism
- Hypothyroidism
- Adrenal insufficiency
- Pheochromocytoma
- VIPoma
- Acromegaly

Granulomatous diseases
- Tuberculosis
- Sarcoidosis
- Fungal infection
- Leprosy

Exogenous agents
- Calcium
- Vitamin D
- Vitamin A
- Thiazide diuretics
- Lithium
- Milk alkali

Immobilization
- Paget disease
- Familial hypocalciuric hypercalcemia (an autosomal dominant disorder characterized by hypercalcemia, hypocalciuria, none of the complications of hypercalcemia, and a urinary calcium clearance of < 0.010 mmol/24 h)

A definitive diagnosis of hyperparathyroidism is made by documenting an elevated serum intact PTH level by an immunoradiometric or chemiluminescence assay. **With the exception of familial hypocalciuric hypercalcemia, which may be associated with a mild increase in serum PTH levels, all other causes of hypercalcemia are associated with suppressed PTH levels.**

Since the introduction of automated laboratory methods in the early 1970s, in most patients primary hyperparathyroidism is diagnosed after incidental hypercalcemia is detected on routine blood testing. The clinical manifestations of primary hyperparathyroidism are protean (Table 36–2). Most patients admit to nonspecific symptoms such as weakness, fatigue, or constipation. **Kidney stones are the most common metabolic complication,** occurring in 15% to 20% of patients with primary hyperparathyroidism. The potential development of skeletal manifestations such as generalized demineralization, osteoporosis, and pathologic fractures are of particular concern for postmenopausal women. Gastrointestinal manifestations include peptic ulcer disease and pancreatitis. Patients may experience joint manifestations related to gout or pseudogout, as well as a wide variety of psychiatric symptoms. **Hyperparathyroidism is also associated with certain well-described cardiovascular effects including an increased prevalence of hypertension, left ventricular hypertrophy, and calcification of the myocardium and the mitral and aortic valves.**

A hypercalcemic crisis may occur in 1.6% to 3.2% of patients with primary hyperparathyroidism. It is manifested by **marked hypercalcemia,** with serum calcium levels usually > **15 mg/dL** and an **altered mental status.** Patients may present with nausea, vomiting, dehydration, lethargy, and confusion or frank coma. The treatment of hypercalcemic crisis consists of forced diuresis with normal saline infusion and furosemide administration. Saline reduces serum calcium by blocking the proximal tubule calcium absorption and furosemide works by blocking the distal tubule calcium absorption.

Long-Term Effects

Untreated hyperparathyroidism reduces patient survival by approximately 10% when compared to age- and gender-matched control subjects without hyperparathyroidism. **This increased risk for premature death is primarily related to cardiovascular disease** and less commonly to malignancy or renal failure, and it can be reversed with parathyroidectomy.

Indications and Preparation for Parathyroidectomy

Currently, the **only definitive treatment for primary hyperparathyroidism is parathyroidectomy. An NIH Consensus Panel in 2002 identified the following criteria as indications for parathyroidectomy: symptomatic patients** and **asymptomatic patients younger than 50 years** with one or more of the following: a serum **calcium level greater than 11.5 mg/dL,** a **24-hour urine**

Table 36–2 CLINICAL MANIFESTATIONS OF PRIMARY HYPERPARATHYROIDISM

SYMPTOMS	METABOLIC CONDITIONS
Skeletal Bone pain Pathologic fractures Joint pain Joint swelling	Osteitis fibrosa cystica Osteopenia Osteoporosis Gout Pseudogout Hyperuricemia
Renal Colic Hematuria Polyuria Polydipsia Nocturia	Nephrolithiasis Nephrocalcinosis Hypercalciuria Reduced creatinine clearance
Gastrointestinal Constipation Abdominal pain Nausea Vomiting	Peptic ulcer disease Pancreatitis
Psychiatric Lethargy Memory loss Confusion Hallucinations Delusions	Depression Psychosis Coma
Neuromuscular Fatigue Muscle weakness Malaise	
Cardiovascular	Hypertension Left ventricular hypertrophy Heart block Cardiac calcifications
Dermatologic Brittle nails Pruritus	

Reproduced, with permission, from McHenry CR. The parathyroid glands and hyperparathyroidism: II. *Hospital Physician.* 2001;4(1):1-11. (General Surgery Board Review Manual). Turner white Communications, Inc., www.turner-white.com. Used with permission.

calcium excretion greater than 400 mg, a creatinine clearance reduction greater than 30% for the age group in the absence of another cause, or a bone mineral density greater than two standard deviations below normal for age-, gender-, and race-matched controls. Because parathyroidectomy may improve the vague nonspecific symptoms and render survival benefits in patients with primary hyperparathyroidism, many experts advise that in the absence of prohibitive operative risk, all patients with primary hyperparathyroidism be treated with parathyroidectomy.

Surgical Treatment

The 2002 NIH Consensus Workshop recommended that all patients under consideration for parathyroidectomy undergo preoperative localization studies to determine the feasibility of minimum invasive parathyroidectomy or unilateral explorations. In various institutions, the preferred localization modality can vary based on local expertise and technology availability. Some of the common localization modalities that have been applied are ultrasonography, nuclear imaging (sestamibi scan), MRI, and CTs. With unilateral parathyroid exploration or the minimum invasive approach, intraoperative parathyroid hormone assay is generally used to verify removal of the parathyroid gland(s) responsible for the hyperparathyroidism.

Published results show that a greater than 95% cure rate can be expected for primary hyperparathyroidism when parathyroid exploration is performed by an experienced parathyroid surgeon.

Comprehension Questions

36.1 A 60-year-old postmenopausal woman with osteoporosis has a serum calcium level of 11.4 mg/dL, a serum phosphorus level of 2.0 mg/dL, and a 24-hour urine calcium excretion of 425 mg. Which of the following serum tests is most likely to establish the cause of her hypercalcemia?

A. Chloride/phosphorus ratio
B. PTH-related polypeptide
C. Urine calcium clearance
D. Intact PTH level

36.2 You are asked to evaluate a patient in the hospital with hypercalcemia. A diagnosis of hyperparathyroidism has been excluded. Which of the following is the most likely cause?

A. Familial hypocalciuric hypercalcemia
B. Sarcoidosis
C. Induced by medication
D. Malignancy

36.3 Which of the following is the most common metabolic complication of primary hyperparathyroidism?
A. Kidney stones
B. Osteoporosis
C. Pancreatitis
D. Gout

36.4 Which of the following abnormalities is most likely to be caused by hyperparathyroidism?
A. Hypocalciuria
B. Hyperphosphatemia
C. Hyperchloremia
D. Elevated serum bicarbonate

ANSWERS

36.1 **D.** An intact PTH level is highly specific for hyperparathyroidism. A chloride/phosphorus ratio greater than 33:1 is only suggestive of hyperparathyroidism, while an elevated PTH is confirmatory.

36.2 **D.** Malignancy is the most common cause of hypercalcemia encountered in patients in the hospital setting, particularly when hyperparathyroidism is ruled out.

36.3 **A.** Kidney stones are the most common metabolic complications associated with hyperparathyroidism, occurring in 15% to 20% of patients with the disease.

36.4 **C.** Hyperparathyroidism is associated with a high secretion of calcium in urine (hypercalciuria), low serum phosphate, high serum chloride, and low serum bicarbonate levels.

Clinical Pearls

- Support for parathyroidectomy in an asymptomatic patient is based on the increase in cardiovascular complications and 10% survival reduction associated with patients with untreated primary parathyroidism.
- The two most common causes of hypercalcemia are hyperparathyroidism and malignancy.
- Hypercalcemia with hypophosphatemia is suggestive of hyperparathyroidism. The diagnosis is confirmed by an elevated PTH level.
- The best treatment for primary hyperparathyroidism is surgery.

REFERENCES

Biliezikian JP, Potts JT, Fuleihan EH, et al. Summary statement from a workshop on asymptomatic primary hyperparathyroidism: a perspective for the 21st century. *J Clin Endocrinol Metab*. 2002;87:5353-5361.

Roman S, Udelsman R. Primary hyperparathyroidism. In: Cameron JL, ed. *Current Surgical Therapy*. 9th ed. Philadelphia, PA: Mosby Elsevier; 2008:626-630.

Case 37

A 66-year-old woman is seen in the outpatient clinic for an evaluation of weight loss. The patient says that 6 months ago her weight was 155 lb (70.5 kg) but over the past several months has steadily declined to 105 lb (47.7 kg). The patient attributes her weight loss to an inability to eat. She indicates that whenever she tries to eat a meal, she develops intense abdominal pain that is severe and diffuse throughout the entire abdomen. To avoid this pain, the patient has limited herself to small meals and soups. She denies any fever, malaise, nausea, vomiting, or constipation. Her past medical history is significant for hypertension for which she takes an angiotensin-converting enzyme inhibitor. She smokes approximately 1 pack of cigarettes per day and consumes 2 glasses of wine per day. The physical examination reveals a thin woman in no distress. Her skin and sclera are nonicteric, and bilateral carotid bruits are present. The results of her cardiopulmonary examination are unremarkable. The abdomen is scaphoid, nontender, and without masses. Her stool is Hemoccult negative. Her femoral pulses are diminished, with audible bruits bilaterally. The pulses are diminished in both lower extremities. Laboratory evaluations are obtained revealing a normal complete blood count and normal electrolyte levels. The serum urea nitrogen, creatine, and glucose values are within the normal range, as are the results from a urinalysis. The 12-lead electrocardiogram reveals a normal sinus rhythm.

- What is the most likely diagnosis?
- What is the most likely mechanism causing the problem?
- What is the best treatment?

ANSWERS TO CASE 37: Mesenteric Ischemia

Summary: A 66-year-old woman with carotid and femoral artery bruits presents with signs and symptoms consistent with mesenteric angina leading to "food fear" and massive weight loss.

- **Diagnosis:** Postprandial abdominal pain, massive weight loss, and signs of advanced atherosclerotic changes suggest possible chronic mesenteric ischemia.
- **Mechanism causing the problem:** Occlusion of the mesenteric arteries related to atherosclerotic changes.
- **Best treatment:** Aortomesenteric bypass grafting.

ANALYSIS

Objectives

1. Learn the causes, presentations, diagnosis, and treatment of mesenteric ischemia.
2. Learn the diagnosis and treatment of patients with mesenteric angina related to mesenteric occlusion.

Considerations

The patient presents with the classic symptom complex of **food fear with postprandial pain and significant weight loss,** which are the hallmarks of **chronic mesenteric ischemia.** However, a thorough workup for other conditions causing abdominal pain is important because mesenteric revascularization is a procedure associated with some morbidity. When more common causes of upper and lower intestinal sources of abdominal pain are ruled out (either by strong clinical impression, endoscopy, or imaging studies), the mesenteric arteries can be studied. At centers with high-quality vascular laboratories, duplex ultrasonography is an excellent screening test. In this setting, **a normal study performed both before and after a food challenge can accurately rule out proximal mesenteric artery vascular disease.** Magnetic resonance angiography can give an accurate assessment of the superior mesenteric and celiac artery origins. Selective arteriography with lateral aortic projections remains the gold standard for definitive diagnosis and therapy planning. **The best treatment for chronic mesenteric ischemia is operative revascularization.**

APPROACH TO Mesenteric Ischemia

CLINICAL APPROACH

Chronic Mesenteric Ischemia

The most common cause of chronic mesenteric ischemia is atherosclerotic occlusive disease of the mesenteric arteries. Typically, a patient has occlusion of two of the three vessels (Table 37–1), with significant disease in the remaining mesenteric vessel. In atherosclerotic mesenteric ischemia without atherosclerotic disease, arteriography can be useful in guiding the therapy. Rarely, patients develop celiac artery compression causing an ischemic syndrome.

In selected high-risk patients, angioplasty can be a useful treatment. However, definitive revascularization with antegrade aortomesenteric bypass or perivisceral aortic endarterectomy is the best option. In the face of higher operative risks or complicating aortic atherosclerosis, a retrograde bypass from an alternative arterial source (such as the iliac artery) has a role. Advanced age, the presence of typical cardiovascular comorbidities, and severe nutritional depletion are factors contributing to the increase in morbidity and mortality associated with open mesenteric reconstructions. Given the high-risk profile of patients with chronic mesenteric ischemia, endovascular reconstruction is being applied by some groups; the results reported have demonstrated reduced complication rates in comparison to open revascularization and 2-year primary patency rates of 70%-95%.

Acute Mesenteric Ischemia

Acute mesenteric ischemia is a surgical emergency. It can be caused by an acute embolus in the superior mesenteric artery (SMA) or the celiac arteries (Figure 37–1). There is usually no history of chronic symptoms. **Arteriography can aid in the diagnosis but may lead to treatment delay;** thus, clinical judgment should be exercised in deciding whether imaging should be performed prior to emergent laparotomy. On laparotomy, the bowel

Table 37–1 VISCERAL BLOOD SUPPLY

Celiac artery	Hepatic, splenic, left gastric artery
Superior mesenteric artery	Small bowel, ascending and transverse colon
Inferior mesenteric artery	Distal colon

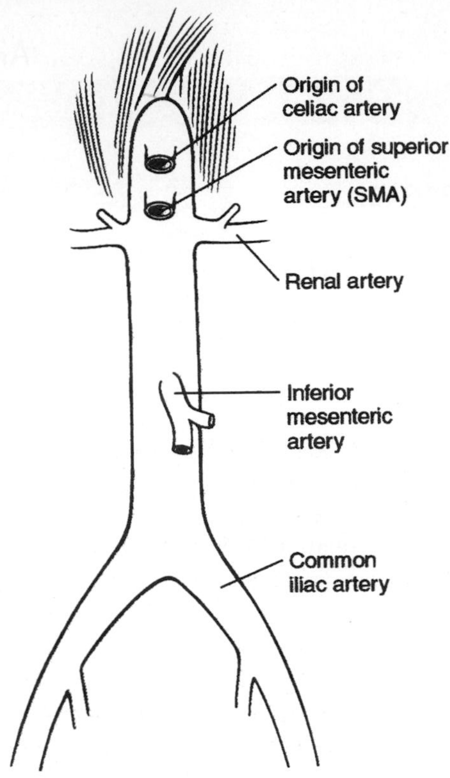

Figure 37–1. Origins of the visceral arteries arising from the abdominal aorta.

can range in appearance from frankly necrotic (a late presentation) to dusky and nonmotile. With an embolus, the proximal jejunum is spared because of small proximal collaterals. The embolus tends to lodge in the more distal main SMA trunk. Embolectomy may be all that is required. However, a **second-look laparotomy** should be strongly considered if the resultant bowel does not appear perfectly viable. In selective cases of acute SMA embolism without clinical evidence of bowel ischemia, a trial of catheter-directed thrombolytic therapy may be attempted; however, the surgeon should be prepared to proceed with prompt abdominal exploration if worsening abdominal symptoms develop or clot lysis fails to occur.

Less Common Causes of Mesenteric Ischemia

Nonocclusive mesenteric ischemia, associated with low-flow states, can develop in a setting of critical illness or as a result of vasospastic medications. Mesenteric venous thrombosis is uncommon and can occur as the result of advanced infectious processes related to gastrointestinal tract pathology, such as appendicitis and diverticulitis. Also, mesenteric venous thrombosis has been seen as a manifestation of a hypercoagulable state.

Comprehension Questions

37.1 A 66-year-old man is admitted to the coronary care unit because of new-onset atrial fibrillation. After 24 hours, he develops the acute onset of abdominal pain and distension, and on examination he is found to have diffuse peritonitis. The patient undergoes exploratory laparotomy with resection of necrotic bowel. Which of the following is the most important postoperative treatment for this patient?

A. Intra-arterial thrombolytic therapy with streptokinase
B. Cardioversion
C. Systemic heparinization
D. Early oral feeding to stimulate intestinal lengthening

37.2 Which of the following clinical presentations is the most typical of mesenteric angina?

A. Diarrhea that occurs following fatty meals, steatorrhea, and chronic epigastric and back pain
B. Daily postprandial abdominal pain, associated with a 40-lb weight loss
C. Recurrent, intermittent epigastric abdominal pain that occurs approximately 1 hour after meals
D. Chronic, persistent abdominal and back pain of 1-month duration and a 10-lb weight loss

37.3 Ligation of the inferior mesenteric artery during aortic aneurysm repair is most likely to produce ischemia in which segment of the intestine?

A. Transverse colon
B. Low rectum
C. Splenic flexture colon
D. Right colon

37.4 A 69-year-old woman with cardiogenic shock following an anterior wall myocardial infarction develops diffuse abdominal pain. On physical examination she is noted to have BP 85/50 mm Hg, pulse 90 beats/min, non-tender abdomen, cool extremities, with skin mottling in the lower extremities. Which of the following is the best management approach at this time?

A. Exploratory laparotomy
B. Dobutamine drip
C. Mesenteric angiography
D. Heparin drip

ANSWERS

37.1 **C.** This patient likely has a mural thrombus of the left atrium, which has embolized to the SMA, leading to bowel necrosis. Initiation of intravenous heparin is important to stabilize and prevent further extension of the clot. Other important steps include antibiotic therapy to prevent sepsis, echocardiography to assess for an intracardiac thrombus, and possibly a second-look laparotomy to evaluate the viability of the remaining bowel. Thrombolytic therapy is not indicated in this case.

37.2 **B.** Mesenteric angina produces symptoms after an increase in GI tract workload such as meals, and weight loss because the patient learns to avoid this challenge. Answer A is more consistent with chronic pancreatitis with pancreatic exocrine insufficiency. Answer C is more typical of biliary tract disease, and answer D correlates with pancreatic malignancy.

37.3 **C.** Splenic flexture colon. The SMA supplies the bowel from distal duodenum to the mid-transverse colon. The IMA supplies the descending colon down to the upper rectum. The "Water-shed" areas of the GI tract include the splenic flexture of colon and distal sigmoid colon/upper rectum.

37.4 **B.** Dobutamine drip. The patient described appears to have a systemic low flow state related to poor left ventricular output, resulting in inadequate mesenteric and lower extremity blood flow. The patient's physical examination does not suggest frank necrosis of the bowel at this point, therefore exploratory laparotomy is not indicated. In fact, given the patient's current cardiac condition, unnecessary exploration of the abdomen could be a fatal insult.

Clinical Pearls

- A patient with chronic mesenteric ischemia almost always has significant unexplained weight loss. If there is no weight loss, the diagnosis should be questioned.
- An abdominal bruit is a very nonspecific finding. It does not pay to be dogmatic about its presence or absence.
- Acute mesenteric ischemia is a surgical emergency.
- Exposure of the SMA for embolectomy is accomplished via the root of the small bowel mesentery.

REFERENCES

Hassoun HT. Acute mesenteric ischemia. In: Cameron JL, ed. *Current Surgical Therapy*. 9th ed. Philadelphia, PA: Mosby Elsevier; 2008:884-889.

Johansen KH, Parikh S. Management of chronic mesenteric ischemia. In: Cameron JL, ed. *Current Surgical Therapy*. 9th ed. Philadelphia, PA: Mosby Elsevier; 2008:889-891.

Case 38

A 72-year-old man undergoes evaluation for the treatment of an 8-cm abdominal aortic aneurysm. His past medical history is significant for unstable angina that was treated by coronary artery angioplasty and stenting 8 months ago. Since that time, he has been doing well without angina. His other medical problems include hypertension and gout. His medications are metoprolol, allopurinol, and aspirin. Recently, he has been active and walks 1 mile daily. He had a 60-pack-year smoking history but quit 8 months ago, and he consumes alcohol socially. He denies any nocturnal dyspnea or pulmonary symptoms. On physical examination, he appears well-nourished. His blood pressure is 138/82 mm Hg, and his heart rate is 66 beats/min. There is no jugular venous distension or carotid bruits. The lungs are clear bilaterally, and the heart sounds are normal. A nontender, pulsatile mass is present in the abdomen. No cyanosis or edema is noted in the extremities. Laboratory evaluations reveal a normal complete blood count and normal electrolyte levels. The serum urea nitrogen and serum creatinine levels are 40/1.4 mg/dL. The urinalysis reveals trace proteinuria. The electrocardiogram (ECG) reveals a normal sinus rhythm and left ventricular hypertrophy.

- What are the risks associated with surgical treatment of this patient's problem?
- What can be done to optimize the patient's condition?

ANSWERS TO CASE 38:
Preoperative Risk Assessment and Optimization

Summary: A 72-year-old man with a large abdominal aortic aneurysm, hypertension, coronary artery disease, gout, and mild chronic renal insufficiency requires risk assessment and optimization prior to elective abdominal aortic aneurysm repair.

- **Surgical risk factors:** The risks include the usual procedural risks and postoperative pulmonary, renal, and cardiac complications.
- **Optimizing the status of the patient:** A complete cardiac risk assessment should be made to define the current cardiac status and identify and quantify any end-organ dysfunction caused by hypertensive and cardiac disease. Optimization of patient status can include pharmacologic therapy, coronary revascularization, and perioperative hemodynamic monitoring.

ANALYSIS

Objectives

1. Learn the general approach to preoperative cardiac risk assessment.
2. Learn the principles of optimization of the medical problems of surgical patients.

Considerations

The goals of preoperative patient evaluation are to prevent perioperative complications, avoid unnecessary delays in surgical therapy, and avoid unnecessary risks to patients from testing procedures. **Elective repair of abdominal aortic aneurysms** is associated with a **postoperative mortality rate of 2% to 6%, with cardiac and renal complications the most common causes of death.** This patient has a history of coronary artery disease and hypertension and subtle evidence of chronic renal insufficiency (proteinuria). It is vital to assess his cardiac and renal status thoroughly prior to surgery. A favorable factor in the history is that his cardiac symptoms have resolved since the coronary artery stent placement. The **risk of perioperative cardiac death or myocardial infarction is extremely low** when a patient has **completed surgical coronary revascularization within 5 years or has undergone coronary angioplasty from 6 months to 5 years prior, and** if the clinical status of the patient has remained stable **without recurrent symptoms of ischemia.** Further formal cardiac evaluation may not be required in this setting.

For this patient, the cardiac evaluation begins with a complete history, a physical examination, and direct communication with the patient's cardiologist or primary physician. Other important issues are the adequacy of the hypertension control and the quantification of the renal insufficiency. If not obtained previously, a 24-hour urine collection to determine creatinine clearance may be helpful because the serum creatinine level in an elderly patient may not accurately reflect renal clearance functions because of the smaller muscle mass. This information may prove useful in the perioperative period for dose adjustment of medications. **Control of systolic hypertension reduces perioperative cardiac complications,** and this should be accomplished prior to any elective surgery. Based on the revised cardiac risk index (RCRI), this patient has moderate cardiac risk with a score of 3 (age, coronary artery disease, and major surgery). Patients with **moderate cardiac risks have reduced cardiac complications when adequate beta-blockade** is established during the perioperative period; therefore, if this patient had not been taking a β-blocker (metoprolol), one would have been prescribed preoperatively. Recent evidence suggests that high-risk vascular surgery patients may also benefit from perioperative use of statins, therefore strong considerations for perioperative statins therapy should be given. Further preparations during the perioperative period include preoperative hydration to prevent hypotension during anesthesia induction, monitoring of blood pressure by an arterial line, monitoring of intravascular volume status by central venous pressure measurement, and monitoring of cardiac status by a pulmonary artery catheter or transesophageal echocardiography.

In general, the guiding principle for the majority of asymptomatic patients with cardiac risks or cardiac disease is optimization of medical comorbidities and the initiation of pharmacologic prophylaxis in patients with high-risk profiles. When considering additional testing or interventions for patients in the perioperative setting, it is vital to consider the risk-benefit ratio of the tests and interventions.

APPROACH TO Preoperative Assessment of High-Risk Patients

DEFINITIONS

REVISED CARDIAC RISK INDEX (RCRI): A six-point scoring system that has been shown to help stratify the risk for perioperative cardiac morbidity in elective surgery patients. (1) Ischemic heart disease, (2) Congestive heart failure, (3) Cerebral vascular disease, (4) High-risk surgery (abdominal, thoracic, vascular, major orthopedic procedures), (5) Insulin-dependent diabetes, (6) Serum creatinine more than 2mg/dL. **Perioperative beta-blockade appears to significantly reduce cardiac morbidity in moderate- and high-risk patients with RCRI > 2.**

METABOLIC (MET) DEMAND: An arbitrary measure of the aerobic demands of specific activities. The perioperative cardiac and long-term risks are increased for patients unable to meet a 4 MET demand during most of their daily living. (eg, activities of daily living such as dressing and cooking require from 1 to 4 MET; climbing a flight of stairs, walking at 6 mph, and scrubbing the floor require from 4 to 10 MET).

RESTING LEFT VENTRICULAR FUNCTION: Generally assessed by echocardiography. A patient with a left ventricular ejection fraction (LVEF) of less than 35% has a significantly increased risk of perioperative cardiac complications; however, a LVEF greater than 35% does not reliably rule out the development of cardiac complications.

DOBUTAMINE STRESS ECHOCARDIOGRAPHY: Provocative testing under a controlled setting involves the administration of high-dose intravenous dobutamine to evaluate the cardiac status of patients who are unable to undergo an exercise stress test. Test results are positive when the patient develops symptoms and/or wall motion abnormalities as revealed by echocardiography. Vascular surgery patients with positive test results have a 7% to 23% risk for a perioperative myocardial infarction (MI) (high false-positive rate/low specificity). A dobutamine stress test with negative results is associated with a 0% to 7% risk of perioperative MI (low false-negative rate/high sensitivity).

CLINICAL APPROACH

When preparing a patient with significant medical conditions for elective surgery, the **patient's comorbidity problems must be clearly defined and addressed during the perioperative period.** An assessment of comorbidity has been found to be **particularly important** for patients undergoing **vascular surgery procedures.** Advanced vascular disease is frequently associated with long-standing diabetes, atherosclerosis, and hypertension, and these factors may cause multiple end-organ damage and reduce the patient's physiologic reserve. The assessment of cardiac risk consists of the eight steps listed in Table 38–1. Several major, intermediate, and minor clinical predictors can be used to determine patient risks (Table 38–2). Clinical history, the **patient's current symptoms, and the level of physical activity** are important in determining the patient's risk. Notably, in vascular surgery patients, **coronary artery disease may be clinically silent because of limited activity and/or coexisting diabetes mellitus.** The other major component in risk assessment is stratification of the cardiac risk associated with the proposed operative procedure. The combination of patient risk and procedural risk is used to determine if additional testing, pharmacological intervention, coronary intervention, or perioperative monitoring is indicated.

Additional cardiac evaluation ranges from noninvasive tests such as 24-hour Holter monitoring, echocardiography, exercise stress testing, pharmacologic stress testing, and invasive examinations such as cardiac catheterization. Generally, patients with **moderate clinical risks** who are to undergo moderate- to high-risk procedures may benefit from **noninvasive stress testing.** The role

Table 38–1 CONSIDERATIONS IN PREOPERATIVE CARDIAC RISK ASSESSMENT

Step 1	What is the urgency of the surgical procedure? (If emergent, short-term medical optimization and perioperative monitoring may be indicated.)
Step 2	Has the patient undergone coronary revascularization during the past 5 y, and if so, have the symptoms resolved? (If yes, low risk.)
Step 3	Has the patient undergone an adequate cardiac evaluation during the past 2 y? (If yes and the results are favorable, then repeated studies are unnecessary.)
Step 4	Does the patient have an unstable coronary syndrome or a major clinical predictor of risk? (If yes, the elective procedure should be postponed until these issues can be addressed.)
Step 5	Does the patient have an intermediate predictor of risk? (If yes, consideration of functional capacity and procedural risk are important in identifying patients who may benefit from further noninvasive testing.)
Step 6	(a) Intermediate-risk patients with moderate or excellent functional capacity generally undergo intermediate-risk procedures with low cardiac morbidity. (b) Further noninvasive testing may benefit patients with poor to moderate functional capacity undergoing high-risk procedures.
Step 7	Patients with neither major nor intermediate clinical predictors and those who have moderate to excellent functional capacity (≥ 4 MET) can generally tolerate noncardiac surgery; additional noninvasive testing is performed on an individual basis.
Step 8	(a) The results of noninvasive testing often identify the need for preoperative coronary intervention or cardiac surgery. (b) In general, cardiac intervention is undertaken if the morbidity associated with these interventions is less than that of the planned surgery. (c) If the morbidity of cardiac preoperative intervention exceeds the morbidity of the planned surgical procedures, coronary intervention is indicated only if it also significantly improves the patient's long-term prognosis.

of prophylactic coronary revascularization for high-risk vascular surgery patients has been addressed in a randomized controlled trial, and the results did not demonstrate short-term or long-term advantages to revascularization; in addition, patients undergoing preoperative coronary revascularization had significant delays in receiving their intended therapies.

Table 38–2 CLINICAL PREDICTORS OF CARDIAC RISK

MAJOR CLINICAL PREDICTORS	INTERMEDIATE CLINICAL PREDICTORS	MINOR CLINICAL PREDICTORS
Unstable coronary syndrome Decompensated CHF Significant arrhythmias Severe valvular disease	Mild angina pectoris Prior myocardial infarction Compensated CHF or prior CHF Diabetes mellitus	Advanced age Abnormal electrocardiogram Rhythm other than sinus Low functional capacity History of stroke Uncontrolled systemic hypertension

Abbreviation: CHF, congestive heart failure.

Comprehension Questions

38.1 A 63-year-old man desires elective repair of an asymptomatic inguinal hernia because it interferes with his golf game. He has a history of hypertension controlled with an angiotensin-converting enzyme inhibitor and suffered an MI 4 years ago. He underwent coronary artery bypass 4 years ago and has been asymptomatic since that time. Which of the following is the most appropriate preoperative plan?

A. Review of the history, physical examination, ECG, and routine laboratory tests prior to surgery
B. Review of the history, physical examination, ECG, laboratory tests, and a stress test prior to surgery
C. Review of the history, physical examination, ECG, laboratory tests, and coronary angiography to document the patency of bypass grafts
D. Review of the history, physical examination, ECG, laboratory tests, and ventilation-perfusion (V/Q) scan prior to surgery

38.2 A 55-year-old patient with a history of unstable angina presents with acute abdominal pain. He is found to have diffuse peritonitis, tachycardia, and chest pain. The ECG shows ischemic changes in the anterior leads. An upright chest radiograph reveals a pneumoperitoneum. Based on these findings, a perforated peptic ulcer is suspected. Which of the following is the most appropriate treatment?

A. Antibiotics therapy and immediate cardiac catheterization
B. Antibiotics therapy and nonoperative care
C. Antibiotics therapy, invasive monitoring, maximal treatment for his cardiac disease, and surgery when he is stabilized in 48 hours
D. Antibiotics therapy, invasive monitoring, and early surgical intervention

38.3 A 46-year-old man is being considered for a very symptomatic hernia surgery. He has intermittent chest pain, and due to an ankle injury, he is unable to perform optimal stress testing. Dobutamine echocardiography is ordered. Which of the following is most accurate of dobutamine echocardiography?

A. It is highly specific in identifying patients who will develop perioperative cardiac complications.
B. It is highly sensitive in identifying patients who will develop perioperative complications.
C. When positive, it reliably predicts the occurrence of perioperative complications.
D. It is of limited use in patients with moderate clinical risk who have poor functional capacity and are undergoing high-risk procedures.

38.4 Which of the following statements regarding perioperative cardiac risk-assessment and risk-modification is most accurate?

A. Preoperative coronary artery revascularization is beneficial in preventing perioperative cardiac complications in patients with "silent" coronary artery disease.
B. Beta-blocker application during the perioperative period should be applied for all elective surgery patients over the age of 60.
C. Coronary angiography is a evaluation tool that should be applied liberally to identify asymptomatic patients who might be at risk for the development of perioperative cardiac complications.
D. Perioperative cardiac-risk assessment should lead to risk-modification during and beyond the perioperative period.

38.5 A 66-year-old man with a history of symptomatic, reducible left inguinal hernia is undergoing evaluation for elective hernia repair. He has a history of hypertension, elevated total cholesterol level with unfavorable LDL/HDL ratio. He denies any history of chest pain or shortness of breath associated with exertion. His blood pressure in the office is 150/90 mm Hg. Which of the following is the best next step?

A. Refer patient for exercise stress test.
B. Place patient on a beta-blocker for one-week prior to scheduling his hernia repair.
C. Discuss with patient regarding long-term cardiac risk reduction benefits and work with the patient's primary care physician to help improve these risk factors.
D. Place patient on a beta-blocker for 1 week and then schedule the patient for an elective hernia repair under local anesthesia.

ANSWERS

38.1 **A.** History, physical examination, laboratory tests, and an ECG are sufficient evaluation for this patient who underwent surgical revascularization of the coronary vessels 4 years ago and has had no recurrence of symptoms.

38.2 **D.** A perforated ulcer is a surgical emergency. Early supportive care, invasive monitoring, and operative therapy are indicated for this patient with intra-abdominal sepsis and evolving cardiac ischemia because the underlying septic process is presumably contributing to the cardiac complication.

38.3 **B.** Dobutamine echocardiography has a sensitivity of 93% to 100% in identifying patients with coronary artery disease, but perioperative MI is seen in only 7% to 23% of patients with positive stress test results (low specificity).

38.4 **D.** Evaluations and preparation of a patient for elective surgery offers an opportunity to assess a person's fitness for surgery but also is an opportunity to identify risk factors that may affect the person's longevity and quality of life subsequent to the operation. Perioperative beta-blocker use has been shown to reduce cardiac morbidity and mortality among individuals with revised cardiac index scores (RCRI) > 3, and the application of this strategy in patients with lower risks may be associated with increased morbidity related to medication side-effects. Aggressive pursuit of silent coronary artery disease preoperatively is not indicated for most patients, since routine preoperative revascularization of asymptomatic patients has not been demonstrated to reduce cardiac morbidity and mortality.

38.5 **C.** Counseling and modification of cardiac risk factors including more optimal control of hypertension is important for this patient. The preoperative setting is a great opportunity to perform a comprehensive review of risk factors and initiate long-term cardiac risk-reduction strategies.

Clinical Pearls

- Most body surface operations (eg, hernia repair, breast surgery) can be safely completed with minimal physiologic stress to patients.
- Perioperative beta-blockade has been shown to reduce cardiac morbidity in high-risk patients; at the same time, this intervention has also been shown to produce complications including bradycardia, hypotension, and cardiac arrests, therefore this therapy should be applied toward moderate- and high-risk patients.
- Perioperative cardiac risk is low when patients have completed surgical coronary revascularization within 5 years or have undergone coronary angioplasty from 6 months to 5 years prior and have no symptoms of ischemia.
- The benefits of obtaining a thorough history and physical examination and adjusting medications prior to any planned elective procedures should never be overlooked.

REFERENCES

Eagle KA, Berger PB, Calkins H, et al. ACC/AHA guideline update for perioperative cardiovascular evaluation for noncardiac surgery—executive summary: a report of the American College of Cardiology/American Heart Association Task Force on Practice Guidelines (Committee to Update the 1996 Guidelines on Perioperative Cardiovascular Evaluation for Noncardiac Surgery). *Circulation*. 2002;105:1257-1267.

Poise Study Group. Effects of extended-release metoprolol succinate in patients undergoing noncardiac surgery (POISE trial): a randomized controlled trial. *Lancet*. 2008;371(9627):1839-1847.

Schanzer A, Hevelone N, Owens CD, et al. Statins are independently associated with reduced mortality in patients undergoing infrainguinal bypass graft surgery for critical limb ischemia. *J Vasc Surg*. 2008;47:774-781.

Case 39

A 45-year-old man presents with a 2-month history of epigastric abdominal pain. He describes the pain as burning and says that it occurs at night or early in the morning. The patient has found that eating food generally improves these symptoms. The patient admits to having had similar symptoms intermittently during the past several years, and over-the-counter H_2 antagonists have always resolved his symptoms. He denies any weight loss, vomiting, or melena. He has no family history of significant medical problems. The patient's physical examination reveals a normal head and neck, and cardiopulmonary examinations show no abnormalities. The abdomen is nondistended, minimally tender in the epigastrium, and without masses. A rectal examination reveals Hemoccult-negative stool. Laboratory studies reveal normal values for the white blood cell (WBC) count, hemoglobin and hematocrit levels, platelet count, electrolyte levels, serum amylase level, and liver function tests.

- ➤ What is your next step?
- ➤ What is the most likely diagnosis?
- ➤ What are the treatment options?

ANSWERS TO CASE 39:

Peptic Ulcer Disease

Summary: A 45-year-old man has signs and symptoms consistent with peptic ulcer disease (PUD). The patient has self-medicated with H_2-receptor antagonists in the past with success, but the symptoms are currently unrelieved with medication.

- **Next step:** Perform diagnostic esophagogastroduodenoscopy (EGD).
- **Most likely diagnosis:** Peptic ulcer disease.
- **Treatment options:** Testing for *Helicobacter pylori* should be performed, and if positive results are obtained, treatment should be administered. If the *H pylori* status is negative, conventional treatment for PUD should be administered (see below).

ANALYSIS

Objectives

1. Be familiar with the five types of gastric ulcers and their implications in pathogenesis and treatment.
2. Be able to discuss the relationship between *H pylori* and PUD.
3. Become familiar with the mechanisms of action and the efficacy of medications used for the treatment of PUD.
4. Become familiar with the indications for surgery in the treatment of ulcer disease.

Considerations

The case involves a 45-year-old man with "burning" epigastric pain that improves with eating. This scenario suggests a diagnosis of PUD that is refractory to medical management. However, whenever such a patient is encountered, the initial step should be to evaluate for other disease processes (ie, pancreatitis, gastric malignancy, biliary colic). In this case, upper gastrointestinal (GI) endoscopy is indicated to assess the ulcer disease, as well as the esophagus, stomach, and duodenum. When indicated, ultrasonography and computed tomography (CT) imaging of the abdomen may be useful. When it is confirmed that the patient is indeed suffering from PUD, it is important to question the patient to see if he has been compliant with the medical therapy. Failure of optimal medical therapy may be influenced by the presence of *H pylori*, high gastrin levels, or noxious stimuli such as nonsteroidal anti-inflammatory drugs (NSAIDs).

APPROACH TO Ulcer Disease

CLINICAL APPROACH

Despite advances in medical therapy for the inhibition of acid secretion and the eradication of *H pylori*, surgery remains important in treating patients suffering from PUD. Moreover, the introduction of more effective antiulcer medications has not decreased the mortality from PUD, which has remained stable or risen slightly. Furthermore, with the high recurrence rate of ulcers following the discontinuation of medical therapy, a renewed interest in operative therapy has emerged. There has been a change in the type of surgery performed on patients with PUD in the *H pylori* era. Specifically, gastric resections are less frequently used, and **vagotomy procedures with or without drainage seem to be most effective.**

Pathophysiology of Peptic Ulcer Disease

Benign Gastric Ulcer

The number of hospitalizations and operations for patients with benign gastric ulcers may be increasing slightly because of the greater use and abuse of NSAIDs, particularly in women. As shown in Table 39–1, there are five types of gastric ulcers. **The most common, accounting for 60% to 70% of these ulcers, are type I ulcers located on the lesser curvature at or proximal to the incisura.** Hypersecretion of acid is generally not a causative factor, but acid likely plays a permissive role in ulcer development and accentuates their progression once they occur. Evidence also suggests that *H pylori* has a role in ulcer pathogenesis, although the etiologic role is not as strong as in the case

Table 39–1 TYPES OF GASTRIC ULCERS

TYPE	LOCATION	ACID SECRETION
I	Gastric body, usually lesser curvature	Low
II	Gastric body, in association with a duodenal ulcer	High
III	Prepyloric region	High
IV	High on lesser curvature	Low
V	Anywhere in the stomach	Nonsteroidal anti-inflammatory drugs

of duodenal ulcers. In general, hemorrhage is infrequent in this setting, although penetration with or without perforation is not uncommon. **Type II ulcers** account for approximately 20% and are in the **same location as type I lesions** but **are also associated with duodenal ulcer disease and excessive acid secretion.** Hemorrhage, obstruction, and perforation are frequently seen with this type of gastric ulcer. **Type III gastric ulcers are** located **within 2 cm of the pylorus (ie, prepyloric) and are also associated with excess acid secretion.** Again, hemorrhage and perforation are frequent with this type of gastric ulcer. **Type IV gastric ulcers are rarely encountered** but are situated **within 2 cm of the gastroesophageal junction,** are associated with **hypochlorhydria,** and carry a **significant operative mortality risk.** Hemorrhage is uncommon in this type of ulcer, although penetration is frequent. Type V **gastric ulcer can occur anywhere in the stomach and is a direct result of chronic ingestion of aspirin or NSAIDs.**

Duodenal Ulcers

The number of hospitalizations and elective operations for duodenal ulcer disease has decreased dramatically over the past three decades. However, the number of urgent operations appears to be increasing; also, because patients tend to be older than previously, there is increased perioperative morbidity and mortality. Duodenal ulcer disease has multiple etiologies. The most common contributing mechanisms to PUD are acid and pepsin secretion in conjunction with an *H pylori* infection or the ingestion of NSAIDs. Gastric acid secretory rates are usually increased in patients with duodenal ulcer disease. There is strong evidence for an association between gastric antral infestation with *H pylori* and duodenal ulcer disease, particularly in ulcers that are resistant to or recur after standard antisecretory therapy. Moreover, in patients infected with *H pylori*, complete eradication of the organism results in extraordinarily high healing rates and low recurrence rates of approximately 2%.

Treatment of Uncomplicated Peptic Ulcer Disease

Following a review of the patient's history, a physical examination, and routine laboratory studies, endoscopy is generally performed (Figure 39–1). Testing for *H pylori* should be performed because *H pylori* is present in most gastric ulcer patients (60%-90%), and those who are not infected tend to be NSAID users. *H pylori* is found in more than 90% of patients with duodenal ulcer disease. Nearly all of the currently available tests for detecting *H pylori* have good sensitivity and specificity. Noninvasive testing includes a serologic study and a urea breath test. Useful invasive tests include the rapid urease assay or a histologic study and cultures in conjunction with endoscopy. For an initial diagnosis without endoscopy, a serologic study is the test of choice. With endoscopy, the rapid urease assay and a histologic examination are both excellent options, although the rapid urease test is less expensive.

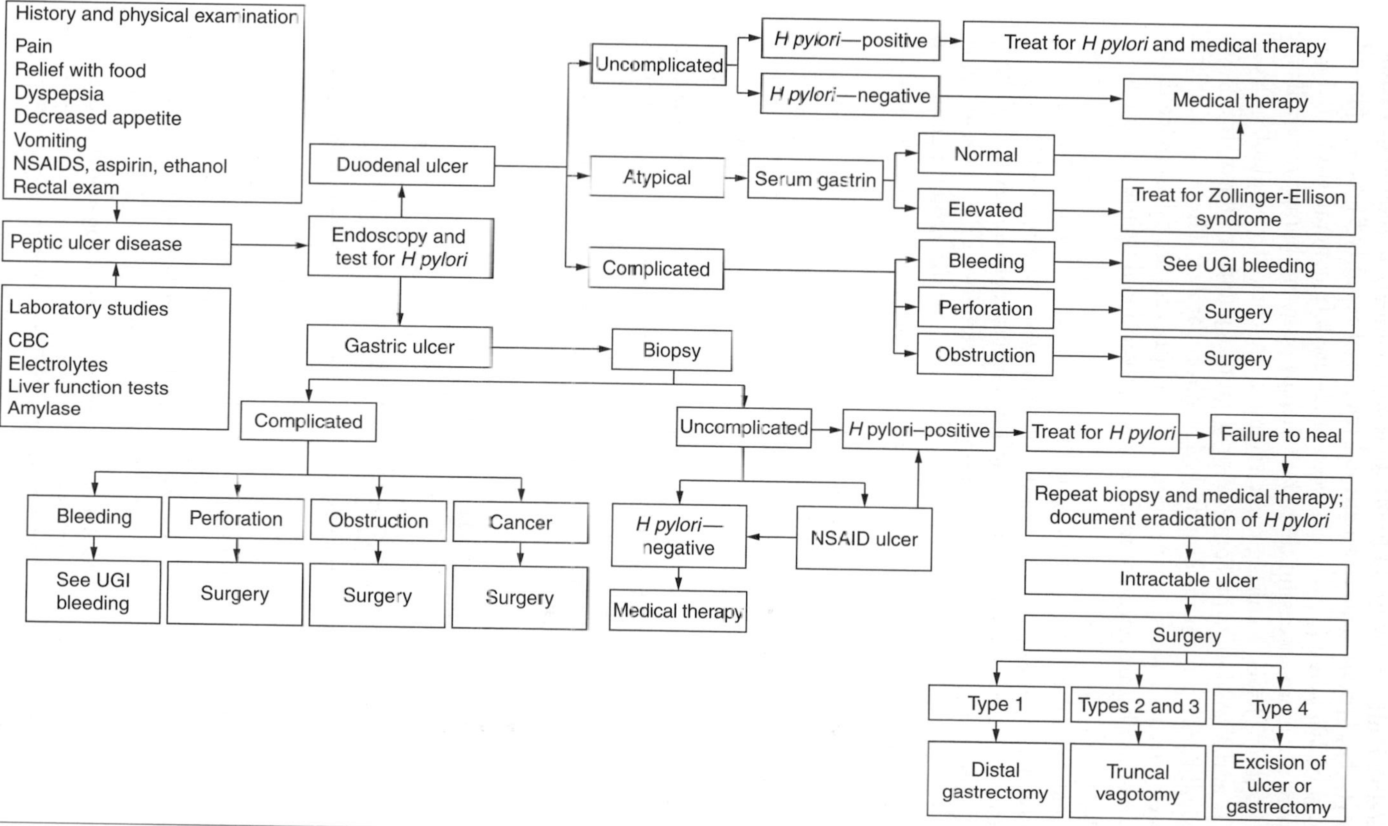

Figure 39–1. Algorithm for the management of peptic ulcer disease. NSAIDs, nonsteroidal anti-inflammatory drugs; UGI, upper gastrointestinal; CBC, complete blood count.

If patients test positive for *H pylori*, treatment should be instituted. **Failure to eradicate *H pylori* leads to an annual relapse of roughly 58%, as opposed to roughly 2% when *H pylori* has been eradicated.** In general, triple therapy regimens are more successful than dual therapy or monotherapy for eradicating *H pylori*. Three promising triple regimens are currently available: OAC, OMC, and OAM (O, omeprazole or a proton pump inhibitor [PPI]; A, amoxicillin; C, clarithromycin; and M, metronidazole). These medications are used for 1 to 2 weeks, do not contain bismuth, and are taken twice daily. For patients who are negative for *H pylori*, conventional treatment should be administered.

Table 39–2 shows the agents available for the medical treatment of gastric ulcers along with their mechanism of action. In general, drugs can heal ulcers by neutralizing acid secretion or by restoring mucosal defenses. Although both H_2-receptor antagonists and PPIs inhibit acid secretion, PPIs block all types of acid secretion because of their direct inhibition of the proton pump. As a result, they also produce more prolonged inhibition of acid secretion than H_2 blockers.

A gastric ulcer should be treated for 8 to 12 weeks and then evaluated for healing. If it has not healed, a biopsy should be repeated to rule out malignancy. If it has healed, maintenance therapy should be considered provided the patient is not taking NSAIDs and does not have *H pylori* infection.

In the setting of NSAID use, it is best to discontinue these drugs if possible while the ulcer is being treated. Ulcer therapy is still initiated with an antacid secretory agent, preferably a PPI. *H pylori* infection should also be treated if present. For NSAID-dependent patients, cotherapy with misoprostol, a prostaglandin analogue, should be considered, or switching to a safer NSAID that selectively inhibits the inducible isoform of cyclo-oxygenase (ie, COX-2).

Table 39–2 MEDICAL THERAPY FOR PEPTIC ULCER DISEASE

AGENT	MECHANISM OF ACTION
Antacids	Neutralize gastric acidity and decrease activity of pepsin
H_2 antagonist	Blocks H_2 parietal cell H_2 receptor
Proton pump inhibitors	Inhibits H^+-K^+-adenosine-triphosphatase pump
Sucralfate	Complexes with pepsin and bile salts and binds to proteins in mucosa
Prostaglandins	Inhibit acid secretion, increase endogenous mucosal defense

Surgical Therapy

In both gastric and duodenal ulcer disease, surgery is indicated for the complications of PUD. Gastrointestinal hemorrhage, perforation, intractable pain, and obstruction are indications for surgical intervention. Ulcer is considered **intractable** if **it persists for more than 3 months despite active drug therapy,** the **ulcer recurs within 1 year after initial healing despite maintenance therapy,** or if the ulcer disease is characterized by **cycles of prolonged activity with brief remissions. Gastric ulcers should undergo biopsy** early in the evaluation process because of **the risk for carcinoma.** Thus, for intractable gastric ulcers, excision of the ulcer should be performed in conjunction with proximal gastric vagotomy or some type of gastrectomy. For a type 1 gastric ulcer in the setting of intractability, elective distal gastrectomy with gastroduodenal (Billroth I) anastomosis is usually performed. The ulcer should be included in the antrectomy specimen. For type 2 gastric ulcers, antrectomy that includes the gastric ulcer is generally performed in conjunction with a truncal vagotomy to further reduce acid secretion and remove the gastric mucosa at risk for ulcer as well as the ulcer itself. The type of reconstruction, gastroduodenostomy (Billroth I) or gastrojejunostomy (Billroth II), depends on how badly the duodenum is inflamed. An alternative is truncal vagotomy and gastrojejunostomy. A third option is vagotomy and pyloroplasty. For type 3 gastric ulcers, a vagotomy and antrectomy that includes the ulcer is usually performed. As previously mentioned, type 4 gastric ulcers are difficult to treat, and the choice of operation depends on a number of factors. These include the size of the ulcer and the degree of surrounding inflammation, as well as the distance of the ulcer from the gastroesophageal junction. **Type 5 gastric ulcers rarely require surgery,** and if this type of ulcer does not heal rapidly with the standard medical therapy mentioned earlier, malignant disease must be excluded.

For treatment of perforated duodenal ulcers, when there is no prior history of ulcer disease or if the patients are positive for *H pylori*, an omental patch closure may be performed followed by treatment for *H pylori*. If the patient has an underlying history of ulcer disease or is known to be negative for *H pylori* and is hemodynamically stable at the time of the procedure, a highly selective vagotomy is another option in addition to closure of the perforation. For the treatment of perforated gastric ulcers, the possibility of malignancy still must be addressed as well as the possibility of *H pylori* infection. Thus, depending on the type of gastric ulcer, the area requires biopsy with closure of the perforation. Alternatively, the ulcer can also be excised and/or resected with primary repair or a Billroth I or II reconstruction. For an obstruction, the patient can be treated with antrectomy and gastroduodenostomy, although if scarring is so severe as to preclude a safe anastomosis, gastrojejunostomy in conjunction with a truncal vagotomy should be performed.

Comprehension Questions

39.1 A 42-year-old woman has progressive epigastric pain, which has improved somewhat with PPI. She underwent upper endoscopy and a gastric ulcer is diagnosed. Which of the following best describes a characteristic of gastric ulcers?

A. Type 1 gastric ulcers are usually not associated with excess acid secretion.
B. Type 1 gastric ulcers are usually located in the prepyloric region of the stomach.
C. Type 2 gastric ulcers are usually associated with esophageal disease.
D. Type 5 is a gastric ulcer associated with chronic steroid use.

39.2 A 35-year-old stock broker has mid abdominal pain throughout the day, which is relieved somewhat by meals and antacids. A gall gladder ultrasound is negative. He undergoes an upper GI endoscopy which revealed a duodenal ulcer. Which of the following best describes characteristics of duodenal ulcer disease?

A. It is rarely associated with hypersecretion of acid.
B. It is a disease of multiple etiologies.
C. Complete eradication of *H pylori* is difficult and associated with frequent recurrences.
D. *H pylori* infestation usually occurs in the gastric cardia.

39.3 Which of the following is correct regarding medical therapy of peptic ulcer disease?

A. PPIs and H_2 antagonists have approximately equal efficacy in controlling ulcer disease.
B. Prostaglandin compounds such as misoprostol promote resolution of gastric ulcers by decreasing acid production.
C. NSAID-induced ulcers are sometimes associated with *H pylori* and require antibiotic therapy.
D. H_1 receptors are associated with gastric acid secretion.

39.4 A 35-year-old man is diagnosed with a duodenal ulcer. He asks about the indications for surgical therapy versus medical treatment. Which one of the following conditions would necessitate surgical therapy?

A. Development of diabetes mellitus
B. Persistent *H pylori* infection
C. Gastric outlet obstruction
D. Need for taking NSAIDs

39.5 Which one of the following patients is most likely to require surgical intervention for the management of peptic ulcer disease?

A. A 44-year-old man with a 1-cm duodenal ulcer that is causing epigastric pain for 3 weeks. His *H pylori* serology is positive.

B. A 68-year-old woman who has been consuming NSAIDs for osteoarthritis and develops melena. She has remained hemodynamically stable and on endoscopy is found to have superficial ulcerations throughout the body of the stomach.

C. A 40-year-old man with epigastric and coffee-ground emesis. His endoscopy revealed a small ulcer in the gastric antrum, and a second ulcer in the duodenal bulb. His *H pylori* serology is positive.

D. A 57-year-old man with history of gastric ulcer that was biopsied 4 months ago and found to be benign. He has received treatment for *H pylori* and has been maintained on PPI and continues to have pain. Repeat endoscopy demonstrates a persistent gastric ulcer involving the lesser curve of the stomach near the antrum.

ANSWERS

39.1 **A.** Type 1 gastric ulcers are usually not associated with excess acid secretion and are usually located on the lesser curvature of the stomach. Type 5 gastric ulcers are associated with chronic NSAID or aspirin use.

39.2 **B.** Duodenal ulcer disease has multiple etiologies and is commonly associated with acid hypersecretion. Antacid therapy results in a high rate of ulcer resolution, but the eradication of *H pylori* helps maintain a long-term ulcer cure.

39.3 **C.** Patients with NSAID-induced ulcers not uncommonly also have *H pylori* involvement, and when *H pylori* is documented, those affected require antibiotic therapy to promote complete healing. In general, PPIs have superior efficacy over H_2 blockers.

39.4 **C.** Gastric outlet obstruction caused by a chronic duodenal ulcer is an indication for surgical therapy, as is the inability to exclude malignancy, intractable symptoms, and perforation.

39.5 **D.** This man has continued pain and non-healing of his type I gastric ulcer, despite having received a course of therapy for *H pylori* and is maintained on PPI. The patients described in "A" and "C" have duodenal ulcer and type 2 gastric ulcer, respectively. Since both patients are *H pylori* positive, they should respond to medical management that includes *H pylori* eradication. The patient described in "B" has gastric ulcers related to NSAID use. This should respond to the cessation of NSAID and treatment with misopostol.

Clinical Pearls

- Appreciation of the types of gastric ulcers helps in identifying the problem and directing the most appropriate therapy.
- Prevention of ulcer recurrence requires *H pylori* eradication rather than treatment alone in selected cases.
- In general, gastric ulcers should be biopsied to exclude malignancy.
- Type 5 gastric ulcers related to NSAIDs or aspirin use rarely require surgery.
- The indications for surgery for PUD are obstruction, hemorrhage, perforation, and intractable symptoms.

REFERENCES

Dempsey DT. Stomach. In: Brunicardi FC, Andersen DK, Billiar TR, et al, eds. *Schwartz's Principles of Surgery*. 8th ed. New York, NY: McGraw-Hill, 2005:933-995.

Mercer DW, Robinson EK. Stomach. In: Townsend CM Jr, Beauchamp RD, Evers BM, et al, eds. *Sabiston Textbook of Surgery*. 18th ed. Philadelphia, PA: Elsevier Saunders; 2008: 1223-1277.

Case 40

A 23-year-old man was the restrained driver of an automobile involved in a high-speed head-on collision with an 18-wheeler that drifted across the highway divider. According to the paramedics, the front-seat occupant in the patient's automobile was found dead at the scene. Extrication of the patient required approximately 30 minutes. His vital signs at the scene were pulse rate 110 beats/min, blood pressure 90/60 mm Hg, respiratory rate 14 breaths/min, and Glasgow Coma Score (GCS) 6. The paramedics performed endotracheal intubation, placed a peripheral intravenous line and initiated ventilation, and administered intravenous fluids during transportation to your trauma center. His vital signs on arrival at the emergency department are temperature 36.2°C (97.2°F), pulse 112 beats/min, blood pressure 88/70 mm Hg, assisted respiratory rate 20 breaths/min, and GCS 6 (4 + 1 + 1). A forehead hematoma, multiple facial lacerations and abrasions, and a bony deformity of the left cheek are present. The breath sounds are diminished on the left, with soft tissue crepitation in the left anterior chest wall. The abdomen is distended, with diminished bowel sounds. The bony pelvis is stable to palpation. Examination of the extremities reveals a markedly swollen, tender left thigh with a 10-cm laceration over the left knee. The peripheral pulses are present in all the extremities. No spontaneous movements in the lower extremities are identified.

- ➤ What should be the next steps in this patient's treatment?
- ➤ What are the most likely mechanisms causing the patient's current clinical picture?

ANSWERS TO CASE 40:
Blunt Trauma (Multiple)

Summary: A 23-year-old restrained driver is involved in a high-speed motor vehicle crash (MVC). He presents with tachycardia, hypotension, and a GCS of 6. The patient's initial assessment suggests the following injuries: closed head injury, left pneumothorax, possible intra-abdominal injury, and left femur fracture. The exact cause of the hypotension is undetermined at this time.

- **Next steps:** Placement of a left chest tube (tube thoracostomy) should be performed to treat the suspected left pneumothorax, which should improve his breathing and address a potential cause of the hemodynamic instability.
- **Responsible mechanisms:** The possible causes of the tachycardia, hypotension, and unresponsiveness in this patient include hemorrhagic shock and left tension pneumothorax; less likely causes are spinal shock, primary cardiac dysfunction, and severe closed head injury.

ANALYSIS

Objectives

1. Learn the priorities and principles in treating patients with multiple injuries, including blunt chest injury, blunt abdominal injury, closed head injury, orthopedic injury, and spinal cord injury.
2. Learn to recognize the causes of hemodynamic instability in a trauma patient and learn the methods of diagnosis for these problems.

Considerations

A young man is injured in a high-speed MVC and presents with tachycardia, hypotension, a GCS of 6 (see Table 12-1 Glasgow Coma Scale), a clinically suspicious left pneumothorax, and a left femur fracture. It is vital to approach any patient with multiple injuries or the potential for multiple injuries systematically to ensure that serious injuries are identified and treated in the most timely manner. **The evaluation begins by learning the details of collision from the patient, eyewitnesses, or paramedics to gain insight into the injury mechanism and severity.** With an initial **GCS of 6, a severe closed head injury should be strongly suspected, and therefore early airway control is essential for oxygenation, ventilation, and minimizing the effects of secondary brain injury.**

The primary survey should begin with reassessment of the airway to make certain the endotracheal tube has been secured in the correct position. The presence of **left chest wall crepitation, diminished breath sounds, and hypotension is highly suggestive of pneumothorax** or possibly tension pneumothorax; therefore, a **left chest tube should be placed even prior to confirmation** by chest radiography or ultrasonography. If the patient remains hemodynamically unstable following chest tube insertion, the cause of the hypotension is most likely hemorrhage. Treatment should then be directed toward restoring intravascular volume, and simultaneous attempts should be made to identify the source of blood loss. It is important to recognize that other causes of hypotension in the acute traumatic setting are possible but less likely, and these include cardiac dysfunction, cardiac tamponade, and neurogenic shock. Because these other causes of shock are far less common than hemorrhagic shock, **hypotension in a polytrauma patient should be presumed to be the result of hemorrhage until bleeding from all possible sources can be ruled out. The potential locations of major blood loss to be considered include external, pleural space, intraperitoneal, retroperitoneal, pelvic, and soft tissue.** A survey of the patient's body for open wounds and clothing for blood is usually helpful in identifying external blood loss. A chest radiograph or bilateral chest tubes are useful in locating pleural space blood loss. A pelvic radiograph can identify bony fractures and/or dislocations, which are the primary cause of extraperitoneal pelvic blood loss.

Intraperitoneal bleeding can be readily identified by focused abdominal sonography for trauma (FAST) or diagnostic peritoneal lavage (DPL) performed during the secondary survey of unstable patients. Major long bone fractures are the result of large kinetic energy transfers and are associated with destruction and bleeding from the surrounding soft tissue; this type of bleeding is generally identified by physical examination and radiography. Retroperitoneal blood loss without pelvic fracture occurs rarely and can be identified by FAST. **Injuries to the cervical or upper thoracic spinal cord can disrupt sympathetic functions** and lead to **neurogenic shock.** The majority of spinal cord injuries occur in the presence of bony fractures and/or dislocations; therefore, plain radiographs of the spine can be used to screen for these injuries. Rarely, cardiac dysfunction can result from blunt injury, which is generally recognized by echocardiography or elevated right heart filling pressures measured through central venous catheters or pulmonary artery catheters. **In a hemodynamically unstable patient, it is important to identify life-threatening problems in a timely fashion without having to transport the patient to the radiology suite. Therefore, the use of a CT scan is not indicated in the evaluation of unstable trauma patients.**

APPROACH TO Multiple Trauma

DEFINITIONS

FOCUSED ABDOMINAL SONOGRAPHY FOR TRAUMA (FAST): A quick ultrasound examination performed during the secondary survey. The four views examined are subxiphoid, right and left upper quadrant, and pelvic.

The FAST procedure is sensitive in identifying intraperitoneal fluid and pericardial fluid, and it is most useful for the rapid assessment of unstable patients.

DIAGNOSTIC PERITONEAL LAVAGE (DPL): A bedside invasive diagnostic procedure performed during the secondary survey in unstable patients. This study is highly sensitive in identifying intraperitoneal blood. Positive results are defined as 10 mL of gross blood or enteric content aspirate or a red blood cell (RBC) count of more than 100,000/mL or a WBC count of more than 500/mL. The primary limitation of DPL is its lack of specificity. In hemodynamically stable patients, laparotomies performed on the basis of microscopically positive DPL result in nontherapeutic laparotomies in up to 30% of patients.

ABDOMINAL CT SCANS: A sensitive, specific diagnostic modality for solid organ injuries, retroperitoneal injuries, and peritoneal fluid in the blunt trauma setting. Because of the time required for completion and the need to transport patients to an uncontrolled environment, CT imaging is contraindicated for unstable patients.

CLINICAL APPROACH

The **initial treatment** begins with a primary survey consisting of **airway (A), breathing (B), and circulation (C)** assessment and optimization, commonly referred to as the ABCs. The primary survey focuses on immediate life-threatening problems, which should be promptly treated. Once the ABCs are addressed satisfactorily, a **secondary survey** is conducted via a **thorough head-to-toe examination and an inventory of all possible injuries.** Plain nasogastric tubes and urinary catheters are placed as needed. After completion of the primary and secondary surveys, the next step in treating the patient can generally be determined. If the patient is stable, additional radiographic studies can be completed in the radiology suite as indicated. It is important to remember that **whenever a patient develops any significant change in clinical condition, a thorough reevaluation beginning with the ABCs should be performed immediately.** For patients with identifiable bleeding, neurosurgical injuries, and orthopedic injuries, the problem of ongoing bleeding should be addressed first if it causes hemodynamic instability. Damage control operations are abbreviated surgeries to control bleeding and may be useful to allow timely management of severe neurosurgical injuries. Generally, the treatment of major orthopedic injuries not associated with significant bleeding can be delayed until after an initial period of stabilization (> 24-48 hours). **Many hemodynamically stable patients with hemoperitoneum, liver, spleen, or kidney injuries can be successfully managed nonoperatively with close observation; therefore, an initial nonoperative approach is appropriate.**

Comprehension Questions

40.1 A 73-year-old man is seen after falling down a flight of stairs. He arrives on a backboard with a C-collar in place. His initial pulse rate is 70 beats/min, blood pressure 160/80 mm Hg, respiratory rate 10 breaths/min, and GCS 6. He has a large scalp hematoma, a dilated, nonreactive left pupil, and a large bruise over his left flank. Which of the following is the most appropriate treatment?

A. Provide an O_2 face mask and intravenous (IV) fluids, obtain a head and abdomen CT scan, and request a neurosurgical consultation.

B. Perform endotracheal intubation, provide IV fluids, obtain an abdomen CT scan, and request a neurosurgical consultation.

C. Perform endotracheal intubation, provide IV fluids, perform a FAST examination, request a neurosurgical consultation, and prepare to perform bedside decompressive craniectomy.

D. Perform endotracheal intubation, provide IV fluids, perform a FAST examination, obtain a head CT scan, and request a neurosurgical consultation.

40.2 A 34-year-old man, who is an unrestrained passenger, underwent a high speed motor vehicle accident, and experiences a fractured femur as well as blunt abdominal trauma. After stablization of the patient, the ED physician orders a CT scan of the abdomen. Which of the following statements is most accurate regarding abdominal CT scan for blunt trauma patient?

A. Costly and time consuming and thus should not be used when DPL is available.

B. Highly sensitive and specific for solid organ injuries but lacks sensitivity for retroperitoneal and hollow viscus injuries.

C. Highly sensitive and specific for solid organ injuries but lacks sensitivity for hollow viscus injuries.

D. Highly sensitive and specific for solid organ injuries and intraperitoneal blood and useful for both stable and hypotensive patients.

40.3 A 40-year-old unrestrained man who was the driver of a car that crashed into tree when his car apparently veered off the road. He was brought to the emergency department, and after his initial resuscitation and evaluation, he is found to have multiple superficial scalp lacerations, a left subdural hematoma with no associated midline ship and with a GCS of 14, a 60% left pneumothorax, and left tibia and fibular fractures that are associated with diminished pedal pulses. Which of the following is the most appropriate sequence of prioritization for this patient's injuries?

A. Brain injury, pneumothorax, lower extremity injuries, and facial lacerations
B. Pneumothorax, brain injury, lower extremity injuries, and facial lacerations
C. Pneumothorax, lower extremity injuries, brain injuries, and facial lacerations
D. Brain injury, lower extremity injuries, pneumothorax, and facial lacerations

40.4 A 32-year-old man is brought to the emergency center after having been struck by a large branch that broke off a tree and struck the patient on the side of his head and right chest area. He is brought to the emergency center with a large right parietal scalp hematoma, right cheek deformity, and right chest wall deformity associated with diminished left breath sounds. His pulse rate is 110 beats/min, blood pressure is 110/60 mm Hg, respiratory rate is 30 breaths/min, and GCS is 13. Which of the following is the most appropriate next step?

A. Endotracheal intubation
B. Right chest tube placement
C. CT scan of the brain
D. FAST

40.5 Which of the following factors is most likely to contribute to a worse outcome in a patient with a left subdural hematoma associated with a GCS of 9?

A. Blood pressure of 70/50 mm Hg recorded for approximately 10 minutes prior to arrival to the hospital
B. Epidural hematoma
C. Depressed skull fracture
D. Pelvic fracture

ANSWERS

40.1 **D.** In a hemodynamically stable patient with signs of severe closed head injury with a left hemispheric mass effect as demonstrated by the nonreactive and dilated left pupil, immediate airway management with controlled ventilation is essential to minimize secondary brain injury. A CT scan of the head is vital to help the neurosurgeon define the problem so the appropriate surgical intervention can be performed. A blindly performed craniectomy is never indicated.

40.2 **C.** A CT scan of the abdomen is very accurate in identifying solid organ and retroperitoneal injuries, but it lacks sensitivity for hollow viscus injuries. Fortunately, hollow viscus injuries are unusual following blunt trauma and occur in only 1% to 5% of cases.

40.3 **B.** The treatment prioritization for patients with multiple injuries should always consider life-threatening injuries before injuries that may compromise qualities of life and are non life-threatening. In this patient, the pneumothorax needs to be addressed as part of the ABC. The subdural hematoma is potentially life threatening but with the patient's initial GCS of 14, this is not likely to pose a threat to his life at this time. The lower extremity fracutures are serious and may be compromising his lower extremity circulation, but this poses no threat to his life. Similarly, the facial laceration repair has the lowest priority among all his injuries.

40.4 **B.** Right chest tube placement is the most important initial intervention in this patient with chest wall deformity and diminished breath sounds. Endotracheal intubation does not appear necessary at this time in this individual with probable facial fracture but satisfactory airway.

40.5 **A.** Hypotension alone is associated with a 30-60% increase in the mortality associated with brain injury, and this is due to secondary brain injury that occurs as the result of reduced cerebral perfusion.

Clinical Pearls

- Airway, breathing, and circulation should be reassessed whenever clinical deterioration develops in a trauma patient.
- Obtaining a detailed description of the traumatic event helps identify the injury mechanisms and direct the evaluation process.
- A closed head injury is rarely the cause of hemodynamic instability in a trauma patient; therefore, the evaluation should be directed toward identification of the bleeding source.
- A low GCS score in a patient with profound shock may result from inadequate brain perfusion, and the usual sequence of approach should not be altered.

REFERENCES

Burch JM, Franciose RJ, Moore EE. Trauma. In: Brunicardi FC, Andersen DK, Dunn DL, et al, eds. *Schwartz's Principles of Surgery*. 8th ed. New York, NY: McGraw-Hill; 2005:129-187.

Committee on Trauma of the American College of Surgeons. Initial assessment and management. In: *Advanced Trauma Life Support Program for Doctors*, 7th ed. Chicago, IL: Committee on Trauma of the American College of Surgeons; 2004.

McSwain NE. Initial assessment and resuscitation of trauma patients: a practical, efficient, and evidence-based medicine approach. In: Cameron JL, ed. *Current Surgical Therapy*. 9th ed. Philadelphia, PA: Mosby Elsevier; 2008:930-936.

Case 41

A 44-year-old woman is found to have an incidental anterior mediastinal mass as revealed by a preemployment chest radiograph. The patient has no known medical problems, and she denies respiratory and gastrointestinal symptoms. On examination, she is found to have mild bilateral ptosis and no neck masses. The results of the cardiopulmonary examination are unremarkable, and there is no generalized lymphadenopathy. The neurologic examination reveals normal sensation and diminished muscle strength in all the extremities with repetitive motion against resistance. A CT scan of the chest reveals the presence of a 4.5-cm well-circumscribed solid mass in the anterior mediastinum.

➤ What is the diagnosis?

➤ What is the best therapy?

ANSWERS TO CASE 41: Thymoma and Myasthenia Gravis

Summary: A 44-year-old woman has a 4.5-cm anterior mediastinal mass and symptoms suggestive of myasthenia gravis.

- **Most likely diagnosis:** An incidentally identified thymoma in a patient with class IIA myasthenia gravis (MG).
- **Best therapy:** The best treatment for thymoma is complete resection.

ANALYSIS

Objectives

1. Know the pathogenesis and the medical management of MG.
2. Learn the role of thymectomy in the treatment of MG, with and without the presence of a thymoma.
3. Learn the strategies for diagnosing anterior mediastinal masses.

Considerations

MG is a disorder of the neuromuscular junction resulting from autoimmune damage to the nicotinic cholinergic receptor. Symptoms **include weakness that worsens after exercise and improves after rest.** Other symptoms include ptosis, diplopia, dysarthria, dysphagia, and respiratory complications. MG is evidenced by history and physical examination **and can be confirmed by provocative testing (the Edrophonium-Tensilon test).** The Osserman classification is a commonly used system for characterizing the severity of MG (Table 41–1). Medical management of MG varies depending on the response of the patient, including the response to anticholinesterase drugs, glucocorticoids (prednisone), and immunosuppressive drugs (azathioprine, cyclophosphamide). Acute exacerbations or myasthenic crises are treated medically and with plasmapheresis. **Thymectomy should be avoided during an acute crisis.**

Thymomas are the most common mediastinal tumors, and thymomas are considered borderline malignant because of the potential for local invasion and systemic spread. MG is one of the immune disorders that can occur with thymomas. MG is identified in 30% to 50% of patients with thymoma, whereas 15% of myasthenic patients have thymoma. Pathologic staging of thymoma relies on both the surgical assessment at the time of resection and the microscopic evaluation (Table 41–2).

Diagnostic sampling of anterior mediastinal masses suspected to be thymoma is usually unnecessary. Biopsy of anterior mediastinal masses may prove useful for patients with very extensive anterior mediastinal masses causing

Table 41–1 OSSERMAN CLASSIFICATION FOR SEVERITY OF MYASTHENIA GRAVIS

CLASS	SYMPTOMS
I	Occular involvement only (diplopia, ptosis)
IIA	Generalized muscle weakness without respiratory impairment
IIB	More bulbar manifestation than in class IIA
III	Rapid onset and progression of bulbar and generalized weakness including respiratory muscle weakness
IV	Severe generalized weakness, progressive myasthenic symptoms
V	Muscle atrophy requiring mechanical ventilation

invasion of adjacent vital structures and for patients in whom lymphoma is suspected. **The primary treatment of thymoma remains surgical resection via a median sternotomy.** Complete thymectomy includes removal of the entire thymus gland, pericardial fat, and thymoma *en bloc*. If macroscopic invasion of the thymoma is encountered, adjacent structures may be sacrificed (eg, pericardium, lung, a single phrenic nerve [but never both], great vessels), understanding that the best prognosis relies on a complete resection. Adjuvant therapies can be used accordingly.

Table 41–2 STAGING AND PROGNOSIS OF THYMOMA

STAGE	DESCRIPTION	TREATMENT	5-Y PROGNOSIS (%)
I	Completely encapsulated, no invasion	Surgical resection	90
II	Macroscopic invasion to fat or pleura or microscopic invasion through capsule	Radical surgical resection	70-80
III	Macroscopic invasion to adjacent structure: pericardium, great vessels, lung, or intrathoracic metastasis	Radical surgical resection and/or XRT	50-60
IV	Extrathoracic metastasis	Chemotherapy, XRT	20-30

Abbreviation: XRT, radiotherapy.

APPROACH TO
Thymoma and Myasthenia Gravis

DEFINITIONS

MYASTHENIA GRAVIS (MG): An uncommon autoimmune disorder of peripheral nerves in which antibodies form against acetylcholine (ACh) nicotinic postsynaptic receptors at the myoneural junction. A reduction in the number of ACh receptors results in progressively reduced muscle strength with repeated use of the muscle and recovery of muscle strength following a period of rest. The eye muscles tend to be affected.

THYMOMA: The most common type of tumor of the thymus, located in the anterior mediastinum. Most are benign, although they can be malignant. They can cause autoimmune disorders such as myasthenia gravis, red cell aplasia, or hypogammaglobulinemia.

CLINICAL APPROACH

Surgical Outcome

At 5 years postresection, 25% to 30% of patients show complete remission of MG; 35% to 60% have an improvement in symptoms with a decrease in their medication requirement; 20% show no change in status; and 10% to 15% have a worsening of their symptoms.

Evaluation and Treatment of an Anterior Mediastinal Mass

The mediastinum is divided into three compartments: anterior (superior), middle, and posterior. Neurogenic tumors (20%), usually located in the posterior mediastinum, are the most common mediastinal tumor, followed by thymomas (15%-20%), which are located in the anterior mediastinum. An estimated 25% to 40% of mediastinal masses are malignant.

Evaluation of an anterior mediastinal mass always begins with a review of the history, a physical examination, and a screening chest radiograph demonstrating a mediastinal mass. Particular attention should be given to identifying symptoms and findings that indicate thyroid pathology and to detecting the presence of diffuse adenopathy suggesting the possibility of lymphoma. A CT scan of the chest is often helpful in identifying the exact location, the invasion of adjacent structures, associated lymphadenopathy, and intra- or

Table 41–3 EVALUATION AND TREATMENT OF ANTERIOR MEDIASTINAL MASSES

TUMOR	DIAGNOSIS	TREATMENT
Thymoma	Surgical resection	Surgical resection, possible XRT, chemotherapy
Lymphoma	Open mediastinotomy, video-assisted thoracoscopy if fine-needle aspiration biopsy is equivocal	Chemotherapy or XRT, depending on cell type
Germ cell tumor		
Teratoma	Surgical resection	Surgical resection
Seminoma	PE	XRT
Nonseminoma	PE, positive β-human chorionic gonadotropin and α fetoprotein tests	Chemotherapy
Parathyroid adenoma	Hyperparathyroidism, CT scan, Sestaimibi scan	Surgical resection
Aberrant thyroid	CT scan	Surgical resection if symptomatic
Lipoma, hemangioma, thymic cyst	CT scan, magnetic resonance imaging	Surgical resection if symptomatic or to rule out malignancy

Abbreviations: XRT, radiotherapy; PE, physical examination; CT, computed tomography.

extrathoracic metastasis. When germ cell tumors (seminomatous and non-seminomatous) are suspected, serum marker, α-fetoprotein, and human chorionic gonadotropin measurements should be obtained (see Table 41–3 for a summary of treatment recommendations).

Indications for Biopsy

Patients with mediastinal masses are often referred for tissue diagnosis, but fine-needle aspiration (FNA) is seldom helpful. Open resection can be performed directly for most anterior mediastinal masses. If lymphoma or stage III or IV thymoma is suspected, open biopsy via an anterior mediastinotomy or video-assisted thoracoscopy is indicated.

Comprehension Questions

For questions 41.1-41.3, match the following locations (A–C) within the mediastinum to the most appropriate disorders.

A. Anterior
B. Middle
C. Posterior

41.1 Neurogenic tumors

41.2 Thymomas

41.3 Teratomas

41.4 Staging of thymoma is determined primarily by which of the following?
A. Surgical evaluation
B. Pathologic immunohistochemistry
C. Magnetic resonance imaging evaluation
D. CT scan evaluation

41.5 A 25-year old medical student is reading a chapter on myasthenia gravis, and recalls that his grandmother had this disorder. She had a thymectomy for her condition. Which of the following statements is most accurate regarding thymectomy and myasthenia gravis?
A. Thymectomy is indicated for all patients with myasthenia gravis.
B. Anticholinesterase is used in the treatment of myasthenia gravis.
C. Thymectomy is most effective for the treatment of myasthenia gravis when performed during an acute crisis.
D. The indication for thymectomy in the setting of a patient with a 3-cm suspected thymoma is the prevention of myasthenia gravis.

41.6 In which of the following patients is CT-guided biopsy of the mediastinal mass indicated?
A. A 35-year-old man with HIV who develops a large, ill-defined anterior mediastinal mass that appears to closely involve the mediastinal vessels.
B. A 47-year-old man with enlarged cervical lymph nodes, axillary lymph nodes, mediastinal lymph nodes.
C. A 28-year-old man with a left testicular mass, markedly elevated serum alpha-fetal protein level, and a large ill-defined mass in the anterior mediastinum.
D. A 55-year-old woman with a thyroid mass that has been growing over the past 15 years is complaining of compressive symptoms whenever she lies flat. There is also evidence of tracheal deviation in the upper mediastinum as the result of mediastinal extension of the mass.

ANSWERS

41.1 **C.** Neurogenic tumors are usually located in the posterior mediastinum.

41.2 **A.** Thymomas are usually found in the anterior mediastinum.

41.3 **A.** Germ cell tumors (such as teratomas) are also usually found in the anterior mediastinum.

41.4 **A.** Thymoma staging is based on the pathologic and histologic characteristics of the tumor.

41.5 **B.** Myasthenia gravis is an autoimmune disease causing injury to the nicotinic cholinergic receptors, and anticholinesterase is a form of treatment. Thymectomy is indicated for the subset of patients with myasthenia gravis who also have thymomas, and in these patients, the basis for the thymectomy is to remove the thymoma which has the potential for malignant transformation. The likelihood of postoperative complications is dramatically increased when thymectomy is performed in patients with inadequately treated acute myasthenia crisis.

41.6 **A.** A 35-year-old man with HIV, who develops a large, ill-defined, anterior mediastinal mass could have lymphoma that requires tissue diagnosis prior to the initiation of chemotherapy but would not necessarily benefit from surgical resection; even though, percutaneous biopsy may not provide the definitive diagnosis, it is worth trying. The patient described in "B" most likely has lymphoma and has other sites from where tissue biopsies can be performed that would be less invasive. The patient described in "C" most likely has nonseminomatous testicular cancer, and could have the diagnosis established by radical orchiectomy. The woman described in "D" most likely has a symptomatic goiter with mediastinal extension, surgery for removal is indicated to relieve symptoms and a biopsy is not going to alter her treatment plan.

Clinical Pearls

- Anterior mediastinal masses often require surgical resection for diagnosis and treatment.
- Staging of thymoma takes place at the time of surgical resection by macroscopic inspection.
- Proper staging and complete resection determine the prognosis for thymoma.

REFERENCE

Kesler KA. Primary tumors of the thymus. In: Cameron JL, ed. *Current Surgical Therapy*. 9th ed. Philadelphia, PA: Mosby Elsevier; 2008:717-722.

Varghese Jr TK, Lau CL. The mediastinum. In: Townsend CM Jr, Beauchamp RD, Evers BM, eds. *Sabiston Textbook of Surgery*. 18th ed. Philadelphia, PA: Elsevier Saunders; 2008:1677-1697.

Case 42

A 20-year-old man reports that he has had a nontender, heavy sensation in his scrotal area for 2 months. He jogs several miles every day but denies lifting heavy objects. He does not recall trauma to the area and has no urinary complaints. He is healthy and does not smoke. On examination, his blood pressure is 110/70 mm Hg and his heart rate is 80 beats/min; he is afebrile. The results from his heart and lung examinations are normal. There is no back tenderness. His abdomen is nontender and without masses. The external genitalia reveal a 2-cm nontender mass in the right testis. Transillumination shows no light penetration. The findings from a rectal examination are unremarkable.

- What is the most likely diagnosis?
- What is the best therapy for this patient?

ANSWERS TO CASE 42: Testicular Cancer

Summary: A 20-year-old man is noted to have had a nontender heavy sensation in the scrotal area for 2 months. He jogs several miles every day but denies lifting heavy objects. He denies trauma to the area and has no urinary complaints. A 2-cm, nontransilluminating, nontender mass in the right testis is noted. The results from a rectal examination are unremarkable.

- **Most likely diagnosis:** Testicular cancer.
- **Best therapy for this patient:** Surgery (radical orchiectomy) with possible chemotherapy.

ANALYSIS

Objectives

1. Know that a nontender, nontransilluminating testicular mass in a man younger than 40 years should be considered testicular cancer unless proven otherwise.
2. Understand that knowledge of the correct pathologic diagnosis or cell type(s) is crucial in directing therapy.
3. Know that a testicular carcinoma can be cured; however, patient compliance with treatment and surveillance protocols is important.

Considerations

Testicular cancer is the most common malignancy in men between the age of 15 and 35, with an incidence of 3 to 5 per 100,000 men. It is more common in white males than in black males. Thus, this patient matches the most common profile. Although a **painless scrotal mass is the most common presentation,** references are often made to a trivial traumatic event that may have brought the scrotal mass to the patient's attention. Further, an incorrect clinical diagnosis such as varicocele, spermatocele, hydrocele, epididymitis, or testicular torsion may further delay appropriate evaluation and treatment. Regular scrotal self-examination is advocated but rarely performed; rather, an element of **embarrassment often delays presentation.**

The next step for this patient is a complete examination at the time of presentation to search for evidence of metastatic disease. There are tumor markers for many of cell types, most prominently β-human chorionic gonadotropin (β-hCG) and α-fetoprotein (AFP). A radical orchiectomy would be the best therapy. **Tumor cell types** are generally divided into **seminoma and nonseminomatous germ cell tumors.** Treatment protocols rely on an accurate diagnosis of the cell type(s) within the tumor. A skilled pathologist often reviews many slides from the surgical specimen, using special stainings when necessary to obtain a diagnosis.

APPROACH TO Testicular Masses

DEFINITIONS

RADICAL ORCHIECTOMY: A surgical procedure in which an inguinal incision is made over the cord leading to the testicle to be removed. The surgical specimen includes testis, epididymis, and spermatic cord taken at the internal iliac ring. Care is taken not to incise the scrotum itself during the surgical procedure.

RETROPERITONEAL LYMPHADENECTOMY: A surgical procedure performed to remove the lymph nodes draining the testicle. **Testicular cancer often progresses in an orderly fashion up the lymphatic drainage of the testis.** Testicular lymphatics flow from the testis through the spermatic cord following the testicular artery into the retroperitoneum where they drain into nodes around the vena cava and aorta.

GERM CELL TUMOR: **Ninety percent of cancers of the testis are derived from the germinal epithelium** (sperm-forming elements) of the testis. Subtypes include **choriocarcinoma, embryonal carcinoma, seminoma, teratoma, and yolk sac tumor.** The other 10% of testicular tumors are made up of what is known as gonadal stromal tumors, secondary tumors of the testis such as lymphoma, and metastatic tumors to the testis.

CLINICAL APPROACH

When a man presents with a chief complaint of a testicular mass, a detailed examination of the genitalia should be performed, delineating the **character of the mass, painful versus painless, hard versus soft, and transilluminating versus nontransilluminating.** Palpation of the **lymph nodes,** examination of the male breasts, and a general survey of the signs and symptoms related not only to the genitourinary system but also to the **endocrine and neurologic systems** are important.

Radical (inguinal) orchiectomy should be performed when it is confirmed that the lesion within the scrotum is a **solid mass.** An **ultrasound of the scrotum is helpful** in making this determination. Preoperative testing should also include tumor markers such as **β-hCG** and **AFP, which are elevated in 80%-85% of the patients with nonseminomatous germ cell tumors.** Lactic acid dehydrogenase and placental alkaline phosphatase are also useful tumor markers. A **chest radiograph** should be obtained preoperatively to rule out metastatic disease that may influence the anesthetic method.

Once the diagnosis of testicular cancer is confirmed, further metastatic evaluation such as a CT scan of the abdomen and chest is warranted. Therapeutic decisions depend first on an accurate pathologic diagnosis of the cell type(s) within the tumor. **Often there is more than one cell type, hence the term "mixed germ cell tumor."** Other important factors determining therapeutic decisions include the extent of disease (tumor stage), risk factors (known characteristics of the tumor type or extent that are often associated with an aggressive prognosis), and compliance of the patient.

Although testicular cancer has played a part in one of the modern medical success stories, where the terms "cure" and "cancer" can be used honestly in the same sentence, it does strike men at a time when they are otherwise healthy and are not used to medical intervention. **Compliance with the aggressive regimens of chemotherapy, radiation therapy, and/or surgery is key to avoiding tumor relapse and to detecting disease progression as early as possible.**

Pure seminoma is treated differently from other nonseminomatous germ cell tumors primarily because of its **exquisite sensitivity to radiation therapy and its response to chemotherapy** when the disease is bulky and advanced. Residual testicular tumor following chemotherapy is treated with surgery, most often retroperitoneal lymphadenectomy. After successful treatment of a testicular tumor, patients need lifelong surveillance of their remaining testicle because the incidence of carcinoma becomes greater by a manyfold factor.

Comprehension Questions

42.1 A 16-year-old adolescent is being evaluated by the pediatrician for pubertal abnormalities. The physician describes a risk of malignancy of the gonads. Which of the following is most likely to be associated with testicular cancer?

A. XY gonadal dysgenesis
B. Androgen insensitivity
C. Turner syndrome
D. Noonan syndrome

42.2 Physical examination of a young man with testicular cancer during a routine surveillance visit reveals a hard mass just above the left clavicle. Which of the following is the most likely diagnosis?

A. Chemotherapy sclerosis of the subclavian vein
B. Metastatic testicular cancer
C. Second primary cancer of head and neck origin
D. Pathologic fracture of the clavicle

42.3 A 28-year-old man is found to have a mass of the right testicle, which is suspected to be a malignancy. Which of the following best describes the fertility of a patient before treatment for testicular cancer?

A. Below normal on average
B. Same as that of his peers
C. Above average
D. Far worse than average

42.4 A 22-year old man is noted to have a painless scrotal mass. The alphafetoprotein level is elevated. Which of the following statements is most accurate regarding the role of serum alpha-fetal protein in testicular cancer?

A. Marked elevation in man with testicular mass generally indicates seminomatous testicular cancer.
B. Serum levels may be used to determine response to therapy.
C. The development of effective chemotherapeutic agents has eliminated the need for alpha-fetal protein level assessment.
D. The levels of serum alpha-fetal protein does not change following radical orchiectomy in a patient with a 4-cm nonseminomatous cancer of the left testicle.

42.5 Which of the following is an accurate statement regarding testicular seminomas?

A. Seminomas are sensitive to radiation therapy.
B. Orchiectomy is never indicated for treatment.
C. Pain is the most common presentation.
D. Biopsy is best determined by core needle biopsy under sedation.

ANSWERS

42.1 **A.** Intraabdominal male gonads with Y chromosomes tend to become malignant. In androgen insensitivity, the patient is 46 XY genotype but defective androgen receptors do not allow the external genitalia to masculinize. Although both androgen insensitivity and XY gonadal dysgenesis have a propensity to become malignant, the nonfunctional dysgenetic gonad has the greater risk.

42.2 **B.** The Virchow node is palpated in this clinical question. This physical finding indicates a metastatic tumor within the lymph node. This supraclavicular lymph node is a harbinger of more extensive disease and may be the only clinical finding of more extensive retroperitoneal metastases. Palpation of this region is an essential part of the initial and follow-up examinations of men with testicular cancer because of the lymphatic predilections of the disease.

42.3 **A.** For reasons not yet clear, the fertility of men at the time of diagnosis of testicular cancer is abnormal as assessed by a semen analysis. Certainly, surgery, radiation, and chemotherapy greatly further reduce the fertility of men with testicular cancer. The likelihood of reduced fertility and the side effects of treatments on fertility must be discussed with men who receive a diagnosis of testicular cancer.

42.4 **B.** The serum markers such as alpha-fetal protein levels can be useful in assessing the patient's response to chemotherapy for nonseminomatous testicular cancers. Patients with seminomatous testicular cancers generally have normal or mildly elevated serum marker values.

42.5 **A.** Seminomas are sensitive to radiation therapy, therefore extratesticular extension of the disease such as disease involving the inguinal, iliac, and peri-aortic lymph nodes can be treated with radiation therapy following radical orchiectomy. Needle biopsy is contraindicated for patients with testicular masses that are suspicious for testicular cancers.

Clinical Pearls

- Nearly all testicular cancers are of germ cell origin, and approximately half are caused by seminomas. Many cancers have multiple cell types whose delineation is crucial for the therapy.
- Cryptorchidism (undescended testicle) significantly increases the risk of a germ cell tumor even if the maldescended testicle is surgically corrected.
- An inguinal incision is made for a radical orchiectomy to avoid disruption of the lymphatic drainage of the testicle, which normally does not involve the scrotum itself.
- A testicular mass that is solid (does not transilluminate) in a young man should be assumed to be testicular cancer until proven otherwise.

REFERENCES

Olumi AF, Richie JP. Urologic surgery. In: Townsend CM Jr, Beauchamp RD, Evers BM, Mattox KL, eds. *Sabiston Textbook of Surgery*. 18th ed. Philadelphia, PA: Elsevier Saunders; 2008:2251-2286.

Tanagho EA, McAninch JW. *Smith's General Urology*. 16th ed. New York, NY: Lange Medical Books/McGraw-Hill; 2005.

Case 43

A 35-year-old man presents with a 3-week history of perianal pain. The patient describes excruciating pain and bleeding produced by defecation. These episodes of pain generally last for 15 to 20 minutes. Because of his pain, the patient has been unable to defecate over the past 3 days. He denies any fever, difficulty with urination, or previous episodes of pain. His past medical history is unremarkable. He does not take any medications. On physical examination, his temperature is 37.7°C (99.9°F), pulse rate 100 beats/min, and blood pressure 140/90 mm Hg. Examination of the perirectal region reveals an anal skin tag located in the posterior 12 o'clock position. There are no masses, erythema, or tenderness in the perianal or buttock region. During an attempted digital rectal examination, the patient had exquisite tenderness, resulting in an inadequate evaluation. The laboratory findings revealed a normal WBC count, normal hemoglobin and hematocrit values, and a platelet count within the normal range.

- What is the most likely diagnosis?
- What is the most likely mechanism for this condition?
- What are your next steps?

ANSWERS TO CASE 43: Anorectal Disease

Summary: A 35-year-old man presents with severe anorectal pain associated with defecation. He has no fever. The examination is incomplete because of patient discomfort and reveals a perianal skin tag but no erythema, mass, or swelling.

➤ **Diagnosis:** Anal fissure.

➤ **Mechanisms:** Causes include trauma to the anal canal from the passage of large firm stool and regional ischemia of the mucosa related to a hypertonic internal sphincter.

➤ **Next steps:** At this juncture, a complete anal examination should be performed. Severe pain frequently prevents this examination from being completed, and most patients require sedation or a topical, regional, or general anesthetic.

ANALYSIS

Objectives

1. Learn the differential diagnosis for anorectal pain.
2. Learn the approach to diagnosis and treatment of common anorectal diseases.

Considerations

The case presented is classic for a patient with an anal fissure. Hemorrhoids, fistula-in-ano, and perirectal abscess are other commonly encountered anorectal complaints seen in clinical practice. These diagnoses are unlikely because hemorrhoids and fistulae are usually painless and an abscess would cause erythema and tenderness in the perianal and buttock region. To treat this patient, a thorough physical examination must be performed either under regional anesthesia or with sedation. An anal fissure may present as an acute or chronic problem. On physical examination, a tear is seen in the anoderm. The tear can also extend into the lining of the anal canal, often to the dentate line. It is produced by trauma caused by the passage of hard stool and the presence of elevated internal sphincter pressures (resting pressures). Anal fissures are commonly found in the posterior midline position and, if chronic, can be associated with a skin tag. The symptom most typical of anal fissures is intense pain accompanying defecation. Bleeding is also very common. Many patients with fissures have constipation, which can contribute to the problem but may develop as the patient refuses to defecate in an effort to avoid the pain. Nonoperative treatment should be attempted for patients with an acute anal fissure, including sitz baths, bulking agents, a stool softener, and topical nitroglycerine ointment. Nitroglycerine ointment acts as a vasodilator and improves blood flow to the ischemic posterior portion of the anal canal. When patients with chronic and recurrent fissures are encountered, local injection of botulinum toxin or operative therapy to reduce the resting sphincter tone (lateral internal sphincterotomy) may be indicated. The risk of incontinence with lateral internal sphincterotomy is as high as 35%. Thus, it should be used as a last resort.

APPROACH TO Anorectal Complaints

DEFINITIONS

HEMORRHOIDS: Abnormal enlargement of the hemorrhoidal venous plexus caused by constipation or diarrhea, obesity, and increased intra-abdominal pressure. Internal hemorrhoids are located above the dentate line; external hemorrhoids are located below the dentate line. Internal hemorrhoids can be classified as follows:

Grade I—prominent hemorrhoids on inspection or on anoscopy
Grade II—hemorrhoids that prolapse but reduce spontaneously
Grade III—hemorrhoids that require manual reduction
Grade IV—nonreducible hemorrhoids

FISTULA-IN-ANO: Abnormal communication between the anal canal and the perineum. Fistulas are draining sinuses that represent the end result of perianal abscesses. Abscesses form when the crypts at the dentate line become obstructed. The crypts lead into anal glands, which then become infected and create abscesses. Most fistulas arise several weeks to months after the abscess is drained and track into different spaces and planes in the perianal region. Fistulas are named based on their relationship to the anal sphincter muscles; intersphincteric, between the internal and external sphincters; transsphincteric, across both the internal and external sphincters; suprasphincteric, above the sphincter complex, originating at the dentate line; and extrasphincteric, above the sphincter complex but originating in the rectum.

GOODSALL RULE: Used to find the internal opening of a fistula. Most fistulas located anteriorly to a transverse anal imaginary line, that is, an anterior hemicircumference of the anus, track straight directly to the dentate line. Fistulas in the posterior portion or hemicircumference track in a curved line toward the posterior midline or commissure of the anal canal.

SETON: A loop of plastic or silicone, commonly a vascular "vessel loop," which is placed through a fistula when there is a significant amount of sphincter muscle involved. The seton spares the sphincter muscle and remains in place for weeks to months until the drainage resolves and the fistula closes.

CLINICAL APPROACH

Most patients with perianal, anal, or rectal disease self-medicate with over-the-counter products. They consult a physician only when the symptoms worsen or become complicated. It is therefore imperative to obtain a thorough, detailed history regarding symptom duration and prior treatments. An anorectal examination can be performed with the patient either in the left lateral decubitus position with knees flexed or in the prone jackknife position. The key is to provide the most privacy and comfort. The examination consists of a careful inspection of the anoderm followed by a digital examination and circumferential anoscopy with or without sedation. When indicated, rigid proctosigmoidoscopy or flexible sigmoidoscopy may provide additional information but generally requires additional preparations and a separate visit to the office or outpatient endoscopy suite. During inspection, one should look for lesions, rashes, discharge, or other defects. Digital palpation is performed to identify any masses, gauge sphincter tone, and establish the presence of bleeding (Table 43–1). Malignancy and inflammatory bowel disease should always be considered in the differential diagnosis when patients present with chronic or recurrent anorectal complaints. Biopsies should be strongly considered during the evaluation. Anoscopy is performed to visualize an anal tear and to inspect and evaluate palpable lesions and hemorrhoids. During anoscopy, visualization of the dentate line marks the division between the rectal and the anal mucosae. The lack of somatic innervation above the dentate line makes lesions above this area less painful.

Table 43–1 EXAMINATION FINDINGS AND TREATMENT

SOURCE	APPEARANCE	PALPATION	ANOSCOPY
Anal fissure	Superficial tear in anoderm, sentinel tag	Tear; increased sphincter tone, hypertrophic anal papilla	Tear, bleeding, hypertrophic anal papilla
Hemorrhoids	Blue or purple mass at anus	Enlarged soft mass	Prominent veins above or below dentate line
Fistula-in-ano	Purulent drainage, erythema, ulcer, fluctuant mass	Fluctuant mass, induration	Small rough areas in anus

Symptoms

Anal Fissure: Severe anal pain with defection, bleeding, itching, and minimal drainage.

Hemorrhoids:

Grade I—asymptomatic or possible painless bleeding
Grade II—possible bleeding and pruritus
Grade III—prolapsing and bleeding
Grade IV—painful, nonreducible hemorrhoids

Perianal Abscess: Painful, fluctuant perianal mass or ulcer associated with fever and/or purulent drainage.

Fistula-in-ano: Drainage of pus or mucus or minimal stool soilage on undergarments.

Treatment

Anal fissure: Sitz baths, stool softeners, suppositories, bulking agents, and nitroglycerin ointment. Chronic fissures can be treated with botulinum toxin injection or internal sphincterotomy (see Table 43–2).

Table 43–2 ANORECTAL DISEASES AND TREATMENT

	SYMPTOMS	FINDINGS	TREATMENT
Fissure-in-ano	Anal pain with defecation, bleeding, itching, drainage	Tear in anoderm, spastic sphincter tone sentinel tag, hypertrophic anal papilla	Sitz baths, stool softeners, suppositories, nitroglycerin; partial internal sphincterotomy
Hemorrhoids Grade I	Painless bleeding	Engorged hemorrhoids	Diet changes
Grade II	Bleeding, pruritus, mild pain	Hemorrhoid prolapses	Diet, band ligation, infrared coagulation
Grade III	Pain, bleeding	Prolapsing hemorrhoids, manual reduction	Rubber band ligation hemorrhoidectomy
Grade IV	Nonreducible hemorrhoids, severe pain	Bleeding, strangulation	Hemorrhoidectomy
Fistula-in-ano	Ulcer, painful fluctuant mass, purulent	Scarred tract from dentate line to external opening	Draining and/or fistulotomy

Hemorrhoids:

Grade I—diet changes (increase bulk and fluid intake)
Grade II—diet changes, rubber band ligation, infrared coagulation
Grade III—rubber band ligation or hemorrhoidectomy
Grade IV—hemorrhoidectomy

Fistula-in-ano: Fistulotomy for superficial fistulae. Seton placement if more sphincter muscle is involved.

Abscess: Incision and drainage under local anesthetic if small or under sedation if large.

Comprehension Questions

43.1 A 44-year-old man is being evaluated for possible anal fissure. Which of the following findings suggest the diagnosis of an anal fissure?

A. Fever, a fluctuant mass, obesity, and diarrhea
B. Painless rectal bleeding, a purple anal mass, and an ulcer
C. Presence of a purulent sinus, erythema, and a fluctuant mass
D. Severe anal pain, a tear in the posterior anoderm, bleeding, and increased sphincter tone

43.2 The differential diagnosis for an anal fissure should include which of the following?

A. Rectocele
B. Condyloma
C. Rectal polyp
D. Crohn disease

43.3 Which of the following is the most appropriate next step after establishing a diagnosis for a patient suspected of having an anal fissure?

A. Obtain a barium enema, followed by a colonoscopy
B. Rectoanal examination under sedation, anoscopy, and proctoscopy
C. Anal biopsy, anoscopy in the office, and a barium enema
D. Rectoanal examination in the office without sedation, anal biopsy, and fissurectomy

43.4 Which of the following is considered the most appropriate treatment for acute anal fissure?

A. Infrared coagulation, sitz baths, and oral antibiotics
B. Rubber band ligation, suppositories, and topical antibiotics
C. Increased dietary bulk, sitz baths, and nitroglycerin ointment
D. Infrared coagulation and fissurectomy

ANSWERS

43.1 **D.** Severe anal pain, a tear in the posterior anoderm, bleeding, and increased sphincter tone are findings compatible with anal fissure.

43.2 **D.** Crohn disease, ulcerated hemorrhoid, and malignancy should be included in the differential diagnosis when evaluating an anal fissure.

43.3 **B.** Examination under anesthesia, anoscopy, and proctoscopy are appropriate steps in evaluating a patient clinically suspected of having an anal fissure.

43.4 **C.** Conservative management of an anal fissure consists of increasing dietary bulk and using sitz baths, stool softeners, and nitroglycerin ointment.

Clinical Pearls

- ➤ Patients may be reluctant to volunteer information regarding bowel habits and duration of symptoms; therefore, it is important to be specific in questioning the patient during the interview.
- ➤ Anorectal carcinoma may manifest as severe perianal pain and tenderness and must be considered part of the differential diagnosis.
- ➤ Patients with anal fissure characteristically have severe anal pain, a tear in the posterior anoderm, bleeding, and increased sphincter tone.
- ➤ A nonhealing anal fissure or a fissure located anywhere other than in the posterior area of the anus should alert the clinician to the possibility of Crohn disease or a malignancy.
- ➤ A thrombosed external hemorrhoid not responding to medical therapy should be treated by excisional thrombectomy instead of incision and drainage.

REFERENCES

Costedio M, Cataldo PA. Anal fissure. In: Cameron JL, ed. *Current Surgical Therapy*. 9th ed. Philadelphia, PA: Mosby Elsevier; 2008:268-271.

Nelson H, Cima RR. Anus. In: Townsend CM Jr, Beauchamp RD, Evers BM, eds. *Sabiston Textbook of Surgery*. 18th ed. Philadelphia, PA: Elsevier; 2008:1433-1462.

Case 44

A healthy 53-year-old woman was involved in a low-speed automobile collision and brought to the emergency department 4 weeks ago. Because the patient's physical examination revealed mild abdominal tenderness, she underwent a computed tomographic (CT) scan of her abdomen that revealed an incidental 3.5-cm solid mass in the left adrenal gland. The patient was discharged from the emergency department with instructions to follow up for an outpatient evaluation of the left adrenal mass. During her office visit, she indicates she is feeling well, and she is asymptomatic. Her heart rate is 70 beats/min and her blood pressure 138/82 mm Hg. Her physical examination reveals no abnormal findings.

- What is the differential diagnosis for an incidental adrenal mass?
- What are the important elements of the history and physical examination in a patient with an adrenal mass?
- What is the most likely diagnosis?

ANSWERS TO CASE 44:
Adrenal Incidentaloma and Pheochromocytoma

Summary: A 53-year-old woman is found to have an incidental 3.5-cm solid adrenal mass.

- **Differential diagnosis:** May include a variety of primary malignant tumors, metastatic tumors, and benign functioning and nonfunctioning tumors.
- **History and physical examination:** The history should describe symptoms of hypertension, previous malignancies, prior endocrinopathies, and previous imaging studies, as well as family medical history. The physical examination should include an abdominal examination and a blood pressure reading, and the patient's general appearance should be noted.
- **Most likely diagnosis:** Nonfunctioning adenoma.

ANALYSIS

Objectives

1. Learn the prevalence of clinically inapparent adrenal masses otherwise referred to as adrenal incidentalomas.
2. Become familiar with nonfunctioning and functioning adrenal tumors as well as the other clinical entities that may manifest as an incidentaloma.
3. Learn the diagnostic evaluation and management of an adrenal incidentaloma.
4. Become familiar with the clinical presentation of a patient with pheochromocytoma.
5. Learn to outline a diagnostic plan for pre-, intra-, and postoperative treatment of a patient with a pheochromocytoma.

APPROACH TO
Adrenal Incidentalomas

CLINICAL APPROACH

The term "adrenal incidentaloma" refers to a clinically inapparent adrenal mass that is discovered inadvertently in the course of diagnostic testing for other conditions. Incidental adrenal masses are found in 0.7% to 4.3% of patients undergoing abdominal CT scans and in 1.4% to 8.7% of patients at autopsy. **Most adrenal incidentalomas are nonfunctioning adenomas,**

accounting for 55% to 94% of all cases. Functioning tumors, which include pheochromocytoma, aldosterone-producing adenoma, and cortisol-producing adenoma, are less common. Other adrenal tumors that can appear as incidentalomas are ganglioneuroma, adrenocortical carcinoma, and metastases. The differential diagnosis also includes myelolipoma, cysts, and hemorrhage, which are entities that can be diagnosed on the basis of CT criteria alone. An adrenal hematoma is not an infrequent finding in a patient who sustains abdominal trauma, and the diagnosis is confirmed with resolution of the mass on follow-up CT scanning.

The evaluation of a patient with an adrenal incidentaloma consists of obtaining a history, performing a physical examination, and making a functional and anatomic assessment of the adrenal mass. **Specific signs and symptoms of excess catecholamines, aldosterone, cortisol, and androgens should be actively sought in the history and on physical examination.** At minimum, patients should be asked about a history of hypertension and whether or not they have been experiencing headaches, palpitations, profuse sweating, abdominal pain, or anxiety. All patients should be questioned about a prior history of malignancy. When present, adrenal masses are metastases in up to 75% of patients. In addition to obtaining a resting heart rate and a blood pressure reading, patients should be examined for features suggestive of Cushing syndrome such as truncal obesity, moon facies, thin extremities, prominent fat deposition in the supraclavicular areas and the nape of the neck, hirsutism, bruising, abdominal striae, and facial plethora.

The functional assessment consists of the following: measurement of plasma-free metanephrine levels; a **24-hour urine collection** for detection of **vanillylmandelic acid (VMA)**, metanephrine, and normetanephrine to evaluate for pheochromocytoma; a serum potassium test; measurement of aldosterone and plasma renin activity to evaluate for an aldosterone-producing adenoma; and an overnight 1-mg dexamethasone suppression test to evaluate for hypercortisolism.

Once it has been determined whether an adrenal mass is functioning or nonfunctioning, the next step is an anatomic assessment, preferably with unenhanced CT or magnetic resonance imaging. Positron emission tomography (PET) scanning is used for the evaluation of an adrenal mass in a patient with a known extra-adrenal cancer because it is of value in separating benign lesions from metastases. It is also important in excluding the presence of other metastases. Myelolipomas, cysts, and hemorrhage of the adrenal gland can be identified on the basis of CT criteria alone. CT imaging has been less useful in differentiating benign from malignant lesions. However, certain imaging characteristics are suggestive of adrenocortical carcinoma, including irregular margins, inhomogeneous density, scattered areas of decreased attenuation, and local invasion. Other CT criteria that increase the probability of malignancy include large tumor size and tumor enlargement over time. **Primary adrenocortical carcinomas are rare, and the majority of them are ≥6 cm.**

For nonfunctioning tumors of the adrenal gland, selecting a tumor size for which surgery will be recommended requires a determination of the risks and benefits. The larger the size threshold for surgery, the lower the number of unnecessary operations on patients with benign disease; however, rare patients with small adrenocortical carcinomas will be missed. The smaller the tumor threshold, the greater the likelihood that all carcinomas will be resected but at the expense of performing increasing number of unnecessary operations for patients with nonfunctioning, benign tumors. No consensus exists for a recommended size cutoff for surgery. In patients with adrenal incidentaloma, **surgery is recommended for all functioning tumors, nonfunctioning tumors ≥ 4 cm, tumors** < 4 cm that are **enlarging,** tumors of any size with imaging characteristics **suggestive of carcinoma,** and a **solitary adrenal metastasis.**

Treatment in Patients with Other Malignancies

The adrenal gland is well recognized as a site of metastasis. **The most common tumor metastasizing to the adrenal gland is lung carcinoma.** Other tumors include carcinoma of the breast, kidney, colon, and stomach, and melanoma. The patient with adrenal incidentaloma and a prior history of malignancy should undergo a biochemical assessment to exclude a functioning tumor. Whole-body PET scanning is performed in patients with a nonfunctioning tumor to exclude the presence of other metastases. Surgery is recommended for a solitary lesion ≥ 4 cm. **Fine-needle aspiration biopsy is reserved for a solitary nonfunctioning lesion** smaller than **4 cm because the result will alter treatment.** Patients with negative results from a fine-needle aspiration biopsy are treated nonoperatively. Finally, nonsurgical treatment is recommended for patients with diffuse metastases.

Follow-Up

A patient with a nonfunctioning adrenal incidentaloma smaller than 4 cm usually undergoes follow-up CT scans at 3 and 15 months. If there is no change in the size of the mass, the patient is followed annually by reviewing the history and performing a physical examination. Repeated biochemical testing is reserved for abnormal findings from the history or the physical examination.

APPROACH TO Pheochromocytoma

Pheochromocytoma is a tumor that most commonly arises from the chromaffin cells of the adrenal medulla and secretes catecholamines. **Pheochromocytoma is known as the "10% tumor" because 10% are bilateral, extra-adrenal, multiple, malignant, or familial.** The hallmark clinical manifestation of pheochromocytoma is **hypertension** that can be either paroxysmal or sustained. **Headache, palpitations, and profuse sweating** are other common manifestations. Anxiety and abdominal pain may also occur.

Because of the increasing application of CT imaging, up to half of the patients with pheochromocytoma are identified during biochemical testing for clinically silent incidentaloma.

The diagnosis of pheochromocytoma usually requires a demonstration of excess catecholamine production by one of two methods: **a 24-hour urine collection to test for metanephrine, normetanephrine, and VMA and/or measurement of plasma-free metanephrine levels.** Measurements of plasma-free metanephrine levels have a sensitivity of 99% and a specificity of 89% and as a result have been advocated by some as the initial biochemical test for the diagnosis of pheochromocytoma.

Imaging and Localization

Once a pheochromocytoma has been diagnosed by biochemical studies, tumor localization is the next step. Preoperative imaging studies are also important to exclude multiple, bilateral, or extra-adrenal pheochromocytomas. Abdominal CT imaging and magnetic resonance imaging (MRI) have at least 95% sensitivity in detecting an adrenal pheochromocytoma. A pheochromocytoma usually appears bright on a T2-weighted MRI. Both CT imaging and MRI have a specificity of as low as 50% in some studies related to the high frequency of adrenal masses that are not pheochromocytomas. **An iodine-131 metaiodobenzylguanidine (MIBG) scan is usually obtained for confirmation of pheochromocytoma because of its superior specificity of 90% to 100%.** PET imaging can be used when conventional imaging studies cannot localize the tumor.

Patient Preoperative Preparation

A preoperative chest radiograph should be obtained for all patients because the lung is one of the most common sites for metastasis. An electrocardiogram and an echocardiogram are frequently useful because chronic catecholamine excess may cause cardiomyopathy. **Preoperative blood pressure control is essential to minimize the risk of a hypertensive crisis.** The preferred method is to administer an α-adrenergic blocking agent 1 to 2 weeks before surgery. This allows for relaxation of the constricted vascular tree and correction of the reduced plasma volume, which helps prevent the hypotension that can often occur following tumor removal. A β-adrenergic blocking agent is added to oppose the reflex tachycardia associated with α-blockade. In general, **administration of a β-blocking agent should not be started without prior α-blockade because this may precipitate a hypertensive crisis related to unopposed α-receptor stimulation.**

Traditionally, phenoxybenzamine has been the preferred α-adrenergic antagonist. α-Methyl-*p*-tyrosine, which is often used in combination with phenoxybenzamine, competitively inhibits tyrosine hydroxylase, the rate-limiting enzyme in catecholamine synthesis. Newer, selective α_1-blocking agents have also been used with good results.

Surgical Concerns

The intraoperative management is critical because of **the danger of large fluctuations in blood pressure, heart rate, and fluid balance.** Continuous blood pressure monitoring usually is accomplished with an arterial line, and central venous and Foley catheters are inserted for volume assessment and intravenous fluid replacement. An intravenous nitroprusside continuous infusion is often administered for the control of hypertension, and a short-acting β-blocker, such as esmolol, is used to control any tachycardia. Adrenalectomy can be accomplished either laparoscopically or through an open technique. **Acute hypotension may occur following excision of a pheochromocytoma related to sudden diffuse vasodilatation.** Continuous intravenous Neo-Synephrine is used when the blood pressure fails to respond to fluid administration. Postoperatively, a normotensive state is achieved in approximately 90% of patients following tumor excision.

Follow-Up

Because **histopathologic studies cannot always identify whether a tumor is benign or malignant,** all patients are followed for life. In general, **plasma-free metanephrine levels** are measured 1 month after surgery and at yearly intervals thereafter.

Comprehension Questions

44.1 A 44-year-old otherwise healthy man has a 3-cm left adrenal mass found during CT evaluation for acute appendicitis. Following his appendectomy, a serum metanephrine level during his hospitalization revealed mild elevation in value. Which of the following is the most appropriate next step?

A. 24-hour urine collection for VMA, metanephrine, and normetanephrine
B. MIBG scan
C. CT-guided needle biopsy of the adrenal gland
D. Alpha blockage for one week followed by laparoscopic adrenalectomy

44.2 A 3.5-cm right adrenal mass was discovered incidentally on an abdominal CT scan obtained for a 62-year-old man who was a victim of motor vehicular trauma. His medical history was notable for a right upper lobe lung resection 3 years previously for a stage I carcinoma. He is asymptomatic. Which of the following is the next most appropriate step in the evaluation?

A. Fine-needle aspiration biopsy of the adrenal mass
B. Repeated CT scanning in 3 months
C. A functional assessment of the adrenal mass
D. MRI of the adrenal gland

44.3 Observation alone is appropriate for which one of the following patients?

A. A 53-year-old healthy man with a 8-cm nonfunctioning left adrenal mass
B. A 44-year-old woman with a 8-cm left adrenal mass that appears to be a myolipoma based on CT
C. A 32-year-old woman with elevated serum metanephrines and urinary VMA, metanephrines, and an asymptomatic 2-cm right adrenal mass
D. 66-year-old man with a history of malignant melanoma on the leg at age 50, who presents with a newly diagnosed 4-cm right adrenal mass

44.4 Which of the following is the most appropriate management for an 85-year-old nursing home resident, with severe dementia and CHF, and a 6-cm left adrenal mass?

A. Evaluate for the tumor for functionality and treat with laparocopic adrenalectomy.
B. Evaluate the tumor for functionality and perform CT-guided biopsy.
C. Expectant management.
D. Medically optimize the patient and perform laparoscopic adrenalectomy.

44.5 Which of the following statements regarding adrenalectomy for a pheochromocytoma is most correct?

A. It results in blood pressure improvement but blood pressure rarely normalizes.
B. It corrects hypertension only in patients with benign disease.
C. It may lead to profound intraoperative hypotension.
D. It should be reserved for patients with hypertension refractory to drug therapy.

44.6 Which of the following imaging studies has the *highest specificity* when used to confirm the presence of a pheochromocytoma?

A. MIBG imaging
B. CT imaging
C. MRI
D. PET

ANSWERS

44.1 **A.** 24-hour urinary collection for VMA, metanephrines, and normetanephrines is needed in this patient to confirm the diagnosis of pheochromocytoma. While a normal serum metanephrine level has a high negative predictive value for the absence of pheochromocytoma, elevated serum values do not always indicate the presence of a pheochromocytoma, and the possibility of a pheochromocytoma needs to be further explored with the more specific urinary catecholamine analyses.

44.2 **C.** The initial step in evaluating an adrenal mass is performing functional studies.

44.3 **B.** CT is accurate for the diagnosis of myolipoma of the adrenal gland. To be more complete, it is not unreasonable to obtain biochemical studies to rule out functional adrenal adenoma and pheochromocytoma in this patient. The patient with a prior history of melanoma may have an adrenal metastasis and needs biochemical evaluations first to rule out the usual causes, followed by biopsy of the mass.

44.4 **C.** Expectant management is acceptable for this patient with severe comorbidities and asymptomatic adrenal mass. While the possibility of an adrenocortical carcinoma exists in this patient, the risks of treatment would exceed the potential benefits associated with further diagnostic studies and/or treatment.

44.5 **C.** Excision of a pheochromocytoma may result in immediate intraoperative hypotension.

44.6 **A.** An MIBG scan is highly specific in confirming pheochromocytoma.

Clinical Pearls

- Once a pheochromocytoma is diagnosed, CT imaging is the initial test used to localize the tumor. An iodine-131 MIBG scan is usually obtained for the confirmation of pheochromocytoma because of its superior specificity of 90% to 100%.
- Assessment of functional studies is the first step in the evaluation of any patient with an adrenal mass.
- Biopsy of an adrenal mass is indicated only when the mass is suspected of being a metastatic lesion.
- The most common tumor metastasizing to the adrenal gland is lung carcinoma. Other tumors include carcinoma of the breast, kidney, colon, and stomach, and melanoma.
- The functional assessment consists of evaluation for pheochromocytoma, aldosterone-producing adenoma, and a cortisol-producing tumor.
- Pheochromocytoma is known as the 10% tumor because 10% are bilateral, extra-adrenal, multiple, malignant, or familial.
- During surgery, there is significant danger of large fluctuations in blood pressure, heart rate, and fluid balance. Notably, acute hypotension may occur following excision of a pheochromocytoma related to sudden diffuse vasodilation.

REFERENCES

Brunt LM, Moley JF. Incidentaloma. In: Cameron JL, ed. *Current Surgical Therapy*. 9th ed. Philadelphia, PA: Mosby Elsevier; 2008:597-602.
Thompson GB, Grant CS. Pheochromocytoma. In: Cameron JL, ed. *Current Surgical Therapy*. 9th ed. Philadelphia, PA: Mosby Elsevier; 2008:592-597.

Case 45

A 36-year-old man presents with a 1-day history of right groin pain. The patient indicates that the pain developed during a tennis match the previous evening and on returning home he noticed swelling in the area. His past medical history is unremarkable. The patient denies any history of medical problems or similar complaints. He has not undergone any previous operations. The physical examination reveals a well-nourished man. The results from the cardiopulmonary examination are unremarkable, and the abdominal examination reveals a nondistended, nontender abdomen. Auscultation of the abdomen reveals normal bowel sounds. Examination of the right inguinal region reveals no inguinal mass. There is a 3-cm nonerythematous swelling on the medial thigh just below the right inguinal ligament. Palpation reveals localized tenderness. The lower extremities are otherwise unremarkable. Laboratory findings reveal a WBC count of $6500/mm^3$ and normal hemoglobin and hematocrit levels. Electrolyte concentrations are within the normal range as are the results from a urinalysis. Radiographs of the abdomen demonstrate no abnormalities.

- What is the most likely diagnosis?
- What are the complications associated with this disease process?
- What is the best therapy?

ANSWERS TO CASE 45:
Hernias

Summary: A 36-year-old man complains of a new-onset painful mass in the groin region present since he played tennis the previous day.

- **Diagnosis:** Incarcerated femoral hernia.
- **Complications:** Strangulation of the hernia sac contents with resulting sepsis.
- **Best therapy:** Operative exploration of the right groin to evaluate, reduce the hernia sac contents, and repair the femoral hernia.

ANALYSIS

Objectives

1. Know the presentations of inguinal, femoral, and umbilical hernias.
2. Recognize the anatomic landmarks of the different types of hernias.
3. Learn the pros and cons of the different approaches to hernia repair.

Considerations

The differential diagnosis of groin pain and/or mass includes inguinal hernia, femoral hernia, muscle strain, and adenopathy. Although many patients believe the sudden development of pain or a mass in the groin is the classic and usual presentation for a groin hernia, this particular clinical picture is in fact more suggestive of muscle injury. Patients with inguinal hernias generally describe a long history of intermittent groin pain or "heaviness" that is more prominent when standing and during physical activity. **The sudden development of a painful groin mass, such as in a patient with a known hernia, suggests hernia incarceration.** In particular, this patient's presentation is compatible with that for an incarcerated femoral hernia. Because a femoral hernia usually is a small, well-defined anatomic defect, there may be few or no long-term symptoms, and acute incarceration may be the initial presenting symptom. The diagnosis in this case can be established on the basis of the history and the results from a physical examination. In the event of clinical uncertainty, ultrasonography or CT imaging may be helpful in differentiating an incarcerated hernia from lymph nodes, hematomas, or abscesses. Once the diagnosis is made, **a patient with an incarcerated hernia should undergo urgent surgical repair to relieve the symptoms and to prevent strangulation of hernia sac contents.**

APPROACH TO Hernias

DEFINITIONS

INDIRECT HERNIA: An inguinal hernia in which the abdominal contents protrude through the internal inguinal ring through a patent processus vaginalis into the inguinal canal. In men, they follow the spermatic cord and may appear as scrotal swelling, whereas in women they may manifest as labial swelling.

DIRECT HERNIA: An inguinal hernia that protrudes through the Hesselbach triangle medial to the inferior epigastric vessels.

FEMORAL HERNIA: A hernia that protrudes through the femoral canal, bounded by the inguinal ligament superiorly, the femoral vein laterally, and the pyriformis and pubic ramus medially. Unlike inguinal hernias, these hernias protrude below, rather than above, the inguinal ligament.

UMBILICAL HERNIA: A hernia resulting from improper healing of the umbilical scar. Eighty percent of pediatric umbilical hernias close by 2 years of age. In adults, defects are often exacerbated by conditions that increase intra-abdominal pressure, such as ascites.

LITTRE HERNIA: A groin hernia that contains a Meckel diverticulum or the appendix.

RICHTER HERNIA: Herniation of part of the bowel wall through a defect in the anterior abdominal wall. Bowel obstruction does not occur, although the constricted bowel wall may become ischemic and subsequently necrotic.

SPIGELIAN HERNIA: A hernia just lateral to the rectus sheath at the semilunar line, the lower limit of the posterior rectus sheath.

OBTURATOR HERNIA: Herniation through the obturator canal alongside the obturator vessels and nerves. This hernia occurs mostly in women, particularly multiparous women with a history of recent weight loss. A mass may be palpable in the **medial thigh,** particularly with the hip flexed, externally rotated, and abducted (Howship-Romberg sign).

SLIDING HERNIA: A hernia in which one wall of the hernia is made up of an intra-abdominal organ, most commonly the sigmoid colon, ascending colon, or bladder.

CLINICAL APPROACH

Abdominal wall hernias are protrusions of abdominal contents through a defect in the abdominal wall. **Incarceration** occurs if the abdominal contents become trapped. **Strangulation** occurs when the blood supply to the trapped contents becomes compromised, leading to ischemia, necrosis, and ultimately perforation. **Intestinal obstruction can occur in an incarcerated or strangulated hernia.** Abdominal wall defects that develop following surgical procedures not related to a hernia are referred to as incisional hernias and addressed elsewhere.

Anatomy

Knowledge of the regional anatomy is essential for the diagnosis and repair of hernias. In the groin, the inguinal ligament divides inguinal hernias from femoral hernias. Inguinal hernias are further divided into indirect and direct hernias based on their relationship to the inferior epigastric vessels. The **Hesselbach triangle, defined by the edge of the rectus medially, the inguinal ligament inferolaterally, and the inferior epigastric vessels superolaterally, is the site of direct hernias (Figure 45–1).** In this triangle, the peritoneum and transversalis fascia are the only components of the anterior abdominal wall. **Indirect hernias are lateral to the inferior epigastric vessels.** The Cooper ligament, or the pectineal ligament, extends from the pubic tubercle laterally and passes posteriorly to the femoral vessels.

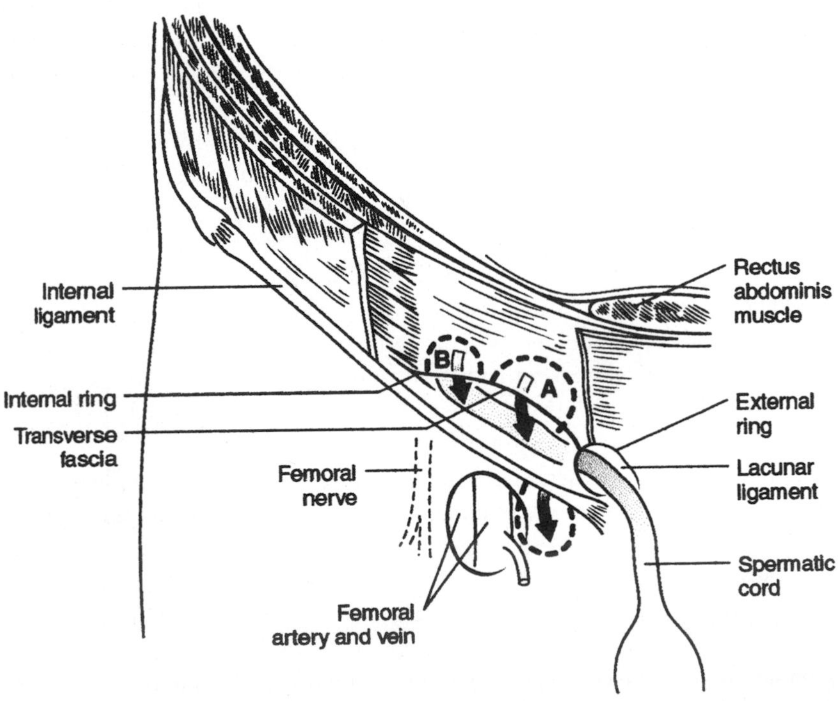

Figure 45–1. Anatomic location of groin hernias. Direct hernia **(A)**, indirect hernia **(B)**, femoral hernia (right groin from an anterior view) **(C)**.

APPROACH TO AN INCARCERATED HERNIA

Reduction should be attempted in a patient with an incarcerated hernia. This procedure is best accomplished by elongating the neck of the hernia sac while judiciously applying pressure to reduce the hernia. **If reduction is unsuccessful, the patient should be prepared for an urgent operation.** In a patient with a bowel obstruction, volume depletion and abnormalities in electrolyte levels are common. These conditions should be corrected before operative intervention. Urgent repair requires an incision over the incarcerated hernia, close inspection of any contents, and **tension-free reapproximation.** For inguinal hernias, the transversus abdominus is sutured to either the Cooper ligament or the shelving edge of the inguinal ligament. For femoral hernias, a Cooper ligament repair must be used. **With a compromised bowel, a prosthetic mesh should be avoided because of the infection risk.**

Indications for Repair

Symptoms produced by hernias are related to the size, location of the hernias, and the activity level of the individual; therefore, it is not uncommon for some patients with small hernias to remain asymptomatic or minimally symptomatic. Until only several years ago, it was the general opinion of the surgical community to recommend that all patients with groin hernias and reasonable life expectancy undergo hernia repairs. This aggressive approach was based on the assumption that these hernias left unattended to would progress to incarceration and/or strangulation. In 2006, the result of the "watchful waiting vs repair" trial was published suggesting that the rate of complications development was low in patients with small, minimally symptomatic, or asymptomatic groin hernias (0.3% over 2 years), and that it was safe and cost-effective to attempt an initial course of nonoperative management.

For individuals with symptomatic hernias, elective repair via an open approach can be performed under local, spinal, or general anesthesia. It can also be done laparoscopically, which requires a general anesthetic. In addition to the elective or urgent/emergent nature of the repair, anesthetic choice, patient preference, and the primary or recurrent nature of the hernia factor into the decision regarding the operative approach. A laparoscopic approach or an open preperitoneal approach is best for recurrent or bilateral hernias (Figure 45–2). For unilateral primary groin hernias, the approaches have similar recurrence rates, similar disability times, and similar costs. Patients who undergo laparoscopy seem to have less pain and may be able to return to work sooner. The recently reported VA Medical Centers Randomized Trial comparing open mesh repairs versus laparoscopic mesh repairs for inguinal hernias found higher complication and recurrence rates for the laparoscopic patients. Although these results are still being debated, the findings seem to suggest no benefits or worse outcome with the laparoscopic approach.

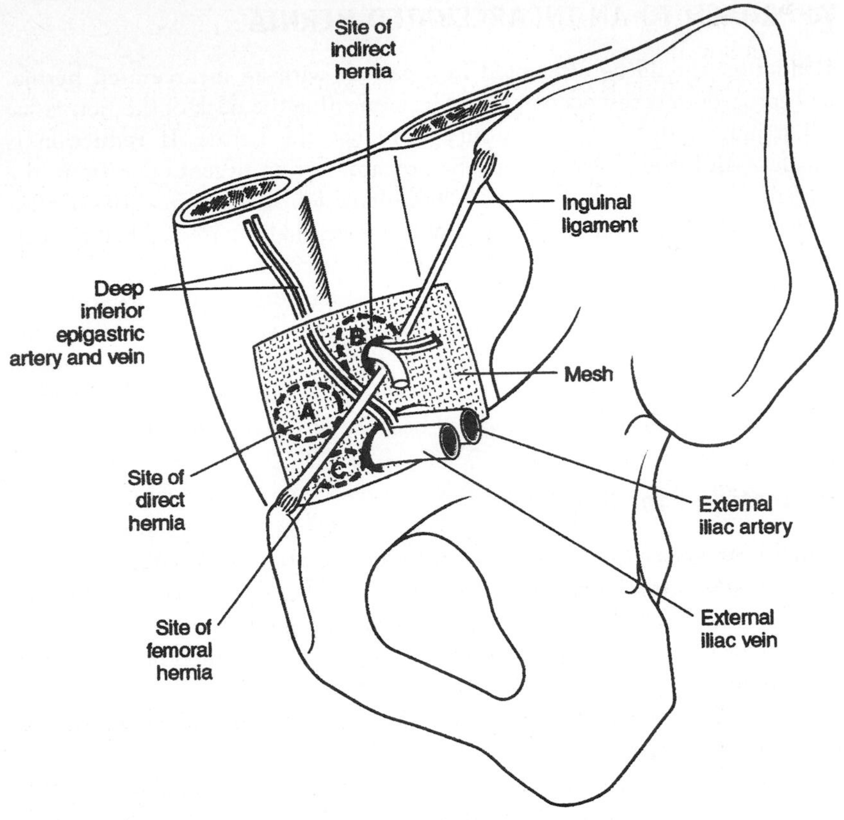

Figure 45–2. Right groin anatomy by preperitoneal view. Operative repair of a direct hernia **(A)**, an indirect hernia **(B)**, and a femoral hernia using a prosthetic mesh in a posterior (preperitoneal) approach **(C)**.

Comprehension Questions

45.1 A 20-year-old construction worker is complaining of pain and intermittent bulge in his left groin. He indicates that the symptoms have been worsening over the past 3 months and beginning to affect his activities. On examination, he appears to have a small indirect inguinal hernia. Which of the following is the most appropriate management?

A. Discuss with the patient potential benefits of "watchful waiting" and re-evaluate the patient in one month.

B. Advise the patient to undergo laparoscopic hernia repair because a large randomized trial showed superior outcome for patients undergoing laparascopic repairs.

C. Perform open left inguinal hernia repair with prosthetic mesh.

D. Perform open left inguinal herniorrhaphy with primary suture repair.

45.2 A 40-year-old man presents with recurrent bulge in the left groin 2 years following open left inguinal hernia repair with mesh. The physical examination showed a moderately dilated external inguinal ring with a small bulge produced by Valsalva maneuver. Which of the following is the most appropriate treatment approach?

A. Obtain a CT to rule out a femoral hernia, followed by elective hernia repair.

B. Schedule patient for left groin exploration and hernia repair with prosthetic mesh.

C. Advise patient to limit his physical activities and re-evaluate in 6 months.

D. Send the patient to an immunologist for evaluation of possible wound healing and tissue collagen defects.

45.3 An 80-year-old woman who resides in a nursing home has several pound weight loss over the past several months. She presents with 3-day history of vomiting and anorexia. Her abdominal examination reveals distension and tympany. There is a firm sot tissue mass measuring approximately 4-cm in the medial aspect of her left upper thigh. Her abdominal CT scan reveals fluid-filled dilated small bowel loops and evidence of decompressed ileum and colon. Which of the following is the most appropriate treatment for this patient?

A. Exploration of the left groin and thigh, repair of her femoral hernia.

B. Exploratory laparotomy.

C. Initial observation of this elderly patient with small bowel obstruction, and if the process fails to resolve in 5 days, proceed with exploratory laparotomy.

D. Comfort care.

45.4 Which of the following is the appropriate treatment for the patient in question 45.3?

A. Schedule her for an elective operation.

B. Request a barium enema.

C. Take her straight to the operating room.

D. Hospitalize her for volume and electrolyte replacement and urgent operation.

ANSWERS

45.1 **C.** Open repair with prosthetic mesh. The study by Neumayer et al (NEJM 2004) was a randomized comparison of laparoscopic vs. open mesh inguinal hernia repair that actually showed increased recurrence rate with laparoscopic repair. There is no definitive evidence to support laparoscopic repair, watchful waiting, or primary open repair in this patient's case.

45.2 **B.** This patient has history and physical findings that are compatible with having a recurrent inguinal hernia, and repair for this recurrent hernia is a reasonable approach. CT evaluation to rule out a femoral recurrence is reasonable only if the patient does not have clinical evidence or history that his recurrent hernia is inguinal in location. "Watchful waiting" is only reasonable if the patient is minimally symptomatic and re-repair of his hernia would not improve his quality of life.

45.3 **B.** This patient has signs and symptoms of high-grade small bowel obstruction. The association of her obstructive symptoms with a newly identified tender medial thigh mass could indicate the presence of an incarcerated femoral hernia or an incarcerated obtrator hernia. In a patient with small bowel obstruction that is likely produced by incarcerated hernia, an initial course of nonoperative management is not appropriate. Comfort care is only reasonable if the patient has extremely limited life expectancy, because the quality of life of the patient is extremely compromised given her bowel obstruction, and effective strategies for long-term palliation of bowel obstruction are not available.

45.4 **D.** Resuscitation and urgent repair are indicated for patients with a bowel obstruction caused by a hernia.

Clinical Pearls

- Recent clinical evidence suggests that hernia incarceration and strangulation rate is quite low in patients with small, asymptomatic, or minimally symptomatic inguinal hernias; therefore, an initial trial of nonoperative care is safe and cost-effective.
- The Howship-Romberg sign refers to obturator neuralgia produced by nerve compression by an obturator hernia. (The sign is produced by thigh extension, adduction, and medial rotation.)

REFERENCES

Fitzgibbons RJ Jr, Giobbie-Hurder A, Gibbs JO, et al. Watchful waiting vs repair of inguinal hernia in minimally symptomatic men: a randomized clinical trial. *JAMA*. 2006;295:285-292.

Khaitan L, McKernan JB. Groin hernia. In: Cameron JL, ed. *Current Surgical Therapy*. 9th ed. Philadelphia, PA: Mosby Elsevier; 2008:561-568.

Neumayer L, Giobbie-Hurder A, Jonasson O, et al. Open mesh versus laparoscopic mesh repair of inguinal hernia. *N Engl J Med*. 2004;350:1819-1827.

Case 46

A 48-year-old man with a history of alcoholism and cirrhosis undergoes evaluation for severe left leg pain and fever. The patient says his symptoms began after he scraped the lateral aspect of his knee at home 3 days ago. During the past 2 days he has had subjective fevers and noticed decreased urinary frequency. The patient has been self-medicating with aspirin for these symptoms. He consumes approximately 16 oz of whiskey per day and smokes 1 pack of cigarettes per day. On physical examination, his temperature is 39.2°C (102.6°F), pulse rate 110 beats/min, blood pressure 115/78 mm Hg, and respiratory rate 28 breaths/min. His skin is mildly icteric. The findings from his cardiopulmonary examination are unremarkable. The abdomen is soft and without hepatosplenomegaly or ascites. The left leg is edematous from the ankle to the upper thigh. The skin is tense and exquisitely tender; however, it is without erythema, fluctuance, necrosis, or vesicular changes. Examination of the other leg reveals normal findings. Laboratory studies demonstrate a WBC count of 26,000/mm^3 and normal hemoglobin and hematocrit values. Other laboratory studies reveal sodium 128 mEq/L, glucose 180 mg/dL, total bilirubin 3.8, and direct bilirubin 1.5 mg/dL. Radiographs of the left leg reveal no bony injuries and no evidence of air in the subcutaneous soft tissue space.

- ➤ What is the most likely diagnosis?
- ➤ What is the best therapy for this condition?

ANSWERS TO CASE 46:
Necrotizing Soft Tissue Infections

Summary: A 48-year-old man with alcoholic cirrhosis presents with necrotizing soft tissue infection (NSTI) following a trivial injury to the left leg.

- **Most likely diagnosis:** Necrotizing soft tissue infection.
- **Best therapy:** Early initiation of appropriate antibiotics and radical surgical debridement of necrotic tissue. The treatment outcome is adversely affected by delays in therapy.

Objectives

1. Learn to recognize the clinical presentation and diagnostic strategies for NSTI.
2. Understand that rapid, aggressive surgical debridement is crucial in the treatment of NSTI.
3. Become familiar with the bacteriology of NSTI and appropriate antimicrobial choices for these conditions.

Considerations

A patient with alcohol-induced cirrhosis, in an immunocompromised state, presents with a high fever, soft tissue edema, and leg pain out of proportion to the physical findings, all of which strongly suggest the possibility of severe soft tissue infection. These findings are not specific for NSTI and may be compatible with a deep-seated abscess. The patient reports receiving minor trauma to his leg prior to the onset of leg pain, which favors the diagnosis of NSTI over that of an abscess. The development of NSTI following trivial soft tissue trauma is typical of infections caused by gram-positive skin flora, including group A β-hemolytic *Streptococcus*. Because NSTI frequently involves mixed bacterial organisms, the initial antibiotic regimen for this patient should include broad-spectrum antibiotics directed against gram-positive, gram-negative, and anaerobic bacteria. Following initial resuscitation, the patient should undergo examination of the leg with exploration of the subcutaneous tissue for infection and tissue viability. Once the bacteriologic findings from the operative drainage/debridement become available, the antibiotic regimen can be modified to cover the specific pathogens identified.

Distant end-organ dysfunction such as acute respiratory insufficiency, acute renal insufficiency, and acute liver insufficiency may occur with NSTI; therefore, most patients should be treated in the intensive care unit with careful monitoring and maximal supportive care. The systemic consequences of NSTI can develop because of overwhelming sepsis and from circulating toxins (associated with *Staphylococcus* and group A *Streptococcus* toxic shock syndrome [TSS]).

Surgical debridement for this patient should begin with an incision over the involved soft tissue and an inspection of the subcutaneous tissue for gross evidence of necrosis and adherence to the underlying fascia. **Easy separation of the subcutaneous tissue from the underlying fascia indicates microvascular thrombosis and necrosis** and should be treated by tissue debridement.

Because of the rich blood supply to the skin, patients with NSTI generally do not develop skin necrosis and bullous changes until late in the disease process. **It should be recognized that the absence of skin abnormalities is one of the leading factors contributing to delays in the recognition of NSTI.** When identified, all necrotic tissue should be excised. The fascia commonly serves as a natural barrier to the infectious processes; involvement below the fascia occurs infrequently except during infections by *Clostridium* species. Patients whose conditions do not respond appropriately to supportive care, antibiotics therapy, and surgical debridement should be reassessed; the **lack of improvement may be related to inadequate debridement and/or inappropriate antibiotic selection (source control).**

APPROACH TO Soft Tissue Infection

DEFINITIONS

CELLULITIS: A milder form of soft tissue infection without the association of microvascular thrombosis and necrosis. Clinically, patients do not have evidence of systemic toxicity and can be adequately treated with antibiotic therapy.

NSTI: Soft tissue infection that affects primarily the dermis and subcutaneous tissue.

CLINICAL APPROACH

Early manifestations include the extension of edema beyond the spread of erythema and severe pain. Late clinical manifestations may include crepitation, the formation of skin vesicles, cutaneous anesthesia, and focal necrosis. CT scans and magnetic resonance imaging (MRI) are helpful in differentiating NSTI from cellulitis. The diagnosis of NSTI in most cases can be established on the basis of clinical evaluation (see Table 46–1). Adjunctive imaging studies should not be obtained if they would lead to additional delays

Table 46–1 CLINICAL MANIFESTATIONS OF NECROTIZING SOFT TISSUE INFECTION

CLINICAL SETTING	ORGANISMS	CLINICAL MANIFESTATIONS	ANTIBIOTICS
Acquired after contact with fish or seawater	*Vibrio* species	Rapid progression of soft tissue infection, fever, rigors, and hypotension	Ceftazidime plus quinolone or tetracycline
Mixed synergistic infection; progression of perirectal infection or complications of gastrointestinal surgery	Mixed gram-negative aerobes and anaerobes	Clinical progression over several days; may involve perineum and abdominal wall	Multiple regimens developed to cover gram-negative bacilli, and anaerobes
Gas gangrene may complicate trauma or ischemia	Clostridrial species	Swollen, tense skin, crepitation, and skin vesicles; frequently present with systemic toxic therapy	Penicillin (questionable benefit with hyperbaric therapy)
Necrotizing soft tissue infection related to injectional drug abuse (IDA) or "skin popping"	Clostridial species and other gram-positive anaerobic organisms	Swelling and systemic toxicity due to the release of exotoxins. As the injections are through the fascia and into the muscles during "skin popping," the area of infection is in the muscles and below the fascia. These infections have very high mortality due to sepsis and organ failure	Penicillin, clindamycin, and vancomycin

in surgical therapy. A definitive diagnosis can be achieved on the basis of needle aspiration of the involved tissue, Gram stain evaluation, or exploration and visualization of the subcutaneous tissue under anesthesia. **The infection is associated with spreading thrombosis of the blood vessels in the subcutaneous fat and dermis, leading to tissue necrosis and poor antibiotic penetration into the affected tissue.** NSTI can involve a variety of bacterial organisms. Optimal treatment consists of systemic antibiotic administration, surgical debridement, and supportive care.

Group A β-hemolytic *Streptococcus* Soft Tissue Infection: Referred to in the lay press as the "flesh-eating infection," this form of NSTI frequently occurs in patients with a compromised immune status (alcoholics, diabetic patients, and the malnourished); however, it can also occur in healthy individuals following trivial soft tissue trauma. Approximately 75% of cases are community acquired. Bacteremia and/or TSS develops in approximately 50% of patients. The local process generally spreads rapidly over the course of hours to days. The combination of clindamycin and penicillin has been touted to produce superior results compared to the use of the penicillins alone. There is limited evidence suggesting that therapy with intravenous immunoglobulins (Ig) neutralizes the bacteria-produced superantigens and may improve patient outcome.

Toxic Shock Syndrome: A clinical syndrome caused by pyrogenic toxin superantigens produced by staphylococcal organisms or group A β-hemolytic *Streptococcus*. The binding of superantigens to major histocompatibility complex class III molecules leads to T-cell clonal expansion and a massive release of proinflammatory cytokines by macrophages and T cells. Patients with TSS frequently develop mental obtundation, hyperdynamic shock, and multiple-organ dysfunction syndrome. The systemic findings in TSS frequently do not correlate with the local extent of the soft tissue (vaginal) infection and thus can cause a delay in diagnosis and treatment.

Fournier Gangrene: A specific form of scrotal gangrene first described by Fournier in 1883. Anaerobic streptococci are the predominant causative organisms, with secondary infection caused by gram-negative organisms. Strictly speaking, the term "Fournier gangrene" refers to the anaerobic *Streptococcus*-related scrotal infection but is frequently inappropriately applied to gram-negative synergistic soft tissue infections of the perineum and groin.

Comprehension Questions

46.1 A 55-year-old man with diabetes presents with a swollen, painful right hand that developed 1 day after he sustained a puncture wound to the hand while fishing in the Gulf of Mexico. His temperature is 39.5°C (103.1°F), pulse rate 120 beats/min, and blood pressure 95/60 mm Hg. His right hand and forearm are swollen, and a puncture wound with surrounding ecchymosis is present on the hand. There is drainage of brown fluid from the wound. Which of the following therapies is most appropriate?

A. Supportive care, penicillin G, and hyperbaric treatment
B. Supportive care, penicillin G/tetracycline/ceftazidime, and surgical debridement
C. Supportive care, penicillin G/tetracycline/ceftazidime, surgical debridement, and hyperbaric treatment
D. Supportive care, penicillin G plus clindamycin, and intravenous Ig

46.2 A 62-year-old man with diabetes returns to the emergency department 3 days after undergoing incision and drainage of a perirectal abscess. The patient is complaining of fever and malaise. Evaluation of the perirectal area reveals an open, draining wound with a 20-cm area of surrounding induration, erythema, localized areas of blister formation, and skin necrosis. The infection has extended to involve the perineum, scrotum, and anterior abdomen. The process in this patient most likely represents which of the following?

A. Fournier gangrene
B. Clostridial gas gangrene
C. NSTI caused by group A β-hemolytic *Streptococcus*
D. Polymicrobial synergistic NSTI

46.3 A 33-year-old house painter sustained an abrasion and superficial laceration of the left shoulder 2 days ago. He presents to the outpatient clinic with an area of erythema extending 3-cm along the area of skin abrasion and superficial laceration. There is an area of fluctuence beneath the area, and the tenderness does not appear to extend beyond the area. His temperature and vital signs are normal. Which of the following is the most appropriate treatment?

A. Incision and drainage of the area, followed by one-week course of oral antibiotic therapy
B. Incision and debridement of the soft tissue infection
C. Oral antibiotics therapy for one week
D. Topical antibiotic ointment application and dressing changes

46.4 A 38-year-old man with a history of injection heroine abuse presents to the emergency center with circumferential tender and tense swelling over his left upper arm. The entire area is minimally erythematous but exquisitely tender. He indicated that he had injected some "black tar heroine" into the area six days ago. His temperature is 39.5°C, his heart rate is 125 beats/min, and his WBC is 46,000/mm^3. Ultrasound of the upper extremity revealed no evidence of venous thromboses or soft tissue fluid collections. Which of the following is the most appropriate treatment?

A. Admit the patient to the hospital for IV antibiotics therapy for his severe cellulites, and if this does not improve, repeat the ultrasound to look for an abscess.

B. Perform radical debridement of the affected area.

C. Perform an trans-esophageal echocardiography to rule out endocarditis and treat with systemic IV antibiotics.

D. Perform radical debridement of the affected area, followed by IV antibiotics therapy.

ANSWERS

46.1 **B.** Supportive care, penicillin G/tetracycline/ceftazidime, and debridement are appropriate initial treatment for a patient who develops severe NSTI in an injury with the potential for *Vibrio* infection (acquired while fishing).

46.2 **D.** Polymicrobial synergistic infection is the most likely diagnosis based on the duration of events and the distribution of soft tissue infection.

46.3 **A.** This patient's history and clinical presentation are compatible with having a superficial soft tissue abscess and some surrounding cellulites. Incision and drainage of the abscess should adequately address the abscess and the course of antibiotics therapy should be enough to address the surrounding cellulitis. Either drainage alone or antibiotics alone may not be sufficient to address the problems this patient has.

46.4 **D.** This patient has a classic presentation of necrotizing soft tissue infection. That is pain and soft tissue changes beyond skin erythema. Based on history, the cause of the NSTI is related to the injection of illicit drugs that may be contaminated with soil or skin bacterial flora, and this form of NSTI is commonly associated with systemic inflammatory changes that this patient has already manifested. Treatment for this individual would consist of debridement of the affected soft tissue in addition to systemic antibiotics.

Clinical Pearls

- The most common findings in a patient with NSTI are local edema and pain in the presence of systemic signs such as high fever (hypothermia in some patients), tachycardia, and frequently mental confusion.
- NSTI should be suspected when pain and tenderness extend beyond the area of skin erythema.
- When NSTI is strongly suspected, exploration of the wound through a limited skin incision may help establish the diagnosis in a rapid fashion.
- Rapid, aggressive surgical debridement is the most important treatment for NSTI.
- Lack of improvement after treatment of NSTI may be related to inadequate debridement and/or inappropriate antibiotic selection (source control).

REFERENCES

Hansen SL, Mathes SJ, Young DM. Skin and subcutaneous tissue. In: Brunicardi FC, Andersen DK, Dunn DL, et al, eds. *Schwartz's Principles of Surgery*. 8th ed. New York: McGraw-Hill; 2005:429-452.

Manahan MA, Milner SM, Fresswick P, Harmon JW. Necrotizing infections of the skin and soft tissue. In: Cameron JL, ed. *Current Surgical Therapy*. 9th ed. Philadelphia, PA: Mosby Elsevier; 2008:11128-11131.

Case 47

A 4-year-old boy informed his mother that he had just passed some blood in his urine. Hematuria was confirmed by the mother who brought the boy in for evaluation. The child denied any significant recent trauma, and he had been in good health. His past medical history is unremarkable. He is in the 56th percentile in height and in the 43rd percentile in weight. On physical examination, the patient appears healthy and has normal vital signs. Findings from the cardiopulmonary examinations are within normal limits. A 10-cm mass is identified in the left upper quadrant of the abdomen. This mass is firm and non-tender. No abnormalities are noted in the extremities. Laboratory studies reveal a normal complete blood count (CBC) and electrolyte levels in the normal range. The urinalysis reveals 50 to 100 red blood cells per high-power field.

- What is the most likely diagnosis?
- What is the best therapy?

ANSWERS TO CASE 47: Wilms Tumor (Pediatric Abdominal Mass)

Summary: A 4-year-old boy presents with hematuria and an abdominal mass.

- **Diagnosis:** Wilms tumor involving the left kidney.
- **Best therapy:** The management of a Wilms tumor depends on the findings from the imaging studies. If the tumor is massive or bilateral and an intracaval extension of tumor extends proximally to the hepatic veins, preoperative multiagent chemotherapy is used initially. These findings are uncommon, and the majority of Wilms tumors, even if large at the initial presentation, can be completely resected prior to chemotherapy. Almost all patients receive chemotherapy following nephrectomy. Radiation therapy is given if there has been tumor spillage, either from a preoperative capsular rupture or from an intraoperative tumor spill.

ANALYSIS

Objectives

1. Become familiar with the common presentation, differential diagnosis, and initial evaluation of an abdominal mass in newborns and pediatric patients.
2. Understand the management and outcome of a Wilms tumor and neuroblastoma.

Considerations

Wilms tumors are renal embryonal neoplasms that occur with a peak incidence in children between 1 and 5 years of age; thus, at 4 years of age this patient is within this group. These tumors usually manifest as asymptomatic abdominal or flank masses, although hematuria is often seen. Before surgery, imaging evaluation is important to determine the extent of the tumor, and in this patient it should include abdominal ultrasonography and a CT scan of the abdomen and chest. If the tumor is unilateral and appears that it can be safely removed, surgical exploration and resection should be attempted.

APPROACH TO An Abdominal Mass in the Pediatric Patient

The etiology of an abdominal mass in a pediatric patient depends to a large extent on the age of the patient at presentation. Knowing the age of the patient, the details of a directed history obtained from the child and the parents, and the results from a routine physical examination allow one to develop a focused differential diagnosis. Based on this list of possible etiologies, imaging studies and selected laboratory findings will then allow a more definitive diagnosis to be made. Table 47–1 lists the most likely etiologies of an abdominal mass for neonates (< 1 month of age) and Table 47–2, the most likely etiologies for older infants and children.

CLINICAL APPROACH

With the information in Tables 47–1 and 47–2, the etiology of the majority of abdominal masses can usually be determined with a high degree of certainty. A careful history should be obtained from the patient and the family that includes the length of time the mass has been present (or noticed), associated

Table 47–1 ABDOMINAL MASSES IN NEONATES (BIRTH TO 1 MONTH)*

Renal
- Hydronephrosis, eg, from obstruction (ureteropelvic junction, obstruction, posterior urethral valves, other)
- Multicystic dysplastic kidney
- Polycystic kidney disease
- Mesoblastic nephroma
- Wilms tumor

Genital
- Hydrometrocolpos
- Ovarian mass, simple cyst, teratoma, torsion

Gastrointestinal
- Duplication cyst
- Complicated meconium ileus
- Mesenteric or omental cyst

Retroperitoneal
- Adrenal hemorrhage
- Neuroblastoma
- Teratoma
- Rhabdomyosarcoma
- Lymphangioma
- Hemangioma

Hepatobiliary
- Hemangioendothelioma
- Hepatic mesenchymal hamartoma
- Choledochal cyst
- Hepatoblastoma

*The most common etiologies of an abdominal mass in a neonate can be categorized as shown here (from most common to least common).

Table 47–2 ABDOMINAL MASSES IN INFANTS AND CHILDREN (1 MONTH TO 18 YEARS)*

Renal
- Wilms tumor
- Hydronephrosis, eg, from obstruction (ureteropelvic junction, obstruction, posterior urethral valves, other)
- Rhabdoid tumor
- Clear cell sarcoma
- Polycystic kidney disease

Retroperitoneal
- Neuroblastoma
- Rhabdomyosarcoma
- Teratoma
- Lymphoma
- Lymphangioma
- Hemangioma

Gastrointestinal
- Appendiceal abscess
- Intussusception
- Duplication cyst
- Functional constipation
- Hirschsprung disease
- Mesenteric or omental cyst
- Lymphoma

Hepatobiliary
- Hepatoblastoma
- Hepatocellular carcinoma
- Benign liver tumors
- Choledochal cyst

Genital
- Ovarian mass (eg, simple cyst, teratoma, torsion)
- Hydrometrocolpos
- Undescended testicle, neoplasm, or torsion

*Note that although many of the specific etiologies of an abdominal mass are the same as listed for neonates, the most likely causes change with older children.

pain or other symptoms, changes in eating habits, changes in bowel or bladder function, associated fatigue or night sweats, associated bleeding or bruising, and other related conditions. An important consideration for neonates is the maternal prenatal history, especially data from prenatal ultrasound and information about the presence or absence of polyhydramnios. **Maternal polyhydramnios may be the first sign of a neonatal bowel obstruction, which then may appear as an abdominal mass.** The physical examination should document the location, size, consistency, and mobility of the mass, as well as associated lymphadenopathy or tenderness.

Radiographic Evaluations

Initially, plain abdominal radiographs are obtained to rule out gastrointestinal obstruction, to assess bowel gas patterns, and to determine the presence or absence of calcifications. Intra-abdominal calcifications in a neonate with an abdominal mass are often associated with complicated cystic meconium ileus. Calcifications in a different distribution can lead to the diagnosis of neuroblastoma, especially in an older infant. If the findings from plain abdominal radiography are nonspecific, which is often the case, abdominal ultrasound is the next imaging modality of choice. Ultrasonography can usually identify the organ of origin, the mass can be classified as cystic or solid, and vascular flow characteristics can be determined using Doppler ultrasound techniques. Sonographic interpretation is very operator dependent and may be inaccurate in children.

CT scans are typically obtained if the ultrasonogram is either nondiagnostic or shows a solid tumor. CT imaging can provide additional anatomic detail and can be diagnostic. Because many of these conditions ultimately require operative intervention, a CT scan can provide an accurate preoperative assessment of the etiology of the mass and the involvement of adjacent structures; it can also detect the distant spread in case of neoplasms. The disadvantages of obtaining CT scans for children include the need for sedation in many cases and the unknown long-term effects of this level of ionizing radiation.

After the history is recorded, a physical examination performed, and selective imaging studies obtained, a short differential diagnosis is compiled. Very selective laboratory analyses can then be used to verify the diagnosis. For example, if the most likely diagnosis based on imaging is neuroblastoma, a CBC and a urine test for catecholamines should be obtained. If, however, the most likely diagnosis is hepatoblastoma, the level of α-fetoprotein should be evaluated prior to resection of the liver tumor.

Comprehension Questions

47.1 A previously healthy 9-month-old boy is brought to the emergency department with severe, intermittent abdominal pain. During the attacks, which are episodic and occur every 10 to 15 minutes, the child draws his legs up to his abdomen. The child is vomiting and has heme-positive stools. On physical examination, a tender, mobile, sausage-shaped mass is found in the midabdomen. Which of the following is the most likely diagnosis?

A. Intussusception
B. Jejunal atresia
C. Neuroblastoma
D. Intestinal duplication cyst

47.2 A 5-year-old girl presents with a 7-cm, vague, left-sided abdominal mass. The patient has also experienced recent weight loss and failure to thrive. The mass is hard and fixed. A plain radiograph reveals fine calcifications in the region of the mass, and a CT scan shows an irregular, solid mass arising from the left adrenal gland. Which of the following conditions is the most likely?

A. Adrenal hemorrhage
B. Adrenal adenoma
C. Neuroblastoma
D. Wilms tumor

47.3 A 15-year-old boy presents to the emergency department with a fever of 38.9°C (102°F), a firm, fixed mass in the right lower quadrant of the abdomen, and a chief complaint of abdominal pain. The patient has been ill for the past 2 weeks but has not sought medical care until now. Which of the following findings is a CT scan of the abdomen most likely to demonstrate?

A. Neoplasm arising in an undescended testicle
B. Right hydronephrosis
C. Lymphoma
D. Abscess from a perforated appendix

47.4 A 12-year-old girl presents with left lower quadrant pain, pelvic pain, and a vague fullness on physical examination. She is otherwise healthy and has no associated symptoms. Which of the following is the most likely imaging modality that would identify the etiology of the mass?

A. Plain abdominal radiograph
B. Upper gastrointestinal tract contrast study
C. Magnetic resonance imaging of the abdomen and pelvis
D. Ultrasound of the abdomen and pelvis

ANSWERS

47.1 **A.** This is a classic and severe presentation of intussusception (when the bowel telescopes on itself). This infant should be treated with intravenous hydration followed by a barium or air contrast enema to both diagnose the condition and attempt to reduce the intussusception. If it cannot be reduced with the enema, an emergent operation is indicated.

47.2 **C.** Children with neuroblastoma are often symptomatic at presentation and suffer from failure to thrive. This is in contrast to children with Wilms tumor who usually appear healthy. Patients with neuroblastoma usually require tumor biopsy followed by neoadjuvant chemotherapy prior to tumor resection, again in contrast to the situation with Wilms tumor. The outcome with neuroblastoma depends on the biology of the tumor and the stage of disease, but overall is much worse than for Wilms tumor.

47.3 **D.** An abdominal mass in a previously healthy adolescent with fever and signs of systemic illness is most commonly an abscess from a perforated appendix, especially if it is located in the right lower quadrant. CT imaging or ultrasound can readily identify this as the likely diagnosis, and image-guided abscess drainage can be employed with plans for a delayed-interval appendectomy. This management option is preferable to urgent appendectomy and abscess drainage in this inflammatory condition.

47.4 **D.** This patient probably has an ovarian tumor, most likely benign. The most common of these tumors is an ovarian teratoma, which can easily be identified with pelvic ultrasound to fully examine the adnexa. None of the other imaging modalities would be the procedure of choice for this patient.

Clinical Pearls

- The most common cause of an enlarged renal mass in a neonate is hydronephrosis.
- The most common presentation (60%) of a Wilms tumor is an asymptomatic upper abdominal or flank mass in a child 1 to 4 years of age.
- A neonatal evaluation should include a review of the prenatal and delivery records.
- Neuroblastoma is the most common type of retroperitoneal mass in a child older than 1 year.

REFERENCES

Hackam DJ, Newman K, Ford HR. Pediatric surgery. In: Brunicardi FC, Andersen DK, Dunn DL, et al, eds. *Schwartz's Principles of Surgery*. 8th ed. New York: McGraw-Hill; 2005:1471-1517.

Warner BW. Pediatric surgery. In: Townsend CM Jr, Beauchamp RD, Evers BM, et al, eds. *Sabiston Textbook of Surgery*. 19th ed. Philadelphia, PA: Sauders Elsevier; 2008: 2047-2089.

Case 48

A 38-year-old morbidly obese woman presents to the clinic for evaluation and management of venous insufficiency in the lower extremities. During your conversation with the patient, she tells you she has been extremely overweight ever since childhood. She has tried many different dietary modifications, hypnosis, and medications but has not been able to achieve sustained weight loss. She is concerned about her health status because of a recent diagnosis of type II diabetes mellitus and a history of coronary artery disease in several immediate family members. The patient is married and without children. She works as a computer programmer. She does not consume tobacco or alcohol. Her current medications are an oral hypoglycemic agent and NPH insulin. On examination, she is found to be 5 ft 3 in and weighs 280 lb. Her body mass index (BMI) is 47 kg/m^2. Her pulse rate is 95 beats/min and her blood pressure is 158/86 mm Hg. The findings from her cardiopulmonary examination and abdominal examination are unremarkable. Examination of the lower extremities reveals mild edema, diffuse varicosity, and venous stasis dermatitis bilaterally. The patient indicates that she is not interested in surgical therapy for her venous disease but would like your opinion regarding operative intervention for management of her obesity.

- Is surgical therapy a reasonable treatment option in this patient?
- What are the complications associated with morbid obesity?

ANSWERS TO CASE 48: Obesity (Morbid)

Summary: A 38-year-old morbidly obese woman (BMI 47 kg/m^2) with obesity-associated complications (diabetes and venous stasis) is inquiring about the surgical treatment of obesity.

- **Surgical therapy:** Surgical therapy is a reasonable option in this patient.
- **Complications associated with morbid obesity:** Diabetes mellitus, hypertension, hyperlipidemia, atherosclerosis, cardiomyopathy, sleep apnea syndrome, gallstones, arthritis, and infertility are disease processes associated with morbid obesity.

ANALYSIS

Objectives

1. Become familiar with the complications associated with morbid obesity and the effectiveness of bariatric operations on these complications.
2. Become familiar with the short- and long-term outcomes in weight reduction achieved with operative treatment.

Considerations

This patient falls within the National Institutes of Health (NIH) class III (see Table 48–1) category of clinically severe obesity and on the basis of weight-to-height ratio alone is a candidate for surgical therapy. Her comorbidities, diabetes and venous stasis, add further evidence of the advanced nature of her disease. Her blood glucose level should be carefully monitored during the postoperative period, and the venous disease in her lower extremities should be treated prophylactically during surgery with miniheparin and sequential compression stockings.

APPROACH TO Surgical Treatment of Morbid Obesity

DEFINITIONS

BODY MASS INDEX: The ratio of weight in kilograms (kg) to height in meters squared (m^2). It is calculated by dividing the weight (in kg) by the height (in m^2) or by multiplying the weight in pounds (lb) by 704 and dividing by the height in inches squared (in^2).

Table 48–1 NIH CLASSIFICATION OF OBESITY (REVISED)

DESCRIPTION	BMI (kg/m²)	OBESITY CLASS	DISEASE RISK
Normal	18.5-24.9		
Overweight	25.0-29.9		Increased
Obesity			
Mild	30.0-34.9	I	High
Moderate	35.0-39.9	II	Very high
Severe	> 40	III	Extremely high
Superobese	> 50		Extremely high

Data from NIH Conference on Gastrointestinal Surgery for Severe Obesity: Consensus Development Conference Panel. *Ann Intern Med.* 1991;115:956-961.

CLINICALLY SEVERE OBESITY: BMI > 40 kg/m^2.

OBESITY-RELATED COMORBIDITIES: Various diseases are considered to be caused by obesity: hypertension, diabetes, coronary and hypertrophic heart disease, gallstones, gastroesophageal reflux disease (GERD), sleep apnea, asthma, reactive pulmonary disease, osteoarthritis, lumbosacral disk disease, urinary incontinence, infertility, polycystic ovarian syndrome, and cancer. This list attests to the serious nature of this problem.

GASTRIC RESTRICTIVE PROCEDURES: Operations, which involve the creation of a small pouch at the upper end of the stomach that communicates directly with the intestine or the stomach.

MALABSORPTIVE PROCEDURES: Surgeries that decrease the contact of food with the digestive juices and the absorptive surface of the small intestine.

LAPAROSCOPIC ADJUSTABLE GASTRIC BANDING: This procedure (Lap-Band) was approved by the Food and Drug Administration (FDA) for application in the United States in 2001. It involves the placement of a silastic band around the proximal stomach at approximately 1 cm below the GE junction. The band is attached to a subcutaneous port that may be injected with saline to adjust the gastric luminal opening (Figure 48–1)

METABOLIC SYNDROME: Metabolic syndrome puts the patient at risk for cardiovascular disease.

CLINICAL APPROACH

Obesity is increasing in epidemic proportions and qualifies as one of the leading medical problems among Americans. The adverse health effects associated with obesity may reduce patient quality of life and longevity. Because of concerns about the prevalence of obesity and its associated health problems,

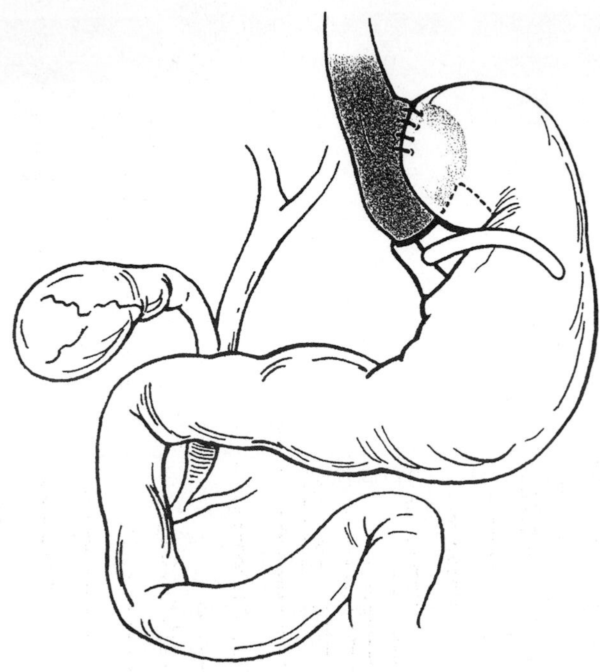

Figure 48–1. Adjustable gastric band. *Reproduced, with permission, from Brunicardi FC, Andersen DK, Dunn DL, et al, eds.* Schwartz's Principles of Surgery. *8th ed. New York: McGraw-Hill; 2005:1004.*

two NIH consensus conferences have taken place to address the surgical treatment of morbid obesity. At the 1991 conference, Roux-en-Y gastric bypass (RYGB) (Figure 48–2) and vertical banded gastroplasty (VBG) (Figure 48–3) were recommended for appropriately selected patients. Based on more current results, an updated statement indicates a **preference for RYGB** compared to VBG because the latter does not result in adequate sustained weight loss and is associated with complications. The treatment goals of any patient with morbid obesity should be focused on weight loss as well as on the reduction of comorbidities (Tables 48–2 to 48–4). It is important for the patient and the physician to have realistic expectations about surgical treatment outcome; **most successfully treated patients achieve a reduction in weight that is frequently sustainable; however, patients rarely achieve the ideal body weight** proscribed in standard height-weight tables. Most patients experience an improvement in obesity-related complications following successful surgery; however, increased longevity has not been demonstrated. The success and the patient satisfaction associated with surgical therapy are further augmented when patients receive proper preoperative counseling and undergo modifications in dietary habits and lifestyle.

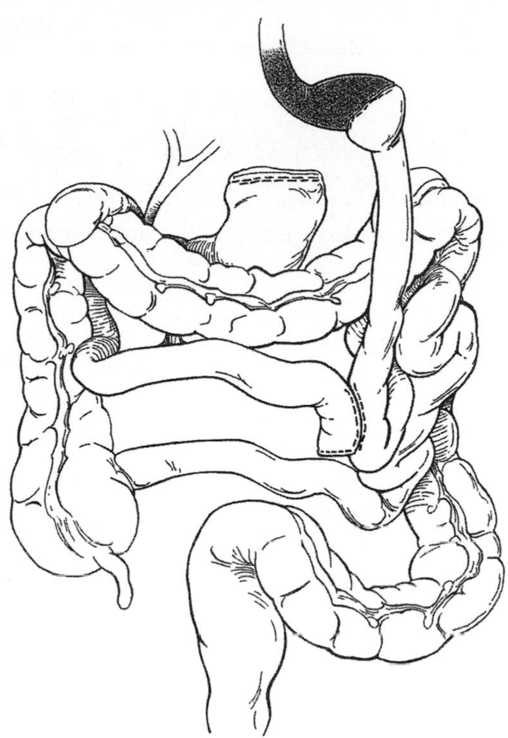

Figure 48–2. Roux-en-Y gastric bypass. *Reproduced, with permission, from Brunicardi FC, Andersen DK, Dunn DL, et al, eds.* Schwartz's Principles of Surgery. *8th ed. New York, NY: McGraw-Hill; 2005:1007.*

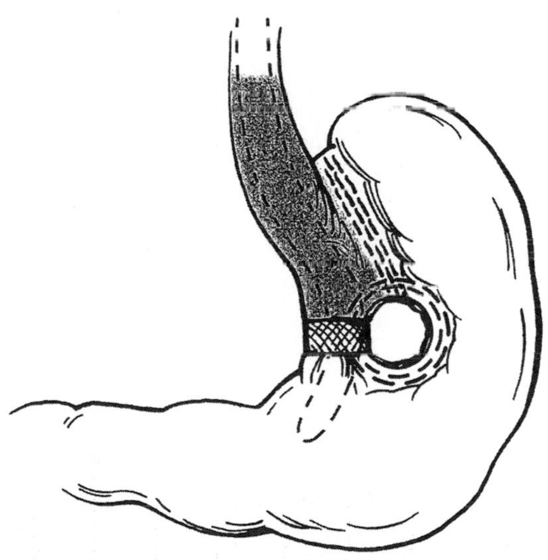

Figure 48–3. Vertical banded gastroplasty. *Reproduced, with permission, from Brunicardi FC, Andersen DK, Dunn DL, et al, eds.* Schwartz's Principles of Surgery. *8th ed. New York: McGraw-Hill; 2005:1003.*

Table 48–2 OPERATIONS USED TO TREAT CLINICALLY SEVERE OBESITY

OPERATION	DESCRIPTION
Roux-en-Y small-pouch gastric bypass	Proximal pouch to Roux limb of jejunum
Vertical banded gastroplasty	Proximal lesser curve pouch to main stomach with circumferential band at communication
Adjustable lap band	Band around upper stomach with circumferential balloon accessible by subcutaneous port
Duodenal switch	Stomach reduction with division of duodenum at the pylorus. The distal small bowel is attached to the gastric tube, and the proximal small bowel is attached to the lower ileum

Table 48–3 TREATMENT RESULTS AND COMPLICATIONS

METHOD	RESULTS	COMPLICATIONS
Vertical banded gastroplasty	Sustained weight loss is difficult, especially with "sweets eaters"	High reoperation rate for stoma erosion; frequent gastroesophageal reflux
Roux-en-Y tric bypass	Sustained results are good; loss of 50%-60% of excess weight	B_{12} deficiency in 15%-20%; iron-deficiency anemia in 20%; marginal ulcer 2%-10%; osteoporosis
Gastric banding	Loss of 33%-64% of excess weight at 3-5 yr	Up to 23% rate of band slippage, resulting in reoperation

Table 48–4 EFFECTS OF SURGERY ON OBESITY COMORBIDITY

Diabetes mellitus	82% of patients cured of type II diabetes at 15-yr follow-up
Sleep apnea	Up to 93% of patients have improvement
Hypertension	Success correlated with the amount of weight loss
Serum lipid abnormalities	Successful gastric bypass is associated with a sustained reduction in triglycerides and low-density lipoproteins and an increase in high-density lipoproteins

Patient Selection

All patients must have unsuccessfully attempted supervised weight-loss programs by diet, exercise, or medications and fulfill minimum weight criteria that include BMI greater than 35 kg/m^2 with comorbidity or BMI greater than 40 kg/m^2 without comorbidity. In addition, all patients must be willing to comply with postoperative lifestyle changes and dietary restrictions, exercise, and follow-up programs. Traditionally, bariatric surgery is offered to patients from 18 to 60 years of age; however, more recently, operations have been performed in older patients in some institutions without an increase in morbidity, and appropriately selected adolescents have undergone weight-reduction procedures in some institutions.

Comprehension Questions

48.1 A 23-year-old woman is referred for an opinion regarding the advisability of surgical treatment for obesity. The patient is 5 ft tall and weighs 210 lb. She has no known comorbidities and is free of symptoms. Your best advice would be which of the following?

A. A small-pouch gastric bypass
B. A vertical banded gastroplasty
C. A Lap-Band procedure
D. Further efforts at medical therapy

48.2 A 45-year-old woman, the mother of two adolescents, presents with long-standing, clinically severe obesity (BMI 50 kg/m^2) that is refractory to medical therapy. Which of the following surgical procedures is most likely to provide the best chance of long-term weight reduction with the least morbidity?

A. Vertical banded gastroplasty
B. Small-pouch gastric bypass
C. Adjustable Lap-Band
D. Duodenal switch

48.3 Gastric restrictive procedures lead to weight loss by doing which of the following?
A. Increasing the basal metabolic rate.
B. Enhancing maldigestion and absorption.
C. Producing early satiety.
D. Inducing nausea and vomiting.

48.4 Which of the following is the most common, most serious postoperative complication associated with small-pouch gastric bypass?
A. Pneumonia
B. Leakage of intestinal contents from the gastrojejunal anastomosis
C. Intestinal obstruction
D. Pulmonary embolus

48.5 Late sequelae from gastric restrictive procedures include which of the following?
A. Anemia
B. Osteoporosis
C. Vitamin deficiencies
D. All of the above

ANSWERS

48.1 **D.** The patient is young, free of comorbid medical problems, and has a BMI less than 40. Her BMI is calculated as $210 \times 704/64 \times 64 = 36.1$ kg/m^2. Further attempts at medical management should be made; however, if significant complications such as hypertension and diabetes are already present, a surgical approach might be appropriate.

48.2 **B.** This patient has strong indications for a surgical approach (BMI > 50, superobese). A small-pouch gastric bypass performed by either an open or a laparoscopic technique will provide the best long-term weight reduction with minimal early and late long-term morbidity.

48.3 **C.** Gastric restrictive operations help people lose weight by producing early satiety and decreasing their appetite. To be successful, the patient must simultaneously restrict caloric intake.

48.4 **B.** Leakage from the attachment of the stomach to the intestine can be a devastating complication. It usually is characterized by fever, leukocytosis, and left shoulder pain on postoperative days 3 to 5.

48.5 **D.** A small-pouch gastric bypass can be accompanied by anemia, osteoporosis, and vitamin deficiencies in view of the marked decrease in food intake. Patients need supplemental vitamins, calcium, and oral iron and vitamin B_{12} following the procedure.

Clinical Pearls

- The body mass index represented in kilograms per meter squared body surface area is a common tool in assessing obesity.
- Many diseases are considered to be obesity-related comorbidities such as hypertension, diabetes, coronary heart disease, gallstones, and sleep apnea.
- In general, surgical weight reduction surgeries should be reserved for severe obesity or those obese individuals with comorbidities.

REFERENCES

National Institutes of Health. Clinical guidelines on the identification, evaluation, and treatment of overweight and obesity in adults: the evidence report. NIH Publication No. 98-4083. Bethesda, MD: National Institutes of Health; 1998.

Richards WO, Schirmer BD. Morbid obesity. In: Townsend CM Jr, Beauchamp RD, Evers BM, eds. *Sabiston Textbook of Surgery*. 18th Ed. Philadelphia, PA: Elsevier; 2008:399-430.

Schauer PR, Schirmer BD. The surgical management of obesity. In: Brunicardi FC, Andersen DK, Dunn DL, et al, eds. *Schwartz's Principles of Surgery*. 8th ed. New York: McGraw-Hill; 2005:997-1016.

Case 49

A 32-year-old woman complains of bleeding gums while brushing her teeth and easy bruising of several weeks' duration. She has no significant past medical history, has had no previous surgery, and does not take any medication. She denies consumption of alcohol, tobacco, or illicit drugs. On examination, you notice several petechiae on her legs and bruises over the knees. The results from her head and neck, cardiopulmonary, and abdominal examinations are unremarkable. No masses are palpable in the abdomen. The laboratory evaluation reveals a normal white blood cell count and normal hemoglobin and hematocrit values. Results from serum chemistry studies are within the normal range. Her platelet count is 27,000/mm^3. A bone marrow biopsy is performed, demonstrating the presence of numerous megakaryocytes but no evidence of malignancy.

- What is the most likely diagnosis?
- What is the mechanism associated with this disease process?
- What is your next step in treatment?

ANSWERS TO CASE 49: Immune Thrombocytopenia Purpura (Splenic Disease)

Summary: A 32-year-old woman presents with easy bruisability, gum bleeding and petechiae, and thrombocytopenia. The bone marrow aspirate shows an increased number of megakaryocytes (normal functions).

- **Diagnosis:** Immune thrombocytopenia purpura (ITP).
- **Mechanism responsible for the process:** ITP is associated with the production of antiplatelet immunoglobulin G (IgG) by the spleen.
- **Next step:** The initial treatment is with corticosteroids. Seventy-five percent of patients respond to corticosteroids, but the best long-term results are achieved with splenectomy.

ANALYSIS

Objectives

1. Become familiar with the role of splenectomy in the treatment of ITP.
2. Be familiar with splenic function and the complications associated with the loss of splenic function.
3. Be familiar with indications for splenectomy other than traumatic injuries.

Considerations

This patient exhibits many of the common clinical manifestations of thrombocytopenia, which include ecchymoses, gum bleeding, purpura, excessive vaginal bleeding, and gastrointestinal tract bleeding. Mechanisms producing thrombocytopenia include inadequate production because of primary or secondary bone marrow dysfunction, splenic sequestration (hypersplenism), and increased platelet destruction. ITP is an acquired disorder leading to increased platelet destruction because of the production of antiplatelet IgG by the spleen. The spleen may further contribute to thrombocytopenia by functioning as a primary site of sequestration and destruction of sensitized platelets. ITP is two to three times more common in women than men. The diagnosis of ITP is one of exclusion, which requires a careful search for possible precipitating factors such as medications and infections. **The diagnosis requires demonstration of a normal to hypercellular megakaryocyte count in the bone marrow, indicating a response to the increased peripheral destruction.** Splenomegaly is rare in ITP, and its presence should suggest another source of thrombocytopenia, such as hemolytic disease.

APPROACH TO
Immune Thrombocytopenia Purpura

The spleen has a number of important functions, including a significant although not indispensable role in host cellular- and humoral-mediated immunity and phagocytic activities. It removes old erythrocytes (120 days old) and platelets (10 to 14 days old). It also removes abnormal intracellular erythrocyte particles (Howell-Jolly bodies, Heinz bodies, and Pappenheimer bodies) and erythrocytes with abnormal membranes. The spleen is also a site of opsonins (tuftsin and properdin) and antibodies (particularly IgM) production.

CLINICAL APPROACH

A carefully recorded history and a physical examination are important in the diagnosis of ITP. A bone marrow aspirate is also necessary to confirm the diagnosis. The management of ITP varies according to the severity of the thrombocytopenia, where patients with asymptomatic platelet counts above 50,000 may simply require monitoring, and some asymptomatic patients with platelet counts of 30,000 to 50,000 may also be monitored. The initial treatment for symptomatic patients or those with lower platelet count is corticosteroids, which leads to an increased platelet count in 50% to 75% of patients. Other medical therapies include administration of intravenous immunoglobulins, plasmapheresis, and chemotherapeutic agents.

Splenectomy

Splenectomy is recommended for patients who do not respond to steroids, those who require an excessively high steroid dose, and those who require chronic steroid therapy (> 1 year). The platelet count can be expected to rise shortly after splenectomy, and sustained remissions are seen in more than 80% of cases. The best indication that splenectomy will be of lasting benefit is an increase in the platelet count with corticosteroid therapy. Patients who are refractory to corticosteroid treatment have a lower rate of long-term remission (approximately 60%). Spontaneous remission occurs in most children (85%), and splenectomy is rarely indicated. When splenectomy is needed, it should be delayed until after 4 years of age, at which time the risk of postsplenectomy sepsis is dramatically reduced. Laparoscopic splenectomy has been shown to be safe and effective. Furthermore, patients undergoing laparoscopic splenectomy tolerate feeding sooner, require less pain medication, and are discharged from the hospital sooner than those undergoing open splenectomy. Platelet transfusions generally are not required despite low platelet counts unless bleeding is uncontrollable. Platelet transfusion should be withheld intraoperatively until just after the spleen is removed; if given before this time, they are consumed and confer minimal benefit. A systemic review of articles published between 1996 to 2004 reported complete response of 66% and partial response of 88% following splenectomy for ITP.

Splenectomy Other than for ITP

Traumatic injury has been the most common indication for splenectomy. Other common nontraumatic indications for splenectomy may be categorized as red cell–, white cell–, and platelet-related disorders, and these include congenital hemolytic anemias, such as hereditary spherocytosis and thalassemia major. Myeloproliferative disorders may lead to massive splenomegaly, which can cause symptoms that are best relieved by splenectomy. Splenectomy for myeloproliferative disorders is performed primarily for symptomatic relief.

Because of the loss of splenic immunologic function following splenectomy, postoperative infectious complications may occur, such as wound infections and intra-abdominal abscesses. **Overwhelming postsplenectomy sepsis (OPSS) is an uncommon but well-recognized potential complication associated with splenectomy.** The risk of OPSS depends on the age of the patient and the reason for splenectomy. It occurs in 0.3% of adults and 0.6% of children and is **more common when splenectomy is performed for hematologic disease compared to splenectomy for trauma.** OPSS most commonly develops within the first 2 years after splenectomy, although it can occur later. The typical onset of this clinical syndrome is often insidious and marked by nonspecific symptoms of malaise, headache, nausea, and confusion; it can progress rapidly to shock and death. Early medical evaluation at the first signs of illness is important in decreasing mortality. The mortality of OPSS exceeds 50% in children and is approximately 20% in adults. The most common organisms are encapsulated bacteria such as *Streptococcus pneumoniae*, *Haemophilus influenzae* **B, and** *Neisseria meningitidis*, which are typically killed by the immunologic functions of the spleen. **All patients undergoing planned elective splenectomy should receive a polyvalent pneumococcal vaccination 2 weeks before surgery. Children and all immunosuppressed patients** should be vaccinated against **pneumococcus,** *H influenzae* **B, and meningococcus.**

Comprehension Questions

49.1 A 44-year-old woman has recurrent thrombocytopenia following a 4-week course of corticosteroid therapy for ITP. Her platelet count has decreased from the initial post-treatment level of 120,000 to 75,000. The patient has remained asymptomatic without further treatment for the past 3 months. Which of the following is the most appropriate recommendation for this patient at this time?

A. Laparoscopic splenectomy because she has had a favorable but unsustainable response to steroids treatment
B. Intravenous immunoglobulins
C. Observation
D. Vaccination against pneumococcus, *H influenzae* B, and meningococcus, followed by laparoscopic splenectomy 2 weeks later.

49.2 A 20-year-old man sustained blunt trauma to the spleen when his car crashed into a tree. During his exploratory laparotomy, splenic lacerations were identified and treated with a partial splenectomy. Based on report, approximately one-third of the splenic mass was preserved. Which of the following studies may be helpful to determine if the patient has retained splenic functions following this procedure?

A. A CT scan of the abdomen
B. An MRI
C. A peripheral blood smear
D. PPD skin test

49.3 Fever in which of the following individuals is most likely overwheming post-splenectomy sepsis syndrome (OPSS)?

A. A 30-year-old man who underwent splenectomy for trauma 3 years ago
B. An 8-year-old boy who had underwent splenectomy for complications related to acute lymphocytic leukemia 2 years prior
C. A 60-year-old man with hypercoagulable state and splenic vein thrombosis and partial splenic infarct
D. A 12-year-old boy with history of trauma and partial splenectomy at the age of 8

49.4 Splenectomy for ITP is most likely to provide long-term remission in which of the following patients?

A. Patients with an enlarged spleen
B. Patients with a high reticulocyte count
C. Patients younger than 4 years
D. Patients who respond to corticosteroid therapy

ANSWERS

49.1 **C.** Observation is reasonable in this patient with ITP, initial response to corticosteroids, and current level of thrombocytopenia. Further medical or surgical treatment may be appropriate if the patient's platelet counts drop below the 30,000-50,000 range, or if the patient develops bleeding or bleeding complications.

49.2 **C.** A peripheral blood smear may demonstrate Howell-Jolley bodies, Heinz bodies, and Pappenheimer bodies if the patient's spleen is unable to scavenge old and abnormal RBCs. Whether the presence of these peripheral smear abnormalities indicates the absence of normal immunological functions of the spleen is not clear.

49.3 **B.** OPSS is a rare condition, but pretest probability suggests that this condition occurs more commonly in children in comparison to adults, and the condition is more likely to occur following splenectomy for primary hematological disorders.

49.4 **D.** The patient group that has the best response to splenectomy consists of patients with ITP who respond to corticosteroid therapy.

Clinical Pearls

- Splenomegaly is rare in ITP.
- Splenectomy for ITP is most likely to provide long-term remission in patients who respond to corticosteroid therapy.
- **Overwhelming postsplenectomy sepsis is an uncommon but well-recognized potential complication associated with splenectomy;** it has a higher incidence in children than in adults.
- Bone marrow aspirates from ITP patients typically reveal normal or increased number of megakaryocytes thus indicating normal bone marrow response to low circulating platelet counts.

REFERENCES

Deauchamp RD, Holzman MD, Fabian TC, Weinberg JA. The Spleen. In: Townsend CM Jr, Beauchamp RD, Evers BM, Mattox KL, eds. *Sabiston Textbook of Surgery*. 18th ed. Philadelphia, PA: Saunders Elsevier; 2008:1624-1652.

Kojouri K, Vesely SK, Terrelll DR, et al. Splenectomy for adult patients with idiopathic thrombocytopenic purpura: a systemic review to assess long-term platelet count responses, prediction of response, and surgical complications. *Blood*. 2004;104:2623-2634.

Park AE, McKinlay R. Spleen. In: Brunicardi FC, Andersen DK, Billiar TR, et al, eds. *Schwartz's Principles of Surgery*. 8th ed. New York, NY: McGraw-Hill; 2005:1297-1315.

Case 50

A 26-year-old man with 3-year history of Crohn disease presents to the emergency department with postprandial abdominal pain and vomiting of 2 days' duration. He has been receiving infliximab (Remicade) infusions at 5 mg/kg every 8 weeks for the past 8 months. Before that time, he had taken prednisone 40 mg/day for several weeks intermittently for treatment of disease exacerbation. Also, he had received Asacol (a 5-aminosalicylate [5-ASA] derivative), 2.4 g/day. The patient reports a 15-lb weight loss over the past 2 months. His past surgical history is significant for an appendectomy 4 years ago. On examination, his temperature is 38.0°C (100.4°F), pulse rate 95 beats/min, and blood pressure 130/70 mm Hg. His abdomen is moderately distended and tender in the right lower quadrant. There are no masses or peritonitis. A rectal examination reveals no perianal disease or abnormalities. The remaining results from the physical examination are unremarkable. The complete blood count revealed a white blood cell count of 14,000/mm^3, and his hemoglobin level is 10.5 g/dL. The results from serum electrolyte studies and a urinalysis are within the normal range.

- ➤ What is the most likely diagnosis?
- ➤ What is the next step?

ANSWERS TO CASE 50: Crohn Disease

Summary: A 26-year-old man presents with a history of Crohn disease with disease exacerbation. Despite infliximab therapy, the patient's symptoms have not improved. Currently, he has nausea, vomiting, abdominal pain and distention, and a low-grade fever and leukocytosis, which are suggestive of chronic small bowel obstruction and low-grade sepsis.

- **Diagnosis:** Crohn disease, likely ileocolic, complicated by obstruction and possible intra-abdominal infection.
- **Next step:** The next step is to define the extent of disease involvement, the site of obstruction, and the possible presence of intra-abdominal abscesses. A computed tomography (CT) scan of the abdomen and pelvis, small bowel follow through (SBFT) radiography, and colonoscopy are indicated.

ANALYSIS

Objectives

1. Know the clinical features, diagnosis, and natural history of Crohn disease.
2. Be familiar with the medical therapies and the role of surgery in Crohn disease.

Considerations

A 26-year-old man presents with a 3-year history of Crohn disease, refractory to maintenance therapy with a 5-ASA derivative. Exacerbations required steroid therapy in the past; however, he has now received several doses of infliximab. Despite this, he has progression of disease evidenced by weight loss, GI tract obstructive symptoms, and fever. This patient's bowel obstruction is likely related to chronic fibrotic strictures rather than subacute inflammation. Obstruction from subacute inflammation can be resolved with anti-inflammatory and immunomodulator therapies. In contrast, **fibrotic strictures cannot be resolved with medical management and generally require surgical therapy** to relieve the obstruction. A CT scan is a useful initial imaging study for assessing the severity and extent of the disease and for detecting intra-abdominal abscesses. Crohn disease may involve both the small bowel and colon. Therefore, complete evaluation should include colonoscopy and an SBFT contrast study to visualize the location and severity of small bowel disease. Once the small bowel and colon have been evaluated, this patient should undergo exploratory laparotomy to relieve his bowel obstruction. Surgical options include resection of the obstructed bowel or stricturoplasty.

APPROACH TO Crohn Disease

DEFINITIONS

DISEASE ACTIVITY: Severity can be assessed by histology, endoscopy, radiography, symptoms, or surgical findings. Histologic, endoscopic, radiographic, and surgical criteria frequently do not correlate with clinical criteria and may not correlate with the physiologic impact of the disease on the patient. It is more important to know how the disease is affecting the patient. The histologic finding of granulomas is pathognomonic for Crohn.

DISEASE PATTERNS: Crohn disease can be intra-abdominal, perianal, or both. Intra-abdominal Crohn disease usually results in one of three predominant disease patterns: stricture, perforation, or inflammation. Perianal disease results in anal strictures, fistulas-in-ano, and abscesses.

MEDICAL THERAPY: Pharmacologic therapy can be generally categorized as maintenance therapy (to maintain disease remission) and therapy for active disease (for acute flare-ups).

STRICTUROPLASTY: A surgical option that may be effective for patients with intestinal strictures from Crohn disease. The strictured segment of bowel is divided longitudinally then reapproximated transversely, thus increasing the diameter of that segment without resection. This approach may help preserve bowel length and function for patients with involvement of multiple sites by fibrotic strictures.

CLINICAL APPROACH

Most patients with Crohn disease have distinct patterns of disease distribution: terminal ileum and right colon (35%-50%), ileum (30%-35%), colon (25%-35%), or stomach and/or duodenum (0.5%-4%). Anorectal involvement is frequently found in patients with small bowel Crohn disease and may be the initial manifestation in 10% of patients. Therefore, Crohn disease should be considered whenever recurrent or complex perianal abscesses and fistulas are encountered. The other symptoms related to Crohn disease are often nonspecific, including chronic abdominal pain, postprandial abdominal cramps, weight loss, or fever related to fistulizing disease. It is not uncommon for patients with Crohn disease to have symptoms for months to years before the diagnosis is established. The goals of management are to relieve symptoms and optimize the patient's quality of life. Medical and surgical options should be viewed as complementary therapeutic options rather than competing modalities. Thus, when medical therapy becomes ineffective or significantly compromises the patient's quality of life, surgical interventions should be implemented. Similarly, the role of surgery in Crohn disease is palliative and not curative; therefore, surgical goals should be directed toward symptom relief without exposing patients to excessive short- and long-term morbidity. Whenever an operative procedure is to be implemented, it is vital for the surgeon to coordinate with the gastroenterologist in formulating plans so that the patient will have the best possible outcome.

Medical Therapy

The etiology of Crohn disease remains unknown, but it is in part caused by stimulation of an intestinal immune cascade in genetically susceptible individuals. Severity of disease dictates medical therapy, and gastroenterologists now use a sequential approach, using more aggressive medications for more aggressive disease. Categories of disease severity include mild, moderate, severe, and fulminant (Table 50–1). Medical therapy can be broadly categorized as nutritional, antimicrobial, anti-inflammatory, immunomodulatory, and anti-TNF (tumor necrosis factor) (Table 50–2). Nutritional therapies include bowel rest with total parenteral nutrition (TPN), elemental feeding, or omega-3 fatty acid supplementation. Nutritional therapies produce improvement and cause remission in patients with active disease; however, because of the impact of nutritional therapy on a patient's lifestyle, nutritional therapy has been limited to the short-term treatment of active disease.

Table 50–1 DISEASE SEVERITY OF CROHN DISEASE

DISEASE SEVERITY	CLINICAL PRESENTATION
Mild to moderate disease	Ambulatory, eating and drinking without dehydration, toxicity, abdominal tenderness, painful mass, obstruction or > 10% weight loss
Moderate to severe disease	Failure of response to mild medical therapies or fevers, significant weight loss, abdominal pain or tenderness, intermittent nausea and vomiting (without obstructive findings) or significant anemia
Severe to fulminant disease	Persistent symptoms despite use of corticosteroids as outpatient or high fevers, persistent vomiting, evidence of intestinal obstruction, rebound tenderness, cachexia, evidence of abscess

Data from Friedman S. General principles of medical therapy of inflammatory bowel disease. *Gastro Clin Northam.* 2004, 33: 191-208.

Table 50–2 THERAPY FOR CROHN DISEASE

AGENTS	INDICATIONS	ADVERSE EFFECTS
5-Aminosalicylate derivatives (sulfasalazine, Asacol, Pentasa)	Mild to moderate disease; maintenance therapy	Sperm abnormalities, folate malabsorption, nausea, dyspepsia, headache
Metronidazole	Mild to moderate disease: maintenance therapy	Nausea, metallic taste, peripheral nauropathy, disulfuram-like reaction
Corticosteroids	Moderate to severe disease: induce remission during acute flares	Multiple metabolic side effects
Azathioprine and 6-mercaptopurine	Moderate to severe disease: maintenance of remission after flare	Nausea, rash, fever, hepatitis, bone marrow suppression, B-cell lymphoma
Methotrexate	Moderate to severe disease: induce and maintain remission	Nausea, hepatotoxicity, bone marrow suppression, stomatitis
Cyclosporin A	Severe to fulfilminant disease	Hypertension, tremors, opportunistic infections, nephrotoxicity, paraesthesias, hepatotoxicity, gingival hyperplasia
Anti-tumor necrosis factor	Moderate to severe disease or severe perianal fistulizing disease	Abdominal pain, myalgias, lymphoma, teratogenic effects, delayed hypersensitivity reactions, nausea, fatique

First-line therapy for mild to moderate disease is either antimicrobial or anti-inflammatory. Antimicrobial therapy with metronidazole or ciprofloxacin is effective in the resolution of active intestinal and perianal disease, and long-term metronidazole maintenance therapy is effective in preventing disease recurrence. The mechanisms of antimicrobial therapy are largely unknown and may be in part based on its immunosuppressive effects. Long-term metronidazole therapy is poorly tolerated because of multiple side effects including nausea, metallic taste, disulfiram-like reactions, and peripheral neuropathy. Aminosalicylates (5-ASA) are effective in maintenance therapy and in the treatment of mild active disease. Limitations of 5-ASA derivatives include GI tract and systemic side effects, and hypersensitivity reactions.

Moderate to severe disease refractory to antimicrobials and anti-inflammatory agents is treated with corticosteroids. Corticosteroids are nonspecific anti-inflammatory agents effective in treating small bowel and ileocolic disease. Although beneficial for disease flare-ups, corticosteroids are not efficacious in maintenance therapy. Also, they are associated with many major side effects, including hyperglycemia, fluid retention, fat redistribution, acne, mood changes, and growth retardation in children. Budesonide is a newer agent that is more rapidly metabolized than prednisone and may lead to fewer side effects. However, it is most helpful in patients with mild to moderate disease.

In patients with moderate to severe disease who are in remission after a course of corticosteroids, immunomodulators are effective in maintaining remission. Several immunomodulators have been used in the treatment of Crohn disease. Azathioprine (AZT) and 6-mercaptopurine (6-MP) are most commonly used. The potential toxic effects of AZT and 6-MP include bone marrow suppression, nausea, fever, rash, hepatitis, and pancreatitis. Methotrexate is also effective in the treatment of active disease but associated with many side effects including nausea, headache, stomatitis, bone marrow suppression, hepatitis, and pneumonitis. It is thus reserved for patients unable to take AZT or 6-MP.

Cyclosporin A (CSA) produces significant improvement in severe disease associated with fistulas; however, controlled trials in patients with moderate disease have not demonstrated significant benefits. CSA use is associated with severe side effects including hypertension, hyperesthesias, tremors, and nephrotoxicity. Thus, it has been largely replaced by infliximab, the chimeric monoclonal antibody directed toward the TNF receptor. Infliximab is highly effective in the treatment of patients who are refractory to all other medical therapy. It can potentially delay the need for operative intervention in patients with severe disease. It is also an effective first-line therapy in patients with fistulizing perianal disease. Unfortunately, major drawbacks are associated with anti-TNF therapy, including opportunistic infections and B-cell lymphoma development.

Surgical Therapy

There are two major roles of operative intervention in the management of Crohn disease. One is to relieve symptoms associated with Crohn disease refractory to medical therapy, namely pain, obstructive symptoms, and weight loss. Another is to improve the quality of life of patients who experience severe side effects from medical therapy (eg, growth retardation from corticosteroid therapy). Surgical options include bowel resection, stricturoplasty, and abscess drainage. Approximately 30% of patients may require another operation within 5 years after undergoing resection for Crohn disease. One of the potential long-term complications of repeated bowel resection is the development of short bowel syndrome, that is, malabsorption requiring permanent TPN therapy (approximately 1% of patients). In an effort to prevent this, stricturoplasty is performed whenever possible. Patients with multiple sites of disease involvement have a greater risk for disease recurrence. In addition, nonsteroidal anti-inflammatory use and tobacco smoking are linked to disease recurrences; therefore, patients should be counseled regarding these issues.

Comprehension Questions

50.1 Medical management may be effective in the treatment of which of the following symptoms associated with Crohn disease?

A. Partial bowel obstruction
B. Enterocolonic fistulas
C. Abdominal pain related to an inflammatory mass
D. All of the above

50.2 A 22-year-old woman is newly diagnosed with Crohn disease of the terminal ileum. She complains of significant abdominal pain. Her temperature is 36.7°C (98°F), and HR 90 beats/min. Which of the following is the best management for this patient?

A. Exploratory celiotomy to assess for bowel perforation
B. Medical management and reassessment
C. Radionuclide-tagged leukocyte imaging study to assess location of disease
D. Intravenous morphine for pain control

50.3 Four weeks following appendectomy for presumed acute appendicitis a 23-year-old man returns to the emergency center with drainage of bile-stained fluid from his right lower quadrant surgical site. The patient is afebrile and has been tolerating a normal diet. Abdominal CT revealed postoperative inflammatory changes and no abscess. A review of the pathology report from his previous appendectomy specimen revealed involvement of the appendix with transmural inflammation and granulomatous changes. Which of the following is the most appropriate management at this time?

A. Exploratory laparotomy to identify and remove the segment of intestine responsible for the leakage of enteric contents.
B. CT of the abdomen followed by CT-guided drainage
C. Cortical steroids
D. Infliximab

ANSWERS

50.1 **D.** Medical management may be effective for all these complications associated with Crohn disease. They can include obstruction, fistulas, and inflammation. Surgery is also indicated for all these complications if a patient does not respond to medications or if medications produce unacceptable side effects.

50.2 **B.** Medical management is the appropriate choice in a patient with uncomplicated newly diagnosed Crohn disease. A CT scan of the abdomen should be performed to rule out the possibility of intra-abdominal abscess associated with Crohn disease and rule out alternative pathology such as appendicitis.

50.3 **D.** This patient's clinical presentation is compatible with enterocutaneous fistula presumable related to his Crohn disease. Enterocutaneous fistula in the setting of Crohn disease does not always require surgical treatment. In this patient who appears to have a low output fistula, absence of a septic picture, and no evidence of ongoing intraabdominal septic focus, a trial of nonoperative management that includes the use of infliximab may be appropriate. Fistula closure rates reported with inliximab has ranged from 6-70%.

Clinical Pearls

- With the exception of the treatment of toxic colitis, emergency (unplanned) operative treatment for patients with Crohn disease is rare.
- Fibrotic strictures cannot be resolved with medical management and generally require operative therapy to relieve the obstruction.
- Crohn disease may involve both the small bowel and the colon; therefore, a complete evaluation should include colonoscopy and SBFT to visualize the location and severity of the small bowel disease.
- Repeated resection of the GI tract can result in clinical short bowel syndrome requiring permanent TPN therapy in approximately 1% of patients with Crohn disease.
- In general, the role of surgery in Crohn disease is to relieve symptoms refractory to medical therapy (pain, obstructive symptoms, weight loss) and to improve the quality of life of patients who experience severe medication side effects.

REFERENCES

Friedman S. General principles of medical therapy of inflammation bowel disease. *Gastroenterol Clin North Am*. 2004;33:191-208.

Galandiuk S. Crohn's colitis. In: Cameron JL, ed. *Current Surgical Therapy*. 9th ed. Philadelphia, PA: Mosby Elsevier; 2008:178-183.

Mintz Y, Talamini MA. Crohn's diease of the small bowel. In: Cameron JL, ed. *Current Surgical Therapy*. 9th ed. Philadelphia, PA: Mosby Elsevier; 2008:123-127.

Stein RB, Lichtenstein GR. Medical therapy for Crohn's disease. *Surg Clin North Am*. 2001;81:71-101.

Case 51

A 45-year-old man with a 15-year history of ulcerative colitis (UC) is evaluated in the outpatient office with chronic bloody diarrhea over the past 6 weeks. The patient's vital signs are unremarkable. His hemoglobin level is 11.0 g/dL. His current medications consist of prednisone and mesalamine (a 5-aminosalicylate derivative), and he recently completed a course of cyclosporine therapy 2 months ago for another bout of disease flare-up. The patient has been unable to maintain full-time employment over the past year because of UC. Previous colonoscopy has shown that his disease extends from the rectum to the cecum.

- What should be your next step?
- What is the best therapy?

ANSWERS TO CASE 51:
Ulcerative Colitis

Summary: A 45-year-old man has pancolonic chronic UC that is refractory to medical management and causes significant disability.

- **Next step:** The option of surgical therapy should be presented to this patient. The discussion should explain the benefits and limitations of surgery versus those of continued medical therapy.
- **Best therapy:** Proctocolectomy with ileal pouch-anal anastomosis.

ANALYSIS

Objectives

1. Become familiar with the clinical presentation, natural history, medical management, and complications of UC.
2. Become familiar with the indications for urgent and elective operations for the treatment of UC.
3. Be aware of the surgical options and their outcomes for the treatment of UC.

Considerations

Ulcerative colitis is a chronic disease with variable disease severity and variable involvement of the different colonic segments. The symptoms associated with this disease generally respond to medicated enemas or systemic therapy. When a 45-year-old man presents with a 15-year history of pancolitis and disabling symptoms that have been refractory to medical management, the discussion regarding treatment should explain medical as well as surgical options. Surgical excision of the diseased colon and rectum would lead to resolution of the gastrointestinal (GI) symptoms associated with UC. However, the operation would result in permanent changes in bowel function and body image. It is essential to convey to the patient that surgical excision will not resolve the extraintestinal manifestations of UC. Ongoing medical therapy for these symptoms will more than likely be required. Another important consideration for this patient is cancer risk in the setting of chronic UC. This risk is increased with disease extent and duration. Proctocolectomy with ileal reservoir reconstruction can improve the quality of life and virtually eliminate the colorectal cancer risk in properly selected patients.

APPROACH TO Ulcerative Colitis

DEFINITIONS

FULMINANT COLITIS AND TOXIC MEGACOLON: Fulminant colitis is a condition characterized by abdominal pain, fever, and sepsis that most commonly develops in the setting of UC but occasionally occurs in the settings of Crohn colitis and pseudomembranous colitis. Toxic megacolon occurs when the preceding findings are associated with radiographic evidence of colonic distension (> 6 cm). The cecum is the most frequent site of distension. Patients can become extremely ill with clinical signs of sepsis, and this clinical entity can be highly lethal if not promptly recognized and treated. When identified with either condition, patients require prompt fluid resuscitation and the initiation of broad-spectrum antibiotic therapy, with maximal medical treatment. Colectomy is indicated if the patient fails to respond to medical therapy. A third of patients generally go on to require colectomy for this complication.

DYSPLASIA: Premalignant transformation of the mucosa caused by chronic UC. The risk of cancer associated with dysplasia varies depending on the severity of the dysplastic changes. Roughly 40% of patients with high-grade dysplasia harbor synchronous cancer, and 20% of patients with low-grade dysplasia harbor synchronous cancer.

DYSPLASIA-ASSOCIATED LESION OR MASS: A sessile pseudopolyp arising from dysplastic mucosa affected by chronic UC. Fifty percent of patients with these lesions have carcinoma. Patients with this finding should undergo colorectal resection.

PANCOLITIS: Ulcerative colitis that involves the rectum and the entire colon. Patients with this pattern of disease have a significant risk for the development of subsequent colorectal cancers.

ILEAL J-POUCH: A neorectum created with the terminal ileum in the shape of a J. This is then anastomosed to the anus to form the ileal pouch-anal anastomosis.

POUCHITIS: Idiopathic inflammation of the ileal pouch that can develop following ileal reservoir reconstruction. Patients can present with any number of symptoms including increased stool frequency, fecal urgency, incontinence, watery diarrhea, bleeding, abdominal cramps, fever, and malaise. Bacterial overgrowth can be a contributing factor for pouchitis, and therefore some patients respond to antibiotic therapy.

CLINICAL APPROACH

Ulcerative colitis is an inflammatory condition of unknown etiology. Unlike Crohn, which is a **transmural process,** the disease involvement in UC is limited to the mucosa. The distribution begins in the rectum and extends to the proximal colon, with occasional extension to the terminal ileum (backwash ileitis). With chronic inflammation of the colonic mucosa, there is loss of water absorption and normal motility, leading to watery diarrhea, crampy abdominal pain, tenesmus, and urgency. A number of extraintestinal manifestations are associated with UC, including ankylosing spondylitis, uveitis, scleroderma, sclerosing cholangitis, arthritis, dermatomyositis, and hypercoagulable states. Surgical therapy virtually eliminates the symptoms related to the diseased colon and rectum; however, the benefits of surgery for the extraintestinal manifestations have not been established (Table 51–1). In fact, some reports have suggested that extraintestinal disease can be aggravated by removal of the colon and rectum.

The medical management of UC consists of anti-inflammatory therapies of escalating intensity coupled with the administration of antibiotics. When antibiotics and anti-inflammatory agents fail, steroid agents are the next line of therapy. The long-term use of steroids can be effective in reducing the symptoms associated with UC but can lead to immunosuppression, accelerated bone loss, hirsutism, masculinization, osteoporosis, aseptic necrosis, glucose intolerance, and loss of muscle mass. Short- and long-term steroid use increases the morbidity associated with surgical treatment. Newer studies are examining the role of infliximab, the monoclonal anti-TNF (tumor necrosis factor) antibody, in treating UC.

The **main indications for surgical therapy in UC are fulminant colitis or toxic megacolon, dysplasia or cancer, and intractable disease.** The most commonly performed operation for fulminant colitis is total abdominal colectomy with end ileostomy. Because the **colorectal cancer risk increases with chronic** UC, patients with duration of disease of more than 7 to 9 years should undergo annual or biannual surveillance colonoscopy with biopsies. If a surveillance program is not instituted, they should be considered for total proctocolectomy. The majority of patients with UC undergoing surgery do so because of disease intractability. This is determined on the basis of disease symptomatology and tolerance to medical therapy. In the elective setting, surgical options include total proctocolectomy with permanent end ileostomy, total proctocolectomy with continent ileostomy, or total proctocolectomy with ileal pouch-anal anastomosis. The latter two operations, although restoring continence, are associated with many more complications than the end ileostomy. The decision as to which procedure to perform is ultimately up to the patient after receiving extensive preoperative counseling.

Table 51–1 SURGICAL OPTIONS FOR ULCERATIVE COLITIS

SURGICAL PROCEDURE	INDICATION	ADVANTAGES	DISADVANTAGES
Abdominal colectomy with ileostomy	Acute toxic colitis; less frequently for other indications	Less morbidity under urgent settings	Cancer risk in rectum up to 15%-20% at 25-30 y
Abdominal colectomy with ileorectal anastomosis	For intractability or cancer or dysplasia	Preservation of bowel functions with acceptable results in patients with limited rectal disease	Cancer risk in rectum up to 15%-20% at 25–30 y; patients can have continued symptoms
Tool proctocolectomy with permanent ileostomy	For Intractability or cancer or dysplasia	All colorectal diseases removed with symptom resolution	Permanent ileostomy
Total proctocolectomy with ileal pouch-anus anastomosis	For intractability or cancer or dysplasia	All colorectal diseases removed with symptom resolution and maintenance of transanal continence	4-12 bowel movements per day; some have day or nighttime incontinence; pouchitis (7%-40%)
Total proctocolectomy with continent ileostomy	For intractability or cancer or dysplasia	All colorectal diseases removed with symptom resolution; patients do not require external stoma appliance	High malfunction rate associated with the nipple valve requiring revision or urgent canulation for drainage

Comprehension Questions

51.1 A 35-year-old woman with ulcerative colitis underwent a colonoscopy revealing an area of colonic dysplasia described as high grade. Which of the following is the best management for this patient?

A. Surgical resection of colon and rectum.
B. Intensive medical therapy and reevaluation with colonoscopy in 3 months.
C. Increase surveillance to every 6 months.
D. Add an immunosuppressive agent to the medical therapy.

51.2 A 40-year-old woman with a 15-year history of chronic diarrhea and a diagnosis of UC is referred for consideration for total proctocolectomy with ileal pouch-anal anastomosis to eliminate future cancer risks. During the colonoscopy, you notice that the disease involves the entire colon and terminal ileum, with sparing of the rectum. Which of the following is the most appropriate treatment?

A. Proctocolectomy with ileal pouch-anus anastomosis
B. Total abdominal colectomy with ileal-rectal anastomosis
C. Repeated biopsy of the rectum and involved portions of the colon and ileum
D. Total proctocolectomy with the construction of continent ileostomy

51.3 A 46-year-old woman underwent total abdominal colectomy and ileostomy for a severe bout of colitis and sepsis one year ago. She has recovered and now desires restoration of GI tract continuity. Which of the following findings would be considered a contraindication for completion proctectomy and ilealpouch-anus anastamosis?

A. The finding of high-grade dysplasia in the rectal segment at 10-cm from the anal verge
B. The finding of high grade dysplasia with carcinoma in situ in the previously resected colon
C. The finding of granulomatous changes and transmural inflammation in the previously resected colon
D. A prior history of alcohol-induced acute pancreatitis

ANSWERS

51.1 **A.** High-grade dysplasia found on colonic surveillance in a patient with ulcerative colitis is usually treated with total proctocolectomy to avoid the development of cancer.

51.2 **C.** Noninvolvement of the rectum should raise a suspicion of possible Crohn disease, which is a contraindication to performing total proctocolectomy and ileal pouch-anal reconstruction. Repeated colonoscopy and biopsy are indicated in this case.

51.3 **C.** Ulcerative colitis is a mucosal-bound disease, and these pathological changes described are more compatible with Crohn disease. Patients with Crohn colitis are not candidates for ileal pouch reconstruction because of the likelihood of disease development in the ileal pouches. The presence of cancer or dysplasia in the rectum away from the planned area of resection is not a contraindication to ileal pouch-anal reconstruction.

Clinical Pearls

- The main indications for surgical therapy in UC are fulminant colitis or toxic megacolon, dysplasia or cancer, and intractable disease.
- Extraintestinal manifestations of UC include ankylosing spondylitis, uveitis, scleroderma, sclerosing cholangitis, arthritis, dermatomyositis, and hypercoagulable states for which surgery is not effective.
- Surgical and medical treatments for UC are complementary, not competing, modalities.
- The term "refractory to medical therapy" is not strictly defined and should also refer to the failure of appropriate medical therapy as well as patient intolerance to the adverse effects of medical therapy.

REFERENCES

Hanaver SB. New lessons: classic treatments, expanding options in ulcerative colitis. *Colorectal Dis*. 2006;8(suppl 1):20-24.

Serur A, Caliendo FJ, Angel LP, Procaccino JA. Chronic ulcerative colitis. In: Cameron JL, ed. *Current Surgical Therapy*. 9th ed. Philadelphia, PA: Mosby Elsevier; 2008:170-178.

Case 52

A 55-year-old man complains of a 4-month history of lower back pain that is worsened by walking and relieved by lying down. He denies back trauma, heavy lifting, or urologic abnormalities. He states that at times the pain radiates to the back of his right leg. On examination, his blood pressure is 130/84 mm Hg, and his pulse rate 80 beats/min; he is afebrile. He is slightly overweight. The findings from his heart and lung examinations show no abnormalities. The back is without scoliosis. Raising either leg reproduces the pain, which radiates to the right leg. The results from the neurologic examination are normal.

- ➤ What is the most likely diagnosis?
- ➤ What is the best test to confirm the diagnosis?

ANSWERS TO CASE 52: Lumbar Prolapsed Nucleus Pulposus

Summary: A 55-year-old man complains of a 4-month history of lower back pain radiating to the right leg, which is worsened by walking and relieved by lying down. He denies trauma to the back, heavy lifting, or urologic abnormalities. He is slightly overweight. The back is without scoliosis. Raising either leg reproduces the pain, which radiates to the right leg. The neurologic examination is normal.

➤ **Most likely diagnosis:** Lumbar prolapsed nucleus pulposus.

➤ **Best diagnostic step:** Magnetic resonance imaging (MRI) or myelography.

ANALYSIS

Objectives

1. Know the differential diagnosis for lower back pain.
2. Know the typical clinical presentation of lumbar prolapsed nucleus pulposus.
3. Understand that MRI and myelography are the imaging tests that confirm the diagnosis.

Considerations

This 55-year-old man complains of lower back pain with radiation to the right leg. The pain is worse when walking and during straight leg raising. This is typical of herniated lumbar pulposus related to compression of the intervertebral disk causing impingement of the nerve root, typically at the L4-5 level. There is usually paresthesia or radiation of the pain in the leg, usually posterior and/or lateral. MRI is a very accurate test for evaluating the spinal cord and nerve roots.

APPROACH TO Lower Back Pain

DEFINITIONS

MECHANICAL BACKACHE: Usually chronic and may result in a long-term debilitating illness without any definite or demonstrable cause. Back sprains are usually associated with minor trauma producing ligamentous or muscular injury.

ENTRAPMENT NEUROPATHIES: Involve compression of a nerve, such as that produced in sciatica, when a prolapsed intervertebral disk applies pressure to an adjacent nerve in the lumbosacral plexus.

CAUDA EQUINA SYNDROME: Compression of the sacral nerve bundle, which forms the end of the spinal cord, with symptoms of bladder or bowel dysfunction and/or pain or weakness in the legs. This disorder should be diagnosed at an early stage to avoid permanent injury.

CLINICAL APPROACH

Because lower back pain is so common, it is of fundamental importance to differentiate significant from insignificant pain and thus to prevent the onset of chronicity. Spinal pain can be local or referred or can occur along the distribution of nerves. Osteoarthritis and rheumatoid arthritis are associated with conditions such as spinal stenosis, spondylolisthesis, or ankylosing spondylitis that may cause chronic back pain.

Herniation of the nucleus pulposus, the softer inner part of an intervertebral disk, through the outer tough annulus fibrosus causes **compression of adjacent nerves** emanating from the spinal canal. On occasion, fragmentation of the disk may occur without protrusion of the nucleus pulposus; the annulus itself then protrudes. This condition may cause severe pain, weakness, and sensory loss. The problem may also be caused by the protrusion of osteophytes, bony spurs that occur in osteoarthrosis of the spine. Ultimately, **spinal stenosis** may develop.

With disk prolapse, the severity of symptoms may vary from mild, localized back pain to **urgent cauda equina compression resulting in the loss of motor and sensory function. The L4-5 and L5-S1 intervertebral disks are the most commonly involved; thus, pain down the posterior or lateral leg is characteristic (sciatica).** Back pain frequently radiates into the buttock, posterior thigh, or calf. Coughing, sneezing, or straining tends to increase the pain. Other exacerbating factors are bending, sitting, and getting in and out of a vehicle, whereas **lying flat characteristically relieves pain.** Caudal equina compression may affect **bladder and bowel function,** and spinal stenosis may produce pain that radiates down both legs.

The paravertebral muscles are often in spasm, and there is loss of the normal lumbar lordosis. Straight leg raising is limited on the side of the lesion, and dorsiflexion of the foot at the limit of straight leg raising often exacerbates the discomfort. There may be tenderness to palpation of the central back or buttock. Sensory loss and muscular weakness may be present along the appropriate dermatomes; ankle or knee reflexes may be absent. The differential diagnosis includes fracture; joint subluxation; tumors of the bone, joint, or meninges; abscess; arachnoiditis; ankylosing spondylitis; rheumatoid arthritis; aortic occlusion; and peripheral neuropathies. MRI may demonstrate the disk protrusion, and plain radiographs of the lumbosacral spine may show narrowing of the intervertebral space, but these modalities cannot establish a definitive diagnosis.

Bed rest, the application of either heated pads or ice packs, administration of nonsteroidal anti-inflammatory drugs and muscle relaxants, and/or physical therapy represent the first line of conservative management. A back brace or corset may help the patient through the early stages of mobilization. **The indications for surgical decompression are the development of an acute disabling neurologic deficit (bladder dysfunction) or intractable severe pain. A large multicenter randomized (SPORT) trial failed to show superior efficacy of surgery versus conservative therapy, with a large fraction of patients in both intervention groups improving over the 2-year–study period.**

After the site of the disk prolapse is precisely identified, surgery involves laminectomy and removal of the protruding disk. The overlying stretched nerve may show erythema and narrowing, and great care must be exercised in removing the offending protruding disk from underneath this nerve. If several disk spaces are involved, posterior spinal fusion in addition to removal of the disks may be indicated. This form of surgery has been performed with increasing frequency in recent years, using a minimally invasive approach with short incisions, meticulous and specific removal of the disk, and early mobilization. The results of surgery are excellent. Techniques under review are dissolution of the disk by the injection of chemicals, and sometimes steroid injections in the region of the disk may be helpful in the short term.

Comprehension Questions

52.1 A 54-year-old man has lower back pain of 3 weeks duration which has not diminished with rest. He is diagnosed with a "herniated disk." Which of the following describes the most common location of herniated disks in the lumbar spine region?

A. L1-2
B. L2-3
C. L3-4
D. L4-5

52.2 A 47-year-old woman complains of lower back pain with radiation to the right leg, and she is treated with ibuprofen and bed rest. Over the next 3 weeks, the patient's pain worsens, and she complains of difficulty with voiding and bowel movements. Which of the following is the most likely diagnosis?

A. Spinal stenosis
B. Lumbar neoplasm
C. Cauda equina syndrome
D. Tuberculosis of the spine (Pott disease)

52.3 A 56-year-old mailman is diagnosed with probable lumbar prolapsed nucleus pulposus. Which of the following is most consistent with his diagnosis?

A. Pain in the lower back radiating down the anterior thigh
B. Decreased patellar deep tendon reflex
C. Pain worsened with Valsalva
D. Decreased sensation in the medial thigh and weakness of the adductor muscles of the lower leg

ANSWERS

52.1 **D.** Herniated nucleus pulposus commonly impinges on the nerve roots in the lower lumbar or upper sacral region. Typically the symptoms will improve with bedrest. The L4-5 interspace is most commonly affected.

52.2 **C.** The bowel and bladder complaints are typical of cauda equina syndrome. Cauda equina involvement is usually a surgical emergency since permanent nerve damage can ensue without prompt correction.

52.3 **C.** Pain of lumbar disk disease is worse with Valsalva, straight leg raising, and the sitting position. The pain typically radiates from the back to the posterior or lateral leg, and not typically the anterior leg.

Clinical Pearls

- The most common locations of herniated lumbar disk disease are at the L4-5 and L5-S1 levels.
- Bowel and bladder complaints with lower back pain are suggestive of cauda equina syndrome, which must be diagnosed early to avoid permanent damage.
- The initial treatment for herniated lumbar pulposus is bed rest and the administration of nonsteroidal anti-inflammatory agents.

REFERENCES

Patterson JT, Hanbali F, Franklin RL, Nauta HJW. Neurosurgery. In: Townsend CM, Beauchamp RD, Evers BM, et al, eds. *Sabiston Textbook of Surgery*. 18th ed. Philadelphia, PA: Saunders Elsevier; 2008:2090-2130.

Smith ML, Grady S. Neurosurgery. In: Brunicardi FC, Andersen DK, Billiar TR, et al, eds. *Schwartz's Principles of Surgery*. 8th ed. New York, NY: McGraw-Hill; 2005:1609-1651.

Weinstein JN, Tosteson TD, Lorie JD, et al. Surgical versus nonoperative treatment for lumbar disk herniation. The Spine Patient Outcomes Research Trial (SPORT): a randomized trial. JAMA. 2006;296:2441-50.

Case 53

A 1-month-old girl is evaluated for persistent jaundice. The infant was born at 39 weeks' gestation to a healthy 28-year-old woman with no family history of medical problems. The delivery was cesarean after premature rupture of membranes with a birth weight of 3200 g and Apgar scores of 9 and 9 at 1 and at 5 minutes. She had passage of meconium on the first day of life, and she was mildly jaundiced at the time of discharge from the hospital on day 2 of life. During the past several days, the patient has been having acholic stools and darkly stained urine. On examination, she is deeply jaundiced; the cardiopulmonary examination is unremarkable. The liver is palpable and firm. No other abdominal masses are identified. The laboratory evaluations reveal a normal CBC, total bilirubin and direct bilirubin levels of 28 mg/dL and 24 mg/dL, and serum levels of AST/ALT and alkaline phosphatase of 300/250 U/L and 950 IU/L, respectively.

- What are the differential diagnoses?
- What is your next step(s)?
- Should this be urgently evaluated or electively and definitively diagnosed?

ANSWERS TO CASE 53:
Neonatal Jaundice (Persistent)

- **Differential diagnoses:** Neonatal hepatitis; toxoplasmosis, other agents, rubella, cytomegalovirus, herpes simplex (TORCH) infections; metabolic diseases (α 1-antitrypsin deficiency, cystic fibrosis, and others); biliary atresia; and choledochal cyst.
- **Next steps:** After the initial laboratory studies are performed, the evaluation should simultaneously include TORCH/metabolic studies (as listed in Table 53–1), abdominal ultrasound, and hepatoiminodiacetic acid (HIDA) scan (^{99m}Tc-labeled iminodiacetic acid).
- **Timing:** Hyperbilirubinemia in the neonate that persists beyond 2 weeks of age is rarely physiologic, particularly when it is predominantly conjugated bilirubin. Because surgical correction of biliary atresia is optimally performed before 8 weeks of age (12 weeks maximum), urgent evaluation and potentially preoperative preparation is warranted over 5 to 6 days.

ANALYSIS

Considerations

Jaundice is a common finding during the neonatal period, where it is observed in 60% of term infants and 80% of preterm infants. Newborn jaundice occurs most commonly as the result of "physiologic jaundice," which develops primarily from the combined effects of high circulating levels of hemoglobin and immature mechanism for bilirubin conjugation in newborns. When it occurs, physiologic jaundice is usually evident by day 2 to 3 and resolves by day 5 to 7 of life. By definition, jaundice that persists beyond 2 weeks is considered pathologic, and the mechanisms responsible for pathologic jaundice include biliary obstruction, increased hemoglobin load, and liver dysfunction.

This patient history is fairly typical of those referred for surgical consultation in the evaluation of neonatal jaundice. Usually, the infant has no specific symptoms. Physical findings include acholic stools and, occasionally, a palpable, firm liver. The timing and pattern of jaundice onset can give some clues as to the diagnosis (eg, hemolytic diseases often present early and are more progressive/severe). The degree of conjugated hyperbilirubinemia offers a key distinguishing direction as to how to approach the workup. Table 53–1 lists the causes of neonatal hyperbilirubinemia and some of their distinguishing characteristics. Metabolic and infectious causes should be investigated. A prompt evaluation includes an abdominal ultrasound, HIDA scan, and percutaneous liver biopsy. If the imaging studies do not rule out biliary atresia, then operative exploration with intraoperative cholangiogram is indicated.

Table 53–1 CLINICAL MANAGEMENT OF PERSISTENT JAUNDICE IN CHILDREN

DISEASE	CLINICAL FINDINGS	STUDIES	TREATMENT
UNCONJUGATED HYPERBILIRUBINEMIA			
Hemolytic diseases	Early, severe jaundice	Coombs positive	Phototherapy; exchange transfusion
Metabolic diseases	Disease specific	Disease specific	Disease specific
Physiologic jaundice	Nonspecific	Fractionated bilirubin	Phototherapy
CONJUGATED HYPERBILIRUBINEMIA			
Biliary atresia	Nonspecific	US; HIDA; liver biopsy; IOC	Portoenterostomy
Choledochal cyst	Abdominal mass Rarely, cholangitis	US; HIDA	Cyst excision and hepaticojejunostomy
Biliary hypoplasia (Alagille syndrome)	Cardiovascular, spinal, eye abnormalities and jaundice common	US; HIDA; liver biopsy; IOC; investigate other organ systems	Choleretics
Total parenteral nutrition	Short bowel syndrome (anatomic or functional)	US; HIDA/liver biopsy of diagnosis in question	Enteral feeding
Inspissated bile syndrome	Hemolytic diseases or cystic fibrosis	US	IOC may be diagnostic and therapeutic
Sepsis/infection	Clinically ill	TOCH screen, blood culture	Supportive/specific to disease

Abbreviations: US, ultrasound; IOC, intraoperative cholangiogram; HIDA, hepatoiminodiacetic acid; TORCH, toxoplasmosis, other agents, rubella, cytomegalovirus, herpes simplex.

Surgical reconstruction for biliary atresia is a Kasai portoenterostomy and a hepaticojejunostomy for choledochal cyst.

Objectives

1. Be familiar with the differential diagnosis for neonatal jaundice.
2. Be familiar with the diagnostic approach and initial supportive management of patients with neonatal jaundice.
3. Be familiar with the treatment for biliary atresia and choledochal cyst.

APPROACH TO Neonatal Obstructive Jaundice

DEFINITIONS

CHOLEDOCHAL CYST: Congenital anatomic malformation of a bile duct, including cystic dilatation of the extrahepatic bile duct or the large intrahepatic bile duct.

BILIARY ATRESIA: Congenital or developed stricture or absence of the major bile ducts that drain bile from the liver.

CLINICAL APPROACH

The precise etiology of biliary atresia is unknown. Various theories include viral infections and autoimmune processes. Histologically, the biliary tracts contain inflammatory cells surrounding obliterated ductules. The liver shows signs of cholestasis and, in later stages, fibrosis. Grossly, the most common finding is fibrosis of the entire extrahepatic biliary tree, followed by proximal duct fibrosis with distal duct patency.

Similar to biliary atresia, **the exact etiology of choledochal cysts is unknown.** A widely held theory is that the common bile duct and pancreatic duct share a common channel leading to retrograde reflux of pancreatic juice into the choledochus with subsequent cystic dilation. There are 5 types of choledochal cysts, but the fusiform, or type I, comprises 90% of all lesions.

Preoperative Management and Surgical Treatment of Biliary Atresia and Choledochal Cysts

Prior to surgical intervention, these patients must be evaluated for coagulation abnormalities, anemia, and hypoproteinemia. Correction of coagulopathy usually requires both vitamin K and fresh-frozen plasma. Anemia may be of moderate severity requiring the availability of cross-matched blood. Parents should be made aware of the prognosis of biliary atresia preoperatively. Conversely, the surgical management of choledochal cyst carries an excellent prognosis.

Surgical Treatment

The surgical management of biliary atresia consists of operative exploration of the porta hepatis with intraoperative cholangiogram. If dye does not enter the duodenum, then the limited right upper quadrant incision is extended and the extrahepatic biliary tree is dissected up to the level of the portal plate. The portal plate is transected flush with but not into the liver. This exposes the biliary ductules that drain bile. A Roux-en-Y limb of jejunum is attached to the porta in a retrocolic manner. Jejunal valves, stomas, and other approaches were used previously, but these have fallen out of favor because of complexity and lack of improved outcomes with the more complex procedures. Similarly, choledochal cysts are excised, but instead of fashioning the limb of jejunum to the porta, it is attached to the bifurcating hepatic ducts at their confluence.

Complications

The **three main complications of the surgical management of biliary atresia** are **cholangitis, cessation of bile flow, and portal hypertension. Cholangitis is the most frequent complication** occurring **after portoenterostomy** and is manifest by **fever, leukocytosis, and elevations in the bilirubin. Treatment** includes intravenous **antibiotics** against gram-negative organisms and **steroids.** Cessation of bile flow can be related to progression of the disease, cholangitis, or Roux-limb obstruction (rare). Treatment is based on steroids and other choleretic agents. Portal hypertension is a late complication of portoenterostomy, and it occurs even in those that are successful in terms of bile flow. The complications of variceal bleeding can usually be managed, and the symptoms may progress when cirrhosis worsens.

Outcome

Biliary atresia—before the introduction of the **Kasai procedure,** the survival rates were less than 5% at 12 months. With hepatoenterostomy 30% to 50% of patients have good long-term results. Ultimately, **only 20% of patients undergoing portoenterostomy survive into adulthood without liver transplantation.** Factors that affect early bile flow after operation are age, immediate bile flow (technically sound operation), and degree of parenchymal disease at diagnosis. The presence and size of ductules in the hilum are of controversial prognostic significance. Choledochal cyst—the prognosis for patients undergoing excision of choledochal cyst and Roux-en-Y hepaticojejunostomy is excellent.

Comprehension Questions

53.1 A 2-year-old male child is noted by his pediatrician to have progressive jaundice. There is a suspicion of biliary atresia. Which of the following imaging studies is most definitive in its ability to diagnose biliary atresia?

A. Abdominal ultrasound
B. HIDA scan
C. Intraoperative cholangiogram
D. Magnetic resonance cholangiopancreatography

53.2 A 140-day-old infant with a mixed hyperbilirubinemia undergoes a percutaneous liver biopsy, HIDA scan, and abdominal sonography that are consistent with biliary atresia. Metabolic and infectious evaluations are negative. Which of the following is the best management for this patient?

A. Kasai procedure (portoenterostomy)
B. Listing for liver transplantation
C. Open liver biopsy and cholangiogram
D. Tube cholecystostomy

53.3 An 18-month-old infant who underwent a successful Kasai procedure as an infant returns with fever, leukocytosis, and a new hyperbilirubinemia. Which of the following is the best initial management?

A. Revision of portoenterostomy
B. Corticosteroids and antibiotics
C. Corticosteroids alone
D. Antibiotics alone

ANSWERS

53.1 **C.** Although abdominal ultrasound and HIDA scan are used as suggestive evidence of biliary atresia, they do not definitively rule it in or out. For example, approximately 10% to 15% of biliary atresia cases have visible, normally distended gallbladders. It is not uncommon for patients with biliary hypoplasia (Alagille syndrome) to have no excretion of tracer into the duodenum on HIDA scan. The only definitive way to diagnose biliary atresia is by operative exploration and intraoperative cholangiogram. Magnetic resonance cholangiopancreatography is not routinely used to evaluate the neonatal biliary tract.

53.2 **B.** After 120 days of life, portoenterostomy is rarely indicated. Although there have been occasional successful procedures, these are the overwhelming exception. A cholangiogram and liver biopsy may be useful, but they will not alter the therapy—meaning that a finding of biliary atresia would not prompt a portoenterostomy. Therefore, a standard approach to these infants is referral for liver transplantation after 120 days of life.

53.3 **B.** The child described has a classic clinical presentation of post-Kasai cholangitis. This is a frequent complication of portoenterostomy. Revision of the portoenterostomy is rarely indicated. Occasionally this is done for the functioning Kasai that acutely fails—usually in the immediate postoperative period. The findings of fever, leukocytosis, and rising bilirubin suggest cholangitis. Standard management includes supportive measures, blood cultures, antibiotics against gram-negative organisms, and steroids (function as choleretic and anti-inflammatory).

Clinical Pearls

- Jaundice in the neonate beyond 2 weeks of age is rarely physiologic, especially when involving mainly conjugated bilirubin.
- The most common complication after portoenterostomy is cholangitis.
- Neonates with biliary atresia or choledochal cysts should be assessed for coagulopathy prior to surgery.

REFERENCES

Hackam DJ, Newman K, Ford HR. Pediatric surgery. In: Brunicardi FC, Andersen DK, Billiar TR, et al, eds. *Schwartz's Principles of Surgery*. 8th ed. New York, NY: McGraw-Hill; 2005:1471-1517.

Warner BW. Pediatric surgery. In: Townsend CM Jr, Beauchamp RD, Evers BM, eds. *Sabiston Textbook of Surgery*. 18th ed. Philadelphia, PA: Saunders Elsevier; 2008:2047-2089.

Case 54

A 54-year-old man presents for evaluation of pain and difficulty with swallowing, and weight loss. The patient states that over the past 4 to 5 weeks, he has noticed a decrease in the ability to tolerate solid foods; he has been having pain and discomfort with swallowing, along with a sensation of "the food being stuck in his chest." Because of these symptoms, he has switched over to a liquid diet essentially consisting of soups, juices, and tea that he has tolerated reasonably well. During this period of time the patient has noticed a 20 lb (9.1 kg) weight loss. His past medical history is significant for hypertension, and his medications include metoprolol and proton-pump inhibitor (over the counter). The patient appears thin with significant temporal wasting. His vital signs are normal, there is no evidence of adenopathy, and the remainder of the physical examination is unremarkable. His white blood cell count is normal, hemoglobin is 12 g/dL, and hematocrit is 40%. His serum electrolytes, liver enzymes, and glucose are within normal limits.

- What is the most likely mechanism causing this process?
- What is the most appropriate next diagnostic step?
- What are the risk factors associated with this process?

ANSWERS TO CASE 54: Esophageal Carcinoma

Summary: A previously healthy 54-year-old man presents with dysphagia and weight loss.

- **Most likely mechanism:** Mechanical obstruction from a neoplastic process.
- **Most appropriate next step in diagnosis:** Esophagoscopy with biopsy.
- **Risk factors associated with this process:** Known risk factors associated with squamous cell carcinoma of the esophagus include caustic burns, alcohol consumption, tobacco smoking, and nitrite- and nitrate-containing food. Gastroesophageal reflux disease (GERD) is a known risk factor associated with gastroesophageal junction (GEJ) adenocarcinoma (odds ratio of 7.7), and other suspected risk factors are western diet and acid suppression medications.

ANALYSIS

Objectives

1. Learn the approach to local and systemic staging of esophageal and proximal stomach carcinoma.
2. Learn to apply staging information and clinical assessment to help determine the optimal treatment course for patients with esophageal carcinoma.

Considerations

This patient describes dysphagia to solid foods that has developed over a fairly short time period (several weeks). The timing of symptom progression along with a history of self-medicating with PPI suggests that he may have had a history of GERD and has now developed adenocarcinoma of the distal esophagus. If the patient were to describe a more protracted course (months to years) of dysphagia, the differential diagnoses would also include benign strictures, congenital malformations, and achalasia; however, given the fairly rapid onset and progression of symptoms, a neoplastic process is the most likely cause.

The most important initial evaluation is to determine the nature and location of the blockage, and this can be best accomplished by esophagogastroduodenoscopy (EGD) and tissue biopsy. If the biopsy should demonstrate the presence of esophageal cancer, the next step would be tumor staging, which includes the assessment of local disease with endoscopic ultrasound and evaluation for possible metastatic disease with computed tomography (CT) of the chest and abdomen. In some institutions, positron emission tomography (PET) CT scan has replaced standard CT as the staging modality of choice. It is important to bear in mind that carcinoma of the esophagus and proximal stomach may produce very similar clinical pictures but would require different treatment approaches; therefore, EGD, endoscopic ultrasound, and CTs are extremely important to help pinpoint the tumor location. Precise localization of the tumor is essential not only for the surgical planning but also may influence the selection of palliation for patients who are not candidates for surgery.

Early on during the evaluation process, it is important to assess and optimize the patient's nutritional status. Initial nutritional assessment involves the quantification of weight loss and measurement of serum albumin level. For this individual, who is still tolerating liquids, it would be possible to initiate nutritional supplementation with high-protein, high-calorie liquid supplements to help replenish his losses and meet his ongoing metabolic needs. If this patient is unable to tolerate adequate oral intake, it may be necessary to initiate enteral nutritional support, which can be accomplished with the placement of a feeding access distal to the obstructive process. Since there is no contraindication to enteral nutrition, total parenteral nutrition (TPN) is not indicated.

APPROACH TO Esophageal And Proximal Gastric Cancers

DEFINITIONS

ENDOSCOPIC ULTRASONOGRAPHY (EUS): EUS is currently the most accurate imaging modality for identifying the depth of tumor invasion (T stage) and for identifying regional nodal disease (N stage). In patients in whom lymphadenopathy is visualized, EUS-directed fine needle aspiration of the nodes can help confirm regional nodal metastasis. EUS results can be highly operator dependent.

SIEWERT CLASSIFICATION OF GE JUNCTION ADENOCARCINOMAS (TYPE I-III): Type **I** tumors are located more than 1-cm above the GE junction (surgical treatment would generally consist of esophagectomy); Type **II** tumors are located within 1 cm proximal and 2 cm distal to the GE junction (surgical treatment would consist of esophagectomy with partial resection of the proximal stomach); Type **III** tumors are located more than 2 cm distal to the GE junction (surgical treatment would consist of total gastrectomy).

TRANSTHORACIC ESOPHAGECTOMY (TTE): This resection is traditionally done through an incision in the abdomen (or laparoscopic approach) and a separate incision through the right chest. The proximal esophagus is divided at approximately the level of the azygos vein and distal transection is usually at the level of the proximal stomach. The stomach is then brought into the mediastinum and anastomosed to the proximal esophagus. TTE has the disadvantages of having an anastomosis in the mediastinum and is associated with a high rate of pulmonary complications due to pain from incisions in both the chest and upper abdomen.

TRANSHIATAL ESOPHAGECTOMY: This resection is done through an abdominal incision (or by laparoscopic approach) and a cervical incision. Through the abdominal approach, the stomach is mobilized and the distal esophagus is dissected after enlargement of the hiatal opening. Through the cervical incision, the cervical esophagus is mobilized and the proximal thoracic esophagus is dissected, and the entire thoracic esophagus and the proximal stomach are resected, and the gastric conduit is brought up through the posterior mediastinum and anastomosed to the cervical esophagus in the neck. The major advantages of this approach are reduction in pulmonary complications compared to TTE and reduced mortality and morbidity-associated cervical anastomotic leaks.

CLINICAL APPROACH

The incidence of esophageal cancer has increased sixfold over the past 25 years, where this tumor is the sixth most common malignancy encountered in the United States. Although squamous cell carcinoma continues to account for the majority of esophageal cancers encountered in developing countries, adenocarcinoma is the predominant tumor encountered in North America (~70%).

Curative Therapy

Overall, cancers of the esophagus and GE junction carry a poor prognosis with a 5-year survival of less than 20% for all affected patients, and cancer stage has been established as one of the best determinants of survival (Table 54–1). Because early stage cancers are curable, it is important to identify the disease in the treatable stages, such as by identifying Barrett changes in patients with reflux and the identification of dysplasia or cancerous changes through surveillance. Unfortunately, due to tumor local extension, the presence of metastatic disease, and poor host conditions, fewer than 50% of patients presenting with esophageal cancers are eligible for surgical resection. In the past, palliative resections had been routinely performed for the relief of dysphagia; however, with recent advances in palliative therapy, the majority of surgical resections are now performed with curative intentions. While patients with stage I (T1N0) cancers may require surgical resection only, surgery + chemotherapy ± radiation therapy are the multimodality treatment approaches currently recommended for the majority of patients with potentially curable cancers.

Table 54–1 AMERICAN JOINT COMMITTEE ON CANCER (AJCC) ESOPHAGEAL CARCINOMA STAGING AND SURVIVAL BASED ON STAGING

Primary Tumor (T)	**Tx:** Tumor cannot be assessed **T0:** No evidence of tumor **Tis:** High-grade dysplasia **T1:** Tumor invades lamina propria, muscularis mucosa, submucosa, but does not penetrate through the submucosa **T2:** Tumor invades into but not beyond the muscularis propria **T3:** Tumor invades periesophageal tissue but not adjacent structures **T4:** Tumor invasion of adjacent structures	**5-yr Survival**
Regional Lymph Nodes (N)	**Nx:** Regional lymph nodes cannot be assessed **N0:** No regional lymph node metastases **N1:** Regional lymph node metastases	
Distant Metastases (M)	**Mx:** Distant metastases cannot be assessed **M0:** No distant metastases **M1a:** Upper esophageal tumor with metastases to cervical lymph nodes Midthoracic lesion with metastases to mediastinal lymph nodes Lower thoracic esophageal lesion with metastases to celiac nodes **M1b:** Upper esophageal lesion with metastases to mediastinum or celiac lymph nodes Midthoracic esophageal lesion with metastases to cervical or celiac lymph nodes Lower thoracic esophageal lesion with metastases to cervical or mediastinal lymph nodes	
Stage Groupings	**T N M**	**5-yr Survival**
Stage 0	Tis N0 M0	**100%**
Stage 1	T1 N0 M0	**75-80%**
Stage IIA	T2 or T3 N0 M0	**35-40%**
Stage IIB	T1 or T2 N1 M0	**25-30%**
Stage III	T3 N1 M0 T4 N0 or N1 M0	**10-15%**
Stage IVA	Any T Any N M1a	**0%**
Stage IVB	Any T Any N M1b	**0%**

There have been a number of clinical trials evaluating preoperative chemoradiation therapy + surgery versus surgery alone in patients with stage I and II squamous cell carcinoma, and despite prolongation in survival with preoperative chemoradiation, no long-term survival advantages have been demonstrated. In contrast to the marginal survival difference reported for patients with esophageal squamous cell carcinoma, there is good evidence supporting the use of pre- and postoperative chemotherapy in the treatment of patients with adenocarcinoma of the esophagus and stomach. In a trial reported by Cunningham et al in the *New England Journal of Medicine* in 2006, patients with esophageal (14%), GE junction (12%), and gastric adenocarcinoma (74%) were randomized to pre- and postoperative chemotherapy (epirubicin, cisplatin, 5-FU) versus surgery alone, where the combined therapy patients benefited with higher rate of curative resections and improved survival. It is important to bear in mind that during this trial, the majority of the patients had gastric adenocarcinoma (74%) and esophageal carcinoma and GE junction carcinoma patients made up only 26% of the entire study population; therefore, one must remain cautiously optimistic when extrapolating these study findings to patients with esophagus and GE junction adenocarcinoma.

Palliative Therapy

Palliation for patients with esophageal carcinoma are directed at preserving the quality of life for patients in whom cure would not be possible. Since the most common complaint that affects patients' quality of life is dysphagia, the primary goal of palliative care is rapid relief of dysphagia with minimal hospitalization and with the preservation of swallowing function. Secondarily, palliative care may be directed at the prevention of bleeding, perforation, and tracheoesophageal fistula formation.

In general, palliative modalities include endoscopic therapy (stent placement, laser, and photocoagulation), radiation therapy (external beam or intraluminal), chemotherapy, and feeding tube placement. Factors that determine the selection of palliative therapy for any given patient include the availability of technology, local expertise, patient conditions, tumor location and characteristics, and the expected length of survival. Table 54–2 contains the pros and cons of the available palliative modalities.

Table 54–2 PALLIATIVE MODALITIES FOR ESOPHAGEAL CARCINOMA

PALLIATIVE MODALITY	EFFECTIVENESS, ADVANTAGES, AND DISADVANTAGES
Endoscopic Stent placement	**Advantages:** rapid relief of dysphagia; treatment of choice for tracheoesophageal fistula; short procedural time; outpatient procedure **Disadvantages:** recurrence due to stent migration, tumor overgrowth, food impaction; transient pain following placement; gastroesophageal reflux; and increased risk of late hemorrhage
Photodynamic therapy and Nd:YAG laser	Endoluminal destruction of obstructing lesions **Advantages:** works well with exophytic lesions; generally low complication rates **Disadvantages:** Often available only in specialized centers; special expertise required; repeat treatment every 4-8 weeks is needed
Single-dose Brachytherapy	Intraluminal radiotherapy **Advantages:** Long-term dysphagia improvement is better than stent placement; long term quality of life score was better when compared with stent placement; lower rate of hemorrhage than stent placement **Disadvantage:** dysphagia relief is delayed in comparison to stent placement
Palliative Chemotherapy Epirubicin, cisplatin, and 5-FU (ECF) is the chemotherapy combination that has been established as the optimal palliative chemotherapy regimen at this time	**Advantages:** Treatment improves median survival; responders may have improved quality of life due to relief of obstruction. **Disadvantage:** Response to obstruction is variable; therefore, additional treatment for obstruction may be needed; relief from obstruction may be delayed

Comprehension Questions

54.1 Which of the following is the most appropriate treatment for a 45-year-old man with an exophytic adenocarcinoma of the distal esophagus that penetrates to but does not penetrate through the muscularis propria, providing that the CT scan does not demonstrate evidence of distant metastases?

A. Placement of endoscopic stent to relieve obstruction and initiate chemotherapy
B. Initiate chemotherapy followed by endoscopic resection of the tumor, if tumor shrinkage is achieved
C. Initiate chemotherapy followed by esophagectomy and additional postoperative chemotherapy
D. Nutritional therapy followed by esophagectomy

54.2 Which of the following is a major limitation to endoscopic stent placement for the palliation of esophageal carcinoma?

A. Recurrent esophageal obstruction.
B. Patients often have a several week delay before symptom improvement occurs after the therapy.
C. Endoscopic stent placement eliminates the possibility of later surgery.
D. The presence of tracheoesophageal fistula is a contraindication.

ANSWERS

54.1 **C.** The patient described here most likely has a T2N0M0 (Stage IIA) adenocarcinoma of the esophagus. Given the clinical and radiographic staging information, the patient's tumor is potentially curable, and the recent randomized prospective trial data (Cunningham, *NEJM* 2006) suggest that survival may be improved over surgery alone if this patient is treated with initial induction chemotherapy followed by esophagectomy and postoperative chemotherapy. Stent placement and chemotherapy would be appropriate, if the patient has metastatic disease or if his overall condition precludes operative treatment. Endoscopic ablation or resection as definitive therapy is appropriate only for selective patients with intramucosal lesions.

54.2 **A.** Recurrent obstruction may develop due to tumor progression and stent migration following stent placement. Esophageal obstruction is often immediately improved following endoscopic stenting. Esophagectomy following stent placement is generally not a problem. Tracheoesophageal fistula (TEF) is not a contraindication to stent placement; in fact, TEF is preferentially treated with the placement of endoscopic covered stents.

Clinical Pearls

- The incidence of adenocarcinoma of the esophagus and GE junction is rapidly growing in westernized, developed countries.
- Treatment outcome of esophageal carcinoma is improved with multi-modality treatment.
- Esophagectomy is primarily performed in patients with potentially curable esophageal cancers.

REFERENCES

Cunningham D, Allum WH, Stenning SP, et al. Perioperative chemotherapy versus surgery alone for resectable gastroesophageal cancer. *N Eng J Med*. 2006;355:11-20.

Homs MYV, Kuipers EJ, Siersema PD. Palliative therapy. *J Surg Oncol*. 2005;92:246-256.

Maisch M. Esophagus. In: Townsend CM, Beauchamp RD, Evers BM, Mattox KL, eds. *Sabiston Textbook of Surgery*. 18th ed. Philadelphia, PA: Saunders Elsevier; 2008:1049-1107.

Marsman WA, Tytgat GNJ, Ten Kate FJW, Van Lanschot JJB. Differences and similarities of adenocarcinomas of the esophagus and esophagogastric junction. *J Surg Oncol*. 2005;92:160-168.

Case 55

A 38-year-old man presents to an outpatient clinic with several nonspecific complaints. The patient relates that for the past 3 to 4 months, he has become easily fatigued, unable to concentrate at work, and has developed poor appetite and pain in his thighs, knees, and legs. He has been generally healthy in the past but has not seen a physician in 6 years. Eight years ago, he was informed that his blood pressure was elevated when he visited an emergency center for the treatment of a laceration on his arm. The patient is currently afebrile; his blood pressure is 160/94 mm Hg; pulse is 84 beats/min and regular. He has several areas of skin ecchymosis over his knees and thighs. His white blood cell (WBC) count is 6500, hemoglobin is 9 g/dL, hematocrit is 35%, blood urea nitrogen is 80, his serum creatinine is 8.5, and his serum potassium is 5.0 mEq/L.

- What is the most likely diagnosis?
- How will you assess the severity and stage of his disease?
- What are the treatment options for this patient?

ANSWERS TO THE CASE 55: Renal Failure/Renal Transplantation

Summary: A 38-year-old man presents with new onset renal failure and uremia. The cause of the renal failure is unknown but is suspected to be contributed by poor control of hypertension.

- **Diagnosis:** Probable chronic renal failure (CRF) with uremia.
- **Severity and stage of disease:** The severity and stage of CRF can be estimated based on urinary creatinine clearance.
- **Treatment:** Dialysis and renal transplantation are treatment options in the patient with end-stage disease.

ANALYSIS

Objectives

1. Be able to describe and recognize the stages of chronic renal failure and complications associated with this condition.
2. Learn the principles of hemodialysis and options for dialysis access.
3. Learn the outcome and management principles for patients undergoing renal transplantation.

Considerations

The initial evaluation and management in this patient consists of determining the cause of his renal failure and identifying potentially treatable causes. Because the patient has described symptoms for the past 3 to 4 months and has no recent physiologic insults or medication usage that would predispose him to acute renal insults, this process most likely represents CRF. Renal ultrasonography is useful to assess renal size and number, identify urinary obstruction, renal vascular obstruction, and tumor infiltration. The assessment of creatinine clearance allows for estimation of glomerular filtration rate (GFR), which would help to stage his renal disease. Evaluation and treatment of complications associated with CRF are important, including dietary changes and pharmacological therapy to address metabolic complications such as hyperkalemia and hyperphosphatemia. Cardiovascular complications are common in this population and account for approximately 50% of the annual mortality in CRF patients. Echocardiography is helpful to assess for left ventricular hypertrophy (LVH), which is a strong predictor for future adverse cardiac events. In addition, echocardiography may help identify uremic pericarditis and pericardial effusion. If the evaluations verify (end-stage disease) GFR of less than 15 mL/min/1.73 m^2, hemodialysis should be initiated to improve the patient's quality of life and minimize acute metabolic complications. Ultimately, for a patient with irreversible renal failure, chronic dialysis and renal transplantation are the two long-term options.

APPROACH TO Chronic Renal Failure

DEFINITIONS

CHRONIC RENAL FAILURE (CRF): Classified by the National Kidney Foundation Clinical Practice Guidelines as kidney damage of greater than 3 months duration and/or GRF less than 60 mL/min per 1.73 m^2.

CHRONIC RENAL DISEASE STAGES:

Stage 1: kidney damage with normal or increased GFR (GFR > 90)
Stage 2: kidney damage with mild decrease in GFR (GFR 60-89)
Stage 3: moderate decrease in GFR (GFR 30-59)
Stage 4: severe decrease in GFR (GFR 15-29 predialysis stage)
Stage 5: kidney failure (GFR < 15, usually indication for chronic dialysis).

CLINICAL APPROACH

Management for patients with GFR greater than 15 generally consists of dietary and fluid management, pharmacologic management, and close monitoring of complications. Dietary potassium restriction is important for patients with GRF approaching 20 in avoiding hyperkalemia. The initiation of strategies to prevent secondary hyperparathyroidism are important and should include the control of hyperphosphatemia with dietary phosphate restriction, phosphate binder administration at meal time, administration of synthetic 1,25 dihydroxy vitamin D, and subtotal parathyroidectomy for patients with uncontrolled tertiary hyperparathyroidism.

Because anemia is one of the leading causes of LVH and produces significant morbidity and mortality, anemia should be managed early and relatively aggressively with the administration of recombinant human erythropoietin. Hypertension in the setting of CRF is extremely common and contributes to LVH; therefore, intense therapy using a variety of antihypertensive medications is indicated.

Uremia produces an immunodeficiency state that is not reversible with hemodialysis. The mechanisms causing immunodeficiency in these patients remain undetermined at this time; however, due to this condition, CRF patients are at increased risk of developing bacterial, viral, mycobacterial infections, and anergic states. Close monitoring for infections and aggressive treatment of infections are critical in this patient population.

There are a number of neurologic complications that occur with CRF, and these include uremic encephalopathy, uremic peripheral neuropathy that is a mixed motor and sensory distal neuropathy, and uremic autonomic neuropathy producing postural hypotension and hypotension during dialysis; some of these neurologic conditions improve with dialysis.

Hemodialysis Dialysis Access

Hemodialysis access became the standard for the treatment of renal failure in the 1960s. Essentially, the dialysis machine or dialyzer has two spaces separated by a semipermeable membrane, where blood passes through one side of the membrane and dialysate passes on the other side of the membrane. Through diffusion, excess water and solutes pass from the blood to the dialysate resulting in the elimination of the excess water and waste. Hemodialysis requires the placement of dialysis access that include specialized large bore venous catheters through which blood can be drawn off at a high rate (350-400 mL/min) through one lumen and returned through a separate lumen. Hemodialysis catheters are classified as temporary access (days) or intermediate-term access (weeks to months); intermediate-term catheters contain a cuff barrier and subcutaneous tunneled portion, which are barriers against contamination by skin flora and are associated with lower catheter-related infections and complications than the temporary dialysis catheters.

For critically ill patients, cannulation of the femoral vein for the initiation of dialysis is rapid and safe; however, femoral catheters are associated with increased infections when left in for more than a few days. For most patients, the internal jugular veins are the ideal sites for either temporary or intermediate-catheter insertion. Subclavian vein catheter placement should be avoided because of the potential for thrombosis and stenosis, which would affect venous return and compromise the success of future upper extremity arterial-venous fistulas from that side. Dialysis catheter-related bacteremia and sepsis are major causes of morbidity and mortality in this patient population. In addition, dialysis catheter malfunction are common causes of morbidity and mortality, as thrombosis, formation of fibrin sheath, and malposition can all cause inadequate blood flow for hemodialysis.

Long-term Hemodialysis Access: Arteriovenous fistulas (AVF) constructed by directly connecting native arteries to superficial extremity veins are the first choice for long-term access in all patients. Commonly constructed AVF include the radial artery to cephalic vein fistula (Brescia-Cimino fistula), brachial artery-cephalic vein fistula in the upper arm, and brachial-basilic fistula in the upper arm. The major limitations to AVF creation are inadequate size and quality of the veins. Because injuries to the vein can occur with blood draws and IV insertions, it is extremely important to preserve the upper extremity veins in any patient in whom long-term dialysis is anticipated. Most AVF require approximately 6 weeks to mature before they can be accessed for dialysis; therefore, it is common to place an intermediate-term dialysis catheter for dialysis in the interim period. For individual without adequate veins and requiring long-term hemodialysis, a variety of arterial venous grafts can be placed. Expanded polytetrafluoroethylene is the most common material employed for AV grafts. AV grafts are less desirable than AVF because of increased complications associated with this type of access, and complications associated with AV grafts include infection and pseudointimal hyperplasia on the venous end of the graft-vein connection leading to graft thrombosis.

Peritoneal Dialysis

In peritoneal dialysis (PD), the peritoneal surface and the peritoneal microvasculature are the site of exchange of fluids and solute between the patient and the dialysate. In properly selected patients, this form of dialysis allows the patients to ambulate and carry on some of the activities of daily living during dialysis. Peritoneal infections and peritoneal dialysis catheter-related complications are potential limitations associated with this process. Because the dialysis in most cases occurs at home, the ideal patients for PD need to be functional and capable of performing the dialysis process and troubleshoot when minor problems arise.

Transplantation

Renal transplantation has been demonstrated to offer CRF patients better quality of life and is projected to improve overall survival by 10 years when compared to chronic dialysis. The three most common causes of CRF treated by renal transplantation are diabetes mellitus (27%), hypertension (20%), and glomerular diseases (21%). Currently, patients on the renal transplant waitlist in the United States outnumber the number of kidneys transplanted by a ratio of approximately 4:1; consequently, the median time on the waitlist prior to receiving transplantation has been approximately 39 months. The patient who is an ideal candidate for renal transplantation is a young individual without a systemic disease process that will damage the transplanted kidney and does not have coexisting conditions that will lead to significant morbidity and mortality. In the United States, patients are considered for renal transplantation when their GFR fall below 20 mL/min. Preoperatively, all patients undergo psychiatric evaluation to identify possible conditions that would contribute to poor compliance with immunosuppressive therapy and follow-up, assessment for possible malignant conditions, and evaluation to rule out urinary obstructive process and reflux as a cause of CRF. In addition, all patients undergo evaluation for ABO and HLA typing. All candidates also are evaluated for possible infections that include HIV, hepatitis B and C, CMV, and syphilis. In patients with prior history of cancer, the individual must be at least 2 years without evidence of disease prior to being considered for transplantation. Age alone is no longer a contraindication to organ transplantation, as up to 20% of patients on the waitlist are older than 65 years.

Living Donor versus Cadaveric Transplantation

Living donor transplantation currently accounts for 40% of the kidneys transplanted in the United States. Due to overall better medical conditions of the donors and short cold ischemia time, living donor transplanted kidneys tend to have better early and late graft functions in comparison to cadaveric grafts. With the introduction of laparoscopic donor nephrectomy, the morbidity associated with kidney harvest has been further reduced. Recent reported living donor transplantation results have shown graft survival rates of 95%, 80%, and 56% at 1, 5, and 10 years, respectively.

Traditionally, cadaveric organs are retrieved from brain-dead donors between the age of 3 to 60 years and without systemic degenerative diseases such as hypertension and diabetes, and history of a stroke. However, given the current shortage of cadaveric organs and the aging recipient population, kidneys from expanded criteria donors (ECDs) are now utilized. A donor is considered an ECD if he/she is older than 60 years or between 50 and 60 years of age who died of a stroke, with history of hypertension, diabetes, or elevated serum creatinine. The 1-year and 5-year graft survival rates reported for non-ECD kidneys are 90% and 70%, respectively, and for ECD kidneys, the 1- and 5-year graft survival rates reported are 81% and 53%, respectively.

Posttransplantation Immune Suppression and Acute Graft Rejection

Immunosuppressive agents are administered to all patients following renal transplantation, except for those patients receiving organs from identical twin donors.

Corticosteroid interferes with the immune process at multiple sites and has been one of the traditional agents used in maintenance therapy and for acute rejection. Due to the significant side effects associated with steroid use and the availability of newer agents, many centers now have immune suppression protocols that include steroid withdrawal after weeks to months. **Cyclosporin** leads to the inhibition of calcineurin activity and inhibition in IL-2 production. The introduction of cyclosporine in the 1980s represented a major breakthrough in immune-suppression. Major side effects associated with cyclosporine include nephrotoxicity, gingival hyperplasia, hypertension, and hyperkalemia. **Tacrolimus** is also a calcineurin inhibitor causing inhibition in IL-2. IL-3, IL-4, gamma-interferon production. Tacrolimus is considered a significantly more potent immune suppressive agent than cyclosporinc; however, its application is associated with increased side effects that include nephrotoxicity, hypertension, hyperkalemia, hypomagnesemia, CNS symptoms (headaches, tremors, and seizures), and insulin resistance. **Sirolimus (rapamycin)** is a T-cell inhibitor that acts through a pathway that is different from the calcineurin pathway. Even though sirolimus is less nephrotoxic than cyclosporine and tacrolimus, its application is associated with thrombocytopenia, hyperlipidemia, poor wound healing. **Mycophenolate mofetil (MMF)** and **azathioprine (Imuran)** are inhibitors of B- and T-cell proliferation. MMF is often combined with cyclosporine for the prevention of rejection. Azathioprine is an older agent that is substituted for MMF when intolerance develops. Antilymphocyte antibodies such as *OKT3* (a monoclonal murine antibody against the CD3 receptor complex on T-cells) are effective as part of an induction regimen or for the treatment of steroid-resistant acute rejections. Large doses and prolonged antilymphocyte therapy can produce severe side effects including serious viral infections, thrombocytopenia, and leukopenia.

Acute graft rejection occurs in 10% to 20% of patients during the first few weeks to months after transplantation. Classically, this is manifested as fever, malaise, hypertension, oliguria, increase in serum creatinine, and tenderness and swelling over the transplanted kidney. When clinically suspected or confirmed by biopsy, patients with acute graft rejection are generally treated initially with high-dose corticosteroids, and in steroid-resistant rejection cases, antilymphocytic antibodies are often given.

Infections Following Transplantation

Thirty to sixty percent of patients develop some form of infection during the first year following transplantation, and infections during this period of time contributes to 50% of the mortality during the early post-transplant period. Bacterial infections are the most common infections during the first month following transplantation, and during the subsequent time period, opportunistic infections including CMV, *Pneumocystis carinii*, aspergillosis, toxoplasmosis, cryptococcosis, nocardiosis, and blastomycosis become more common causes of infections. Prophylactic antimicrobial therapy with trimethoprim-sulfamethoxazole for the first 6 months after transplantation has been found to be effective in reducing the risk of *P carinii* infections.

Malignancies Following Transplantation

Suppression of the immune system post-transplantation has been shown to increase the risk of malignancy by 3 to 14 times greater in comparison to the general population. The greatest risks in this population appear to be the development of viral-associated neoplasms, including squamous cell carcinoma (HPV), cervical cancer (HPV), Kaposi sarcoma (EBV), non-Hodgkin lymphoma (EBV), and hepatocellular carcinoma (hepatitis B and C). Lymphomas or post-transplant lymphoproliferative disorders are the most common post-transplant malignancies, and the occurrence is related to the intensity and duration of the anti-T-cell therapy. Fortunately, reduction in immunosuppression often may lead to the regression of post-transplant lymphoproliferative disorders.

Chronic allograft nephropathy refers to chronic fibrotic changes and accelerated loss of renal functions that occurs in the transplanted kidneys. This process generally develops years after allograft transplantation and presents as progressive increase in serum creatinine, proteinuria, and microscopic hematuria. Confirmation of this diagnosis is by biopsy. Currently, there is no effective treatment of this condition, which is the major cause of late graft failure. In general, immunosuppressive treatment is gradually tapered in these individuals to limit the nephrotoxicity associated with calcineurin inhibitors.

Comprehension Questions

55.1 Which of the following is the most likely cause of fever in a patient at 8 months following a successful cadaveric renal transplantation?

A. Methicillin-resistant *Staphylococcus* urinary tract infection
B. Cytomegalovirus infection
C. Chronic allograft nephropathy
D. Cyclosporin-associated fevers

55.2 Which of the following treatment strategies is most appropriate in a 24-year-old man who develops fever to 39°C (102.2°F), increasing serum creatinine, and tenderness over his transplanted kidney 4 weeks following cadaveric renal transplantation.

A. Initiation of broad-spectrum antibiotics directed toward urinary tract infection organisms
B. Re-exploration to treat localized infection associated with the transplanted kidney
C. Begin empiric therapy for CMV
D. Renal biopsy and pulse steroid therapy

55.3 A patient with chronic renal failure is currently underlying hemodialysis. He asks his physician about the possibility of receiving a kidney transplant. The physician informs the patient that he is not a candidate for transplantation. Which of the following is the most likely reason for unsuitability of transplant if present in this individual?

A. Age 66 years
B. Colon cancer treated 3 years ago and in remission
C. GFR of 28 mL/min
D. Urinary obstruction and reflux

ANSWERS

55.1 **B.** Fever in the post-transplant patient can be due to a number of possible processes, including infections and acute rejection. Bacterial infection involving the urinary tract is high on the list of possible infections within the first 4 weeks after transplantation. At 8 months after transplantation, infections are most likely from opportunistic organisms. Cyclosporin is associated with many side effects, but fever is not one of them.

55.2 **D.** Fever, increasing serum creatinine, and graft tenderness are signs of acute rejection. For all patients with this presentation, infections need to be considered and ruled out. Renal graft biopsy is helpful when histological features of acute rejection are seen; however, due to sampling error, clinically suspicious rejection episodes are treated empirically, when other causes are not identified.

55.3 **D.** A condition such as urinary obstruction which will likely damage the transplanted kidney is a criteria that usually disqualifies a patient for transplant. Age above 65 is no longer a contraindication for renal transplant. The GFR threshold for transplant is usually 20 mL/min or less.

Clinical Pearls

- Infections and dialysis access complications are the two major causes of mortality in the chronic dialysis population.
- It is important to take steps to anticipate the potential need for hemodialysis and avoid damages to central and peripheral veins in all patients with chronic renal failure.
- Currently, U.S. patients on the waitlist outnumber the number of kidney transplanted by a ratio of 4:1.
- The median time on the waitlist for recipients in the United States is approximately 39 months.
- Fever, malaise, hypertension, oliguria, and increase in serum creatinine are all manifestations of acute graft failure following renal transplantation.
- 30-60% of patients develop infections during the first year following successful renal transplantation, and infections contribute to 50% of the mortality during the early post-transplant period.

REFERENCES

Dosekun A, Foringer JR, Kone BC. Urine formation: from normal physiology to florid kidney failure. In: Miller TA, ed. *Modern Surgical Care: Physiologic Foundations and Clinical Applications*. 3rd ed. New York, NY: Informa Healthcare; 2006:725-765.

Markmann JF, Yeh H, Naji A, Othoff KM, Shaked A, Barker CF. Transplantation of abdominal organs. In: Townsend CM Jr,. Beauchamp RD, Evers BM, Mattox KL, eds. *Sabiston Textbook of Surgery*. 18th ed. Philadelphia, PA: Saunders Elsevier; 2008:692-733.

Case 56

A 62-year-old man presents to the emergency department with an open wound on his left foot. The patient has a history of non-insulin-dependent diabetes mellitus, which is treated with an oral agent. He states that he has not had prior foot infections, foot problems, and denies any recent trauma to the foot. His wound has not been particularly painful, and he only noticed the wound when yellow-color drainage appeared on his socks over the past several days. The patient's temperature is 37.9°C (100.2°F), and his vital signs are normal. His peripheral vascular examination reveals palpable pulses in both femoral regions and normal pulses in both feet. The left foot is swollen over the plantar region and has a 1.5 cm open wound over the plantar surface of the foot overlying the fourth and fifth metatarsal heads. There is some yellow drainage from the area and the surrounding skin is erythematous and warm. There is no exposed bone appreciated at the base of the ulcer. His white blood cell count is 12,000 cells/m^3 and the serum glucose is 230 mEq/dL.

- ➤ What is the diagnosis?
- ➤ What are the next steps in this patient's management?
- ➤ What are the complications associated with this process?

ANSWERS TO CASE 56:
Diabetic Foot Complications

Summary: A 62-year-old diabetic man presents with a swollen foot, low-grade fever, and a plantar ulcer.

- **Diagnosis:** Diabetic foot infection associated with a neuropathic ulcer, although Charcot neuroarthropathy cannot be ruled out based on the initial evaluation.
- **Next Steps:** Assess the wound and patient for signs of infection. Biopsy the wound for culture and send blood for cultures. Obtain x-rays of the foot to look for Charcot neuroarthropathy and/or osteomyelitis. The patient should be placed on initial bed rest, IV antibiotics therapy, and strict glycemic control.
- **Complications:** Nonhealing wound and progression of infections may lead to limb loss.

ANALYSIS

Objectives

1. Learn to monitor and recognize diabetic foot complications.
2. Learn the principles and strategies applied for the treatment of diabetic foot complications.

Considerations

A 62-year-old diabetic man presents with a new plantar ulcer associated with foot swelling, erythema, and warmth. The initial presentation is highly suspicious for a neuropathic ulcer and diabetic foot infection. The presence of palpable pulses in the foot and location of the ulcer suggest that ischemia is not a contributing factor in this case. The initial ulcer evaluation could be quantified by the PEDIS classification that takes into account **P**erfusion, **E**xtent (area size), **D**epth, **I**nfection, and **S**ensation. Since all open wounds are colonized and not necessarily infected, the diagnosis of infection should be based on the combination of culture results and clinical assessment, rather than wound cultures alone. In this case, the patient has local signs of infection (redness, drainage, and swelling), and systemic signs of infection (hyperglycemia). Documentation of tissue infections should be based on tissue biopsy and not wound swab. Given the most common pathogens involved in diabetic foot infections are *Staphylococcus aureus* and beta-hemolytic *Streptococcus*, amoxicillin-clavulanic acid, ciprofloxacin, cephazolin, and vancomycin are all considered appropriate initial empiric therapy. The possibility of polymicrobial infections with aerobic gram-positive cocci, gram-negative bacilli, and anaerobic organisms is unlikely in this patient, given that he has not received prior treatment for diabetic foot infections and does not have evidence of arterial insufficiency. The optimal duration of antibiotics treatment for diabetic foot infections has not been determined on the basis of randomized controlled trials, and treatment courses often ranged between 7 and 14 days. Glycemic control in patients with diabetic foot infection is an important adjunct to the treatment, as hyperglycemia contributes to leukocyte dysfunction and compromised host response to infections. Given the open wound in this patient, if bony destruction is identified during radiography, it would be very difficult to differentiate osteomyelitis from Charcot neuroarthropathy, and long-term (4-6 weeks) course of IV antibiotics treatment may become necessary. In addition to antibiotics, local wound care is essential to promote healing. Local wound care includes a variety of techniques including sharp debridement, larval therapy with medicinal maggots, topical agent applications, and in some cases the local infections associated with abscesses would require surgical drainage and minor amputations. For many patients with neuropathic ulcers, contact casting to offload pressure from the wound site is an important adjunct in promoting healing. Once healing of the ulcer is completed, the patient should be thoroughly evaluated for contributory conditions (limited joint mobility of the foot and ankle, calluses, bunions, hammer toes, claw toes) and undergo treatment to prevent the development of future neuropathic ulcers.

APPROACH TO Diabetic Foot

DEFINITIONS

DIABETIC NEUROPATHIES: These include motor neuropathy leading to muscle atrophy, altered biomechanics, and foot deformities; sensory neuropathy that increases susceptibility to injuries; autonomic neuropathy leading to decreased sweating, skin dryness, cracks, and increased susceptibility to infections.

CHARCOT NEUROARTHROPATHY: This is a noninfective bone and joint destruction that occurs in well-perfused and insensate foot. The exact mechanism producing Charcot foot is unknown, and one theory is that the findings are produced by repetitive trauma to an insensate portion of the foot. Radiographically, there is extensive bone and joint destruction, fragmentation, and remodeling. Charcot foot is reported in approximately 16% of patients with diabetes and a history of neuropathic ulceration. The clinical presentation of acute Charcot neuroarthropathy includes soft tissue swelling, soft tissue erythema, and increased local skin temperature. Clinically, this can be difficult to differentiate from diabetic foot infections and osteomyelitis especially when an open wound is present.

FOOT ULCER CLASSIFICATIONS: Neuropathic foot ulcers are located over weight-bearing portions of the foot and are associated with normal arterial examination. Vasculogenic ulcers are generally located at the tips of the toes where perfusion is most limited. Ulcers can also develop initially as neuropathic ulcers and persist as the result of decreased blood flow.

CLINICAL APPROACH

Disease of the foot is common and one of the most feared complications associated with diabetes. "Diabetic foot" refers to a number of pathologic conditions encountered in this patient population, including **diabetic neuropathy, ischemic vascular disease, Charcot neuroarthropathy, skin ulceration, soft tissue infections, and osteomyelitis**. The lifetime risk of foot ulcer development in a diabetic individual is reported as high as 25%, and infection related to diabetic foot is responsible for 80% of the nontraumatic amputations performed. The prevention of diabetic foot complications is possible through patient education and close patient surveillance so that conditions predisposing to pressure ulceration and trauma could be avoided, identified early, and treated. The National Institute for Clinical Excellence (NICE) has made the following recommendations for diabetic foot surveillance based on patient risk stratification. Low-risk patients with normal sensation and palpable pulses are recommended to have foot examination annually. Moderate risk patients with neuropathy or absence of pulses are recommended to undergo examinations and maintenance care every 3 to 6 months, and high-risk patients with neuropathy or absence of pulses in addition to foot deformity, skin changes, or prior history of ulcers are evaluated every 1 to 3 months. During these scheduled maintenance evaluations, all patients are thoroughly assessed for neuropathies, structural abnormalities (calluses, bunions, hammer toes, etc), and vascular abnormalities (ankle-brachial index, skin changes). Patients with active foot ulceration are recommended to undergo aggressive treatment by a multidisciplinary foot care team.

A challenge in the evaluation of diabetic foot disease is the asymptomatic nature of disease, and lack of recollection of trauma or injury. Additionally due to the microvascular disease even superficial cellulitis can progress to osteomyelitis if not aggressively treated. Hence, the focus of attention should be toward (1) identifying and intervening for deep infection or osteomyelitis due to their associated increased morbidity and mortality, (2) prevention of superficial infection from progressing to more significant disease, and (3) education of the patient and family in prevention of foot injury or infection. Diabetic ulcers (see Figure 56–1) may be present on pressure points and areas of vascular insufficiency. Pain, induration, and wound drainage of the foot may indicate a deep tissue infection. In general, these infections require prompt surgical drainage and debridement. Osteomyelitis should be considered with deeper ulcers, elevated leukocyte count, and pain. However, fever is an

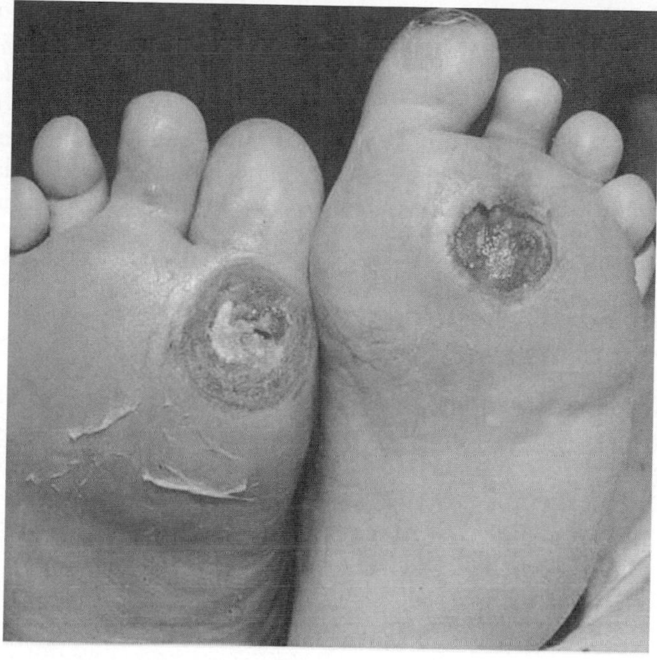

Figure 56-1. Diabetic, neuropathic ulcers on the soles of the feet due to significant long-standing diabetes-associated neuropathy. *Reproduced, with permission, from Wolff K, Johnson RA, Suurmond D.* Fitzpatrick's Color Atlas & Synopsis of Clinical Dermatology. *5th ed. New York, NY: McGraw-Hill; 2005:436.*

unreliable sign, and adenopathy is inconsistent. Radiographic changes may not be present in acute osteomyelitis but usually will be seen in chronic infection. Radionuclide scans such as with gallium are more helpful in the diagnostic evaluation of acute osteomyelitis.

Because atherosclerotic vascular disease occurs commonly in diabetic patients, the contribution of arterial insufficiency to diabetic foot ulcer formation and nonhealing should always be considered. Since the arterial occlusion occurs more commonly in the diabetic population at the level of the tibial-peroneal arteries, the patients often do not experience calf claudication. In the diabetic patient, foot claudication is more common because the decreased blood flow occurs at the tibial-peroneal arteries; however, as the result of concurrent sensory neuropathy, foot claudication would often go undetected. Assessment of blood flow can be quantified with measurement of ankle-brachial indices (ABI), measurement of toe-brachial indices, and duplex ultrasonography; however, it is important to bear in mind that ABI in diabetic patients could be falsely elevated from calcification of the tibial vessels. When arterial insufficiency is identified as a possible cause of ulcerations or nonhealing wounds, the patients should undergo additional arterial evaluation by arteriography or magnetic resonance angiography and consideration for revascularization. Because of the increased frequency of multiple level occlusive disease and tibial level occlusive disease, diabetic patients are generally not good candidates for endoluminal arterial interventions, and revascularization in this patient population often requires open vascular reconstructions.

Comprehension Questions

56.1 Which of the following is the best antimicrobial therapy for a patient who presents with recurrent foul-smelling diabetic foot infection, without ischemia that initially improved after a 2 weeks course of vancomycin treatment?

A. Metronidazole
B. Fluconazole
C. Clindamycin
D. Piperacillin-tazobactam

56.2 Which of the following is the most appropriate treatment for a 55-year-old man presenting with foul-smelling and purulent drainage from a 10-cm left plantar ulcer with bone exposure, fever of 39.4°C (102.9°F), blood pressure of 90/60 mm Hg, WBC of 35,000 cells/m^3, x-ray findings of extensive osteomyelitis involving several metatarsal bones and gas within the soft tissue in the lower leg?

A. Below the knee amputation
B. Piperacillin-tazobactam + clindamycin
C. Piperacillin-tazobactam + vancomycin and wound debridement
D. Below the knee amputation and piperacillin-tazobactam + metronidazole

56.3 A 46-year-old diabetic male is being seen in the office for an ulcer of the right foot and ankle area that appeared approximately 10 days previously. There is some tenderness over the lateral malleolus. An x-ray of the ankle does not show any abnormality. Which of the following would be most likely to help in detecting acute osteomyelitis?

A. Needle aspiration of the region in question
B. MRI of the right ankle
C. Radionuclide scan of the ankle
D. Serum erythrocyte sedimentation rate

ANSWERS

56.1 **D.** Given the prior history of antibiotic therapy directed toward gram-positive organisms and the current foul-smelling drainage associated with this recurrent ulcer, a polymicrobial infection with a combination of gram-positive and gram-negative organism is highly likely; therefore, piperacillin-tazobactam is a good initial empiric antibiotic choice. Anaerobic organisms are less likely to develop in diabetic foot infections without arterial insufficiency. Fungal infection is uncommon in diabetic foot infection.

56.2 **D.** Given the septic presentation of this patient exhibiting advanced diabetic foot infection associated with bone involvement and air-forming organisms in the lower leg soft tissue, the initial management should be directed toward life-saving interventions rather than limb-saving interventions. The most appropriate treatment would include resuscitation, below the knee amputation, and broad-spectrum systemic antimicrobial therapy.

56.3 **C.** With acute osteomyelitis, radiographic changes such as raised periosteum may not be seen until later. Radionuclide scan is often helpful in these circumstances.

Clinical Pearls

- Neuropathic and vasculopathic ulcers may be differentiated based on locations, where neuropathic ulcers occur at pressure and weight-bearing areas of the foot and vasculogenic ulcers occur at the tips of digits.
- Acute Charcot foot is associated with acute pain, soft tissue swelling, erythema, and increased warmth in the foot, and these features are often confused with cellulites, deep venous thrombosis, and osteomyelitis.

REFERENCES

Apelqvist J, Bakker K, van Houtum WH, et al. Practical guidelines on the management and prevention of the diabetic foot. *Diabetes Met Res Rev*. 2008;24(Suppl 1): S181-S187.

Bandyk DF, Stone PA. Diabetic foot. In: Cameron JL, ed. *Current Surgical Therapy*. 9th ed. Mosby Elsevier: Philadelphia, PA. 2008:891-894.

Khanolkar MP, Bain SC, Stephens JW. The diabetic foot. *QJ Med*. 2008;101:685-695.

SECTION III

Listing of Cases

Listing by Case Number

Listing by Disorder (Alphabetical)

INDEX

Page numbers followed by *f* or *t* indicate figures or tables, respectively.

D

E

R